Hot Topics in
General Practice

9th Edition

Hot Topics in General Practice

9th Edition

J. Kilburn MRCGP, FRCS(A&E), DA

Newcastle-upon-Tyne

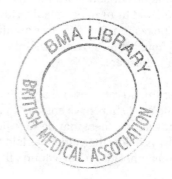

Scion

Ninth Edition © Scion Publishing Ltd, 2009

ISBN 978 1 904842 56 7

Eighth Edition 2007 (ISBN 978 1 904842 37 8)
Seventh Edition 2006 (ISBN 1 904842 35 6)
Sixth Edition 2005 (ISBN 1 904842 05 4)
Fifth Edition first published by Scion Publishing Ltd, 2004 (ISBN 1 904842 00 3)
Fourth Edition 2002 (ISBN 1 85996 073 1); reprinted 2003
Third Edition 2000 (ISBN 1 85996 129 0); reprinted 2001
Second Edition 1998 (ISBN 1 85996 251 3); reprinted 1999
First Edition published by BIOS Scientific Publishers Ltd, 1996 (ISBN 1 85996 210 6); reprinted 1997

A CIP catalogue record for this book is available from the British Library.

Scion Publishing Limited
Bloxham Mill, Barford Road, Bloxham, Oxfordshire OX15 4FF
www.scionpublishing.com

Important Note from the Publisher

The information contained within this book was obtained by Scion Publishing Limited from sources believed by us to be reliable. However, while every effort has been made to ensure its accuracy, no responsibility for loss or injury whatsoever occasioned to any person acting or refraining from action as a result of information contained herein can be accepted by the authors or publishers.

The reader should remember that medicine is a constantly evolving science and while the authors and publishers have ensured that all dosages, applications and practices are based on current indications, there may be specific practices which differ between communities. You should always follow the guidelines laid down by the manufacturers of specific products and the relevant authorities in the country in which you are practising.

Typeset by Phoenix Photosetting, Chatham, Kent, UK
Printed by Biddles Ltd, King's Lynn, UK, www.biddles.co.uk

CONTENTS

PRACTICE ISSUES

CLINICAL ISSUES

ABBREVIATIONS

A&E	accident and emergency
AAA	abdominal aortic aneurysm
ACE	angiotensin-converting enzyme
AF	atrial fibrillation
ARB	angiotensin II receptor blocker
BMA	British Medical Association
BMI	body mass index
BNP	B-type natriuretic peptide
BP	blood pressure
BPH	benign prostatic hypertrophy
CAD	coronary artery disease
CBT	cognitive behaviour therapy
CFS	chronic fatigue syndrome
CHD	coronary heart disease
CHF	chronic heart failure
CK	creatine kinase
COPD	chronic obstructive pulmonary disease
COX	cyclo-oxygenase
CRP	C-reactive protein
CT	computed tomography
DEXA	dual energy X-ray absorptiometry
DMSA	dimercaptosuccinic acid
DVT	deep venous thrombosis
ECG	electrocardiogram
EU	European Union
FOB	faecal occult blood
FPG	fasting plasma glucose
GGT	gamma glutamyl transferase
GI	gastro-intestinal
GMC	General Medical Council
GORD	gastro-oesophageal disease
GP	general practitioner
GUM	genitourinary medicine
HDL	high density lipoprotein
HIV	human immunodeficiency virus
HPV	human papillomavirus
IBS	irritable bowel syndrome
ICD	International Classification of Diseases
IGT	impaired glucose tolerance
IHD	ischaemic heart disease
LDL	low density lipoprotein
LVH	left ventricular hypertrophy
LVSD	left ventricular systolic dysfunction
MCV	mean corpuscular volume
ME	myalgic encephalomyelitis

MI	myocardial infarction
MMR	measles mumps rubella vaccine
MPA	medroxyprogesterone acetate
MRI	magnetic resonance imaging
NHS	National Health Service
NICE	National Institute for Clinical Excellence
NSAID	non-steroidal anti-inflammatory drug
NSF	national service framework
NYHA	New York Heart Association
OGTT	oral glucose tolerance test
POEM	patient orientated evidence that matters
PPI	proton pump inhibitor
PSA	prostate specific antigen
QALY	quality adjusted life year
RA	rheumatoid arthritis
RCGP	Royal College of General Practitioners
RCT	randomised controlled trial
SHO	senior house officer
SMT	spinal manipulative therapy
SSRI	selective serotonin reuptake inhibitor
TNF	tumour necrosis factor
US	ultrasound
UTI	urinary tract infection
VC	virtual colonoscopy

JOURNAL ABBREVIATIONS

Am Heart J	*American Heart Journal*
Am J Cardiol	*The American Journal of Cardiology*
Am J Epidemiol	*American Journal of Epidemiology*
Am J Gastroenterol	*The American Journal of Gastroenterology*
Am J Med	*The American Journal of Medicine*
Ann Intern Med	*Annals of Internal Medicine*
Ann Rheum Dis	*Annals of the Rheumatic Diseases*
Arch Dis Child	*Archives of Disease in Childhood*
Arch Gen Psychiatry	*Archives of General Psychiatry*
Arch Intern Med	*Archives of Internal Medicine*
Arch Neurol	*Archives of Neurology*
Arch Pediatr Adolesc Med	*Archives of Pediatrics and Adolescent Medicine*
Arthritis Rheum	*Arthritis and Rheumatism*
BJU Int	*British Journal of Urology International*
BMJ	*British Medical Journal*
Br J Cancer	*British Journal of Cancer*
Br J Gen Pract	*British Journal of General Practice*
Br J Psychiatry	*The British Journal of Psychiatry*
Clin Infect Dis	*Clinical Infectious Diseases*
Drug Therap Bull	*Drug and Therapeutics Bulletin*
Eur Heart J	*European Heart Journal*
Eur Respir J	*European Respiratory Journal*
Fam Pract	*Family Practice*
J Am Coll Cardiol	*Journal of the American College of Cardiology*
J Am Geriatr Soc	*Journal of the American Geriatrics Society*
J Epidemiol Community Health	*Journal of Epidemiology and Community Health*
J Infect Dis	*The Journal of Infectious Diseases*
J Natl Cancer Inst	*Journal of the National Cancer Institute*
J Neurol Neurosurg Psychiatry	*Journal of Neurology, Neurosurgery, and Psychiatry*
J Rheumatol	*The Journal of Rheumatology*
J Urol	*The Journal of Urology*
JAMA	*The Journal of the American Medical Association*
Mayo Clin Proc	*Mayo Clinic Proceedings*
Med J Aust	*The Medical Journal of Australia*
N Engl J Med	*The New England Journal of Medicine*
Nat Med	*Nature Medicine*
PLoS Med	*Public Library of Science Medicine Journal*
Postgrad Med J	*Postgraduate Medical Journal*
Qual Saf Health Care	*Quality and Safety in Health Care*

PREFACE

When you update a book like this and aim to do it every year you can at times get the feeling that real practical change is actually slower than it is supposed to be. I have on occasions got away with barely touching some chapters when I have not found new high quality evidence in certain areas. This is not one of those years.

Every chapter seems to have needed a major rewrite in order to give the full flavour of recent changes in peer-reviewed knowledge relevant to primary care. I suppose this could be a chance finding but it may also be a sign of the changing times. It seems to me that our best sources of information seem to be getting genuinely better at pointing out where the truth lies. The speed of change, previously glacier-like, now seems to be palpable, even visible.

I have therefore changed the format of the book in order to best accommodate and précis high quality information. Every sentence has been reviewed and revised looking cautiously wherever an apparent 'fact' is claimed while taking great efforts to convey the authors' message from the papers reviewed, regardless of the ultimate fate of that message.

Why not use the new feedback email option if you have constructive comment?

More than ever I have learned in the process where many uncertainties lie and a principal claim of this book is now to assist in pointing out these grey areas. In the past I wonder if I may have naively expected that uncertainties would change with the passage of time into certainties. With this edition I have realised that that process is just as likely to be reversed.

The uncertainty has arisen largely because evidence-based medicine can be manipulated by bias in reporting in so many ways. These may not just be difficult to personally assess but even invisible. Take, for example, unpublished research – sometimes included in a systematic review, sometimes not. Conclusions can flip on such a factor. I highlight these wherever they have been spotted.

Care has also been taken to avoid getting bogged down in semantics and opinion-based zeal. All research is imperfect in some way and paying too much attention to these areas might seem to absolve us from incorporating into daily practice what the research broadly currently says.

There is art in certainty but it is not so easy to find certainty in art. (There is also an 'art nicety' and even an 'Acne – Try it!' contained within 'certainty', but I digress.) Tracking it down is the stuff and story of general practice and we will get closer in this edition to where certainty is and where it is not. The information presented within can quickly be incorporated into a powerful narrative tailored on a patient-to-patient basis. I believe this is key to avoiding the inadequacies in the consultation that doctors who still resist evidence-based medicine may make.

Uncertainty is also a happy hunting ground for the pharmaceutical industry. From the good people who brought you the epidemic of sexual dysfunction comes a new array of precursor conditions that are not quite illness, not quite disease. Whatever you call them, they represent juicy new markets as anyone who wants drugs for their pre-osteoporosis, pre-hypertension or subclinical something-or-other may confirm.

There are other themes to the recent changes too. For example, the place of HRT is agreed more clearly than ever and our latest cure-all, cognitive behavioural therapy, may be losing its shine thanks to modern practicalities and resources limitations.

Still, the refrain that follows all the research efforts is louder than ever. All together now, "More trials are needed......".

Well, bring them on because the modern GP can leave previous prejudices aside. The modern GP can handle the truth. Finding it, however, is not always easy.

Julian Kilburn
September 2008

Feedback

If you have any comments on the content of this book, please feel free to email them to <u>HotTopics@hotmail.co.uk</u>.

Dedication

To Cedric Wylie

A man who loved my mother and was loved by his many patients.

THE CONSULTATION

The Challenge

Delivering personal care involves communication, tailored management and 'whole person' care. It is not the same, however, as continuity of care which is considered more valuable in long-term complex problems, and personal care can still be achieved by a skilled locum in a one-off consultation. The much trumpeted knowledge of social and family factors comes into play only if it is referred to and built upon.

Doctors are just one source of information fighting for the patient's loyalty and people do not think rationally about risk. They overstate the low probability of high consequence risks such as getting killed in a train crash, but underestimate the effect of common risks such as smoking. They worry excessively about unquantified 'virtual' risks, such as catching mad cow disease, and allow the media to feed their fears.

During the MMR controversy, the medical evidence seemed to play little role in parental decisions to vaccinate their children. Even though doctors were usually trusted sources of information, too many concerns over the legitimacy of their role, financial impartiality and political bias got in the way. Trust often does not have to be won but can easily be lost. Patients want to feel that their doctor has expertise but they also want an efficient open manner that makes them feel special. Smiling, the careful use of touch and the odd idiosyncrasy helps.

At the end of the day, how we share and discuss these uncertainties without appearing hesitant might be the greatest challenge of all.

What we know already:

- Uninterrupted, patients conclude their opening monologue in less than 30 seconds in primary care.
- Consultations are more successful where they are perceived to have lasted longer but were not longer. They may be more about quality time than actual time.
- Longer consultations lead to more preventative health care, better recognition of psychosocial problems and less prescribing.
- Patients forget up to 80% of the information from the consultation. Of the information they do recall, half of it is remembered incorrectly.
- Communications skills can be taught but this does not always improve patients' experiences.
- Doctors tend not to elicit patients' expectations or unvoiced agendas. They misconstrue patient pressure resulting in more prescribing and less compliance.
- Using medical terminology can help patients validate their sick role and bestow a sense of greater professionalism on their doctor. Lay labels can result in a greater sense of ownership of the problem which some perceive as blame.
- After controlling for the actual preferences of patients, doctors still perceive non-existent pressure from patients. In one study, doctors felt that there was little or no medical need for 15% of their examinations, 19% of their prescriptions, 22% of their referrals, and nearly half their investigations.
- The patient's life experience makes up the qualitative component of the clinical decision-making.

Recent Papers

COMMUNICATION

Physician scores on a national clinical skills examination as predictors of complaints to medical regulatory authorities
Tamblyn R, Abrahamowicz M, Dauphinee D *et al.*
JAMA, 2007; **298**: 993–1001

> In Canada and the US, part of the requirement of medical registration is a clinical skills test which assesses communication skills. This study looked at nearly 3500 physicians qualifying between 1993 and 1996 and followed them up until 2005.
> - 17% had at least one complaint upheld against them.
> - Doctors performing least well in the communication component of the test were 52% more likely to have a complaint upheld against them.
> - Almost half of these complaints were about poor communication or attitude.
>
> Assessments such as these could be fine-tuned to predict those who generate complaints and establish the need for targeted training.

Effect of providing information about normal test results on patients' reassurance: randomised controlled trial
Petrie KJ, Müller JT, Schirmbeck F *et al.*
BMJ, 2007; **334**: 352
and
Reassuring patients about normal test results
Penzien DB, Rains JC
BMJ, 2007; **334**: 325

> This paper and the accompanying editorial look at the crucial, commonly used yet under-researched area of reassurance. They assessed 92 patients by providing additional information in advance of an investigation, in this case an exercise ECG for investigation of chest pain.
> - Explaining the meaning of normal test results in advance of the investigation improved the success of the reassurance and maintained it at one month.
> - There was also a significant decrease in reported symptoms of chest pain at one month compared to the control group.
> - Making the explanation face-to face was more successful than using a pamphlet alone.
> - The effects were substantial and reliable, confirming that good communication can affect health outcomes.
>
> The paper shows that preparing patients to be reassured strengthened the value of the reassurance. Optimal methods of providing reassurance need to be developed in order to reflect sufficiently the factors known to be at work such as chronicity of symptoms, depth of medical understanding and psychiatric co-morbidities.
>
> Diagnostic testing undertaken mainly to illustrate to patients that symptoms are benign may therefore fail to reassure in the ways anticipated, and may inadvertently end up validating false convictions. Further testing and follow-up of false positives may create a vicious circle of perceived validation for anxious patients.

Effect of patient completed agenda forms and doctors' education about the agenda on the outcome of consultations: randomised controlled trial
Middleton JF, McKinley RK, Gillies CL
BMJ, 2006; **332:** 1238–1242

Two interventions were studied here: patients completing forms detailing their agenda for the consultation and doctors undergoing a one day workshop to help them recognise the layers of the patient's agenda (in terms of ideas, concerns, expectations and reasoning) and then negotiate a management plan.

In this randomised controlled trial of 46 UK practices and nearly 900 patients, using the forms added a minute to the consultation but more problems were identified and patients were more satisfied. Consultations were longer but still only took around five minutes per problem. However, the number of 'by the way, while I'm here' consultations were unchanged.

An accompanying editorial (*BMJ*, 2006; **332:** 1225–1226) comments that the form may be used to expand on the problem, select the desired outcome (prescription, explanation, investigation or certificate), or perhaps most usefully, allow all embarrassing problems to be voiced which may otherwise be the last item to be mentioned.

However, the efficiency gain is unclear from this study as we do not know if there was a successful reduction in future attendances. It is also possible that the extra problems are unnecessarily medicalised, as patients have been shown to have good judgement about whether or not to consult a doctor with their symptoms.

Language proficiency and adverse events in US hospitals: a pilot study
Divi C, Koss R, Schmaltz SP, Loeb JM
Int J Qual Health Care, 2007; **19:** 60–67

A study of adverse events in six US hospitals over 7 months showed that patients who were not proficient in English suffered more adverse events.
- Around 50% of those with a language barrier suffered some physical harm. In half of these the effects ranged from moderate temporary harm to death.
- About 30% of English-speaking patients suffered harm but only one-quarter of those suffered similarly serious adverse events.
- These events were due to communication errors in over half the non-English-speaking patients but only in 36% of the English-speaking patients.

This study illustrates the danger of language barriers, and mentions the paucity of literature on the subject and the need to review current language services.

Shared decision making and the experience of partnership in primary care
Saba GW, Wong ST, Schillinger D *et al.*
Ann Fam Med, 2006; **4:** 54–62

This study in US primary care showed that relationship factors such as trust and perceived respect influence communication as much as style and behaviour. We have to work on relationship dynamics for effective consultation as this study found that shared decision making between patient and physician is frequently a negative experience for the patient.

It can 'look good,' but when it does not also 'feel good', we need to recognise that a purely behavioural model for teaching communication skills appears inadequate

Patients' involvement in decisions about medicines: GPs' perceptions of their preferences
Cox K, Britten N, Hooper R, White P
Br J Gen Pract, 2007; **543**: 777–784

A questionnaire replied to by nearly 500 patients of London-based GPs looked at who should be making the decisions in the consultation and how each party perceived how decisions should be made.

- 39% of patients wanted the GP to share the decisions with them.
- 45% wanted the GP to be the main or only decision maker, but only 16% wanted to be the main or only decision maker themselves.
- GPs accurately estimated patient preferences in 32% of cases.
- GPs overestimated the preference for involvement in 45% of cases.
- GPs underestimated them in 23% of cases.
- Underestimation was more likely with the more intelligent patients, particularly if they had not consulted about a condition before.

RISK

Different ways to describe the benefits of risk-reducing treatments: a randomized trial
Halvorsen PA, Selmer R, Kristiansen IS
Ann Intern Med, 2007; **146**: 848–856

How you describe the anticipated benefit of medication is likely to be reflected in its uptake by patients. This survey of 2754 healthy Norwegians presented two scenarios by describing its statistics in different ways. The scenarios used were the use of statins to prevent heart attacks and bisphosphonates to prevent hip fracture, and they reflected realistic research-based figures.

Describing benefits in terms of NNT – the number needed to treat to prevent one adverse event – was by far the most successful method of achieving compliance.

Offering a postponement of an adverse event for a proportion of the group for several months had an intermediate effect.

Presenting a smaller advantage, such as an average postponement of an event for the entire group by an average of just a few weeks, had the least appeal.

Announcing an NNT of 13 persuaded 93% of the heart attack group to consent to drug therapy, falling by around 10% for each scenario of lesser perceived benefit. Of the hip fracture group, 74% consented to an NNT of 57. This fell by around 20% for each 'lesser' scenario.

The authors explain that people respond with a gambler's instinct. They seem less able or interested in engaging with the concept of disease which has a depressing inevitability when it is merely postponable. But they seem happy to gamble on smaller odds that they are going to be the lucky one and prevent it altogether.

How doctors discuss major interventions with high risk patients: an observational study
Corke CF, Stow PJ, Green DT *et al.*
BMJ, 2005; **330:** 182

We all love role play and this Australian study put 30 junior doctors (not vocationally trained GPs) in a staged no-win scenario (leaking abdominal aortic aneurysm in someone unlikely to survive surgery) to assess their consultation skills. They found that doctors were fine at discussing the medical bits but not so good at engaging with the patient's wishes and fears.

Research estimates at least 75% of patients want their doctor to offer a recommendation when faced with an end-of-life decision. In this study, only 36% of doctors gave advice even when it was directly requested. They suggest this approach is consistent with modern day medical school teaching but proclaim that a role limited to merely providing information is failing our patients. Those that suggested they go and discuss things with their family also came in for criticism, as it was felt such a patient would be too sick to relay all the arguments. Fortunately, they are starting a course to cure the problem.

Personal knowledge
Sweeney K
BMJ, 2006; **332:** 129–130

Research has shown that doctors with personal experience of their warfarin patients undergoing a haemorrhage had lower odds of prescribing warfarin in the future. Yet adverse events associated with underusing warfarin do not exert the same influence.

This editorial expands the discussion that doctors are not simple conduits nor passive recipients for clinical evidence. They undergo an inner consultation where dramatic experiences which are easy to recall add a dimension of personal significance to more scientific evidence.

Two ways of 'knowing' – biomedical and biographical – compete for influence and personal judgements result in sometimes failing to follow through on that which is conventionally known.

CHAPERONES

Chaperones: who needs them?
Richardson C
BMJ Career Focus, 2005; **330:** 175–176

The GMC advise that doctors should always offer a chaperone for intimate examinations.

An accusation of inappropriate behaviour would be devastating for any doctor and would have far-reaching consequences for investigative proceedings and adverse publicity.

The Ayling report publicised in September 2004 provides recommendations on the back of an independent inquiry into a GP from Kent convicted of indecent assault and imprisoned for four years.

They recognise the patient's right to decline a chaperone as many find it intrusive and embarrassing. It recognised that a chaperone may not always be available and you may need to trust your instincts before performing an intimate examination (that is related to breast, genitalia or rectum). Defer examination if there are any concerns.

The report also stated that untrained administrative staff should not be expected to act as chaperones although to train them up would be acceptable. Similarly, family or friends should not be used in a formal chaperoning role. It may worsen embarrassment and lead to inadvertent breaches in confidentiality.

The chaperone should be introduced and the name documented in the notes.

Chaperones for intimate examinations: cross sectional survey of attitudes and practices of general practitioners
Rosenthal J, Rymer J, Jones R *et al.*
BMJ, 2005; **330:** 234–235

A questionnaire answered by over 1200 GPs in England revealed that for intimate examinations:

- only 37% of respondents had a policy on the use of chaperones
- two-thirds of males but only 5% of female GPs usually or always offered a chaperone
- over half the male doctors and only 2% of female doctors usually or always used one
- 8% of males and 70% of females never used one
- although practice nurses were most popular, family and friends were frequently used, as were administrative staff
- most never recorded the offer or the identity of the chaperone in the notes
- although use of chaperones has increased in the last decade, more flexible guidance is needed for GPs other than the universal recommendations from the royal colleges to always use chaperones for intimate examination

CONCORDANCE AND PRESCRIBING

The Challenge

Roughly half of all drugs are not taken as prescribed, creating massive consequences in term of missed benefits and health economics.

Taking medication has an ambiguous yet powerful impact on people's identity. Doctors rarely discuss whether a patient will go along with a treatment plan and mistakenly think they know what their patient's preferences are. They are drawn to prescribing ineffective treatments for a multitude of reasons including a need to act. Their personal clinical experience is at best a poor judge of what works and what doesn't. Patients for their part find it hard to adjust to their new role of drug-taker. The aim is concordance – reaching an agreement with the patient which respects their beliefs and wishes rather than the simple giving of instructions.

Concordance is particularly challenging for preventative therapy in asymptomatic conditions and for those drugs with significant side effects. It is a dynamic concept needing continual exploration and is not necessarily linked to a behavioural outcome. When drugs 'fail', doctors too often look to their own prescribing choices, but it is the desires and beliefs of patients that determine whether medicine will be taken.

Doctors and patients need to recognise the potential conflict between being both patient-centred and evidence-based and, in the absence of a blueprint, learn how to 'do concordance'.

There is also controversy about therapeutically using biologically inert substances known as placebos, yet only about half of all medical treatments are evidence-based. The assumption that use of placebos (from the Latin for 'I will please') has been stamped out by twentieth century medicine is misguided because use is widespread in other countries.

What we know already:

- Many patients want to be involved in prescribing decisions, but not all.
- Most patients would prefer not to take any medicines and many try to minimise their doses.
- As quickly as 10 days after prescription of a new medication, 30% of elderly chronic disease sufferers may not take it as prescribed. This is intentional in almost half of the cases.
- Studies show that patients commonly employ complex strategies of self-regulation to stop, vary or minimise dosage, reflecting a widespread cultural belief that drugs should be used as little as possible.
- Some fear dependency, side effects or interactions, but most acknowledged their need for drugs.
- The same person may take one drug regularly while varying another, illustrating the futility of labelling patients as compliant or non-compliant.
- Low cost prescribers find it easier to refuse patients prescriptions and subscribe more strongly to the importance of a local consensus, a practice formulary and cost-consciousness.
- Both high and low prescribers of new drugs considered themselves to have conservative prescribing behaviour.
- Doctors tend to accept smaller benefits than patients in preventative health care. There is an enormous variation between patients of what is a minimal acceptable benefit of taking a drug long-term. Some would only take a 'perfect' treatment.

- Few doctors or lay people appreciate the statistics enough to realise that increased length of treatment means increased benefit (absolute benefit roughly doubles over double the time).
- Ten year estimates of risk inflate apparent benefits of treatment (assuming 30% risk reduction in patients with a 10 year coronary risk of 30% means 9 out of 10 patients take the drug for 10 years with no benefit).
- Doctors make more confident decisions on medication than patients, but not necessarily more logical or consistent ones.
- In one study in Israel, two-thirds of doctors prescribed placebos and two-thirds of these doctors told patients they were actual medication. Some 94% found them effective and only 5% thought they should be banned.
- A US body recently called for research to optimise use of the placebo phenomenon while attending to the ethical considerations.

Recent Papers

CONCORDANCE

Is it acceptable for people to be paid to adhere to medication? No
Shaw J
BMJ, 2007; **335**: 233

NICE has announced plans to give drug users shopping vouchers to attend treatment programmes and stay clean. This feature argues for and against rewarding patients for compliant drug-taking behaviour.

The cost of wasted drugs and the consequences of not taking them are certainly high to the NHS. Shaw talks of perverse incentives undermining the therapeutic alliances between patients and doctors as well as invasion of personal dignity and privacy.

Payment to take their tablets would presumably be targeted at those who omit to do so intentionally as opposed to those who want to take their drugs but fail to do so for some other reason, e.g. tricky packaging or complex regimes. To ensure we hit our target group we would presumably have to pay everybody. Voluntary adherence would all but disappear and prescriptions with payment attached would surely elevate the request for ever more prescriptions.

Could a case be made with the costs to society of treating a non-compliant case of infectious tuberculosis? Unlikely. People choose not to take drugs for many reasons – lack of trust of doctors or pharmaceutical companies, for example. A cash reward will only reinforce these suspicions, possibly even encouraging people to find a way to fill their pockets without filling their stomachs.

Payment sends a signal that they are doing something inherently not in their own interests. Costly systems of policing or supervised administration would be expensive and unworkable.

Is it acceptable for people to be paid to adhere to medication? Yes
Burns T
BMJ, 2007; **335:** 232

Burns has the tougher sell. As a psychiatrist he focuses on the benefit to society of payment to encourage patients in receiving antipsychotic depot medication and avoiding hospital admission. He notes simplistically that all life's relationships, whether imposed by love, duty or respect, have inherent constraints. He seems to see little conflict with adding cash to our list of weapons to shape behaviour.

He even draws a parallel with the sale of organs in the developing world but finds the sums involved modest enough to appease any irritating conscience about such parallels. Burns claims that studies into cash rewards have had good results with little controversy. As there is a commonly accepted good, he sees the openness as a lack of mystique and therefore a lack of hypocrisy. He defines cash for behaviour as a 'model of respectful and equal exchange'!

A meta-analysis of the association between adherence to drug therapy and mortality
Simpson SH, Eurich DT, Majumdar SR *et al*.
BMJ, 2006; **333:** 15–18

This meta-analysis of nearly 47 000 patients in 21 studies found that good adherence to medication was associated with lower mortality even if the tablets were placebos. This flies in the face of the theory that placebos do not influence health outcomes and supports the 'healthy adherer' theory that speculates that taking your tablets is an overall marker for generally healthy behaviour. This may manifest as better diet, exercise, follow-up, screening, immunisations and use of other drugs.

Mortality of good adherers was half that of patients with poor adherence.

INTERVENTIONS

Interventions to enhance medication adherence in chronic medical conditions: a systematic review
Kripalani S, Yao X, Haynes RB
Arch Intern Med, 2007; **167:** 540–549

This review looked at 37 RCTs between 1967 and 2004 containing at least one thing designed to increase adherence to medication and one clinical outcome.

Around half the interventions used improved adherence to medication but only one-third of interventions improved any of the outcomes.

Almost all of the effective interventions for long-term care were complex, including combinations of more convenience, better information, reminders and reinforcement, self-monitoring, counselling and psychological therapies, crisis intervention and telephone follow-up.

With such improvements still being fairly small, the full benefits of treatment are limited and new methods of achieving concordance are required.

PLACEBOS

Sham device v inert pill: randomised controlled trial of two placebo treatments
Kaptchuk TJ, Stason WB, Davis RB *et al.*
BMJ, 2006; **332:** 391–397

> A study of 270 patients with arm pain compared two placebo treatments – acupuncture with a sham device and inert pills (pretending that they might be amitriptyline). In the long run, there was a larger improvement in reported (subjective) symptoms in those using the sham acupuncture device. The superiority of one placebo over another implies that the rituals involved may be of key importance.

Placebos in practice
Spiegel D
BMJ, 2004; **329:** 927–928

> The concept of placebo responders being healthy, histrionic dimwits is not supported by research. It even has its own industry which incorporates many holistic 'therapies' that harness and market the effect and that are increasingly capturing the public's 'imagination.' Its evil brother – the nocebo effect – describes negative expectations producing negative results. This, so far, has failed to find much of a market share except in a sadomasochistic minority.
>
> Most easy to criticise was the claim that use of placebos helped to differentiate organic pain from psychogenic pain. This involves concepts of pain long since discredited.
>
> New scientific domains such as psychoneuroimmunology and psychoneuroendocrinology are helping to explain the mechanisms of how the mind affects the body and explain associations between, for example, depression and cancer that have been recognised for years.
>
> Deception is not necessary for the placebo effect but ethical considerations need looking at. Can we afford to dispense with any interventions that work?

PHARMACISTS

The Challenge

The pharmacy is the most often visited healthcare outlet and is ideally placed between lay and professional networks. The launch of the recent NHS initiative – *Choosing health through pharmacy, a programme for pharmaceutical public health 2005-2015* – sought to expand the contribution of pharmacists, but the value of such an approach on improving outcomes is mixed at best.

Pharmacists are still viewed as shopkeepers and dispensers of medicines, and GPs express concern and lack of knowledge about their training, activities and primary motivation. For their part, community pharmacists consider themselves to be healthcare professionals and some feel that GPs have no appreciation of their role in healthcare.

Calls have been made for greater collaboration between GPs and community pharmacists in primary care. However, little training exists for the new roles of advice giver or counsellor and very little work has been done to assess its potential or impact.

What we know already:

- Reviewing elderly patients' medication is a requirement of the National Service Framework for Older People but difficult for GPs to prioritise given current pressures.
- In 2006 the Department of Health extended considerable prescribing power to pharmacists.
- A pharmacist could manage an estimated 8% of adult attendances at A&E according to one study from St Thomas' Hospital.
- Community pharmacists given a little training in asthma management can successfully provide self-management plans and basic follow up care.

Recent Papers

EXTENDED ROLES

The role of pharmacists in primary care
Ballantyne PJ
BMJ, 2007; **334:** 1066–1067

So how valuable is the pharmacist likely to be in an extended primary care role?

The studies below used different research methods but came to similar unfavourable findings for the role of pharmacists in primary health care.

It is known that healthcare professionals have the greatest impact when making the effort to meet the patient's own agenda and methods of rationalisation. That is the current emphasis of general practice training. That pharmacists are having difficulty with this intervention, given the complex integration of skills and knowledge base that it requires, can hardly be a surprise.

Pharmacy as a profession has repositioned itself from a clinical service model to a pharmaceutical care model, aligning itself with modern primary care and claiming similar goals.

We may assume they are primarily focussed on patients' drug-related needs but is even this clear anymore? Evidence of their ability to reduce medical and drug costs is lacking and the role seems an unclear as ever.

Effectiveness of visits from community pharmacists for patients with heart failure: HeartMed randomised controlled trial
Holland R, Brooksby I, Lenaghan E *et al.*
BMJ, 2007; **334:** 1098

This large randomised trial of nearly 300 patients admitted to hospital for heart failure looked in more detail at the potential of the community pharmacist. Results were disappointing.

They offered home visits in the weeks after admission to hospital and measured the numbers of re-admissions at 6 months but, unlike specialist nurse intervention, found no benefit. Rather, there was a trend to increasing admissions and mortality and there was no improvement in quality of life or adherence to medication.

The visits seemed popular with patients, but the pharmacists were not heart failure specialists and the patients did have rather advanced disease.

Nevertheless, with the absence of any discernible benefit and a tendency to actually increase use of health services, community pharmacists may not be sufficiently expert to deliver the type of intervention needed to heart failure patients.

Does home based medication review keep older people out of hospital? The HOMER randomised controlled trial
Holland R, Lenaghan E, Harvey I *et al.*
BMJ, 2005; **330:** 293

This interesting study looked at sending in pharmacists to the homes of 872 patients over 80 years old who were on at least two medications and who had been recruited during a recent emergency admission to hospital. The pharmacists visited twice around two and eight weeks after discharge to educate about medication, look for drug interactions and assess adherence to medication.

The NHS advocates such medication review for older patients but this approach resulted in significantly more admission to hospitals, more GP home visits and a worse quality of life while failing to reduce mortality.

This counterintuitive finding might be explained by better help-seeking behaviour or just by creating more dependence through anxiety and confusion, but also may be due to an increase in side-effects with improved compliance causing more iatrogenic illness.

Either way, more research is needed before we go down this line too far.

"I haven't even phoned my doctor yet." The advice giving role of the pharmacist during consultations for medication review with patients aged 80 or more: qualitative discourse analysis
Salter C, Holland R, Harvey I, Henwood K
BMJ, 2007; **334:** 1101

This sub-study from the HOMER trial took place in the homes of a small number of over-80 year olds. It consisted of medication review consultations lasting an average of 45 minutes each undertaken by volunteer pharmacists.

Consultations were observed or transcribed and the pharmacists did not know the elderly patients beforehand. They found many opportunities to offer advice and information but on only one occasion did a patient express a wish to actually ask a question. Advice was often challenged or rejected and difficulties with the dynamic occurred resulting in awkward moments during the consultations.

They advise the need for caution in assuming that measures such as these are bound to lead to improved outcomes. In elderly people at least, such interventions can undermine and threaten the patients' competence, integrity, and self governance.

POLYPHARMACY

Commercial and political pressures raise polypharmacy, so patients suffer
Brewer C
Pharmaceutical J, 2007; **278:** 394

This article notes that a 15 item prescription carries 105 possible drug interactions. Reducing such excessive burdens will require teamwork. So which allies shall we gather on our quest? Well we cannot rely on our sparring partners in the pharmaceutical industry to help us. After all, their motives are hardly clearly aligned with ours. Perhaps our friend the local pharmacist will help. But he is reimbursed per item dispensed and we cannot expect him to put himself out of business.

Doctors don't help themselves as they are driven by the perceived expectation to prescribe and the pursuit of surrogate markers such as blood pressure numbers.

Even the Department of Health seems to love polypharmacy, argues Brewer. How else can they brag about treating more patients than ever before?

Polypharmacy is an insidious disease that advances every time a drug reaction is mistaken for a new symptom.

Free hospital medication reviews may help. The £25 fee for an MUR (medicine use review) delivered by a community pharmacist is also a step in the right direction.

Even putting budgets back under direct responsibility of individual practices as in fundholding could be useful.

But why not dispense with the dispensing fee for pharmacists altogether and give them a vested interest in reducing prescribing and delivering health education?

Treatment reviews of older people on polypharmacy in primary care: cluster controlled trial comparing two approaches
Denneboom W, Dautzenberg M, Grol R, De Smet P
Br J Gen Pract, 2007; **57:** 723–731

It is very important to find the best way to review polypharmacy in the elderly. This controlled trial randomised 738 patients on five or more medicines. It compared written feedback from a pharmacist to a case conference approach with GPs and pharmacists working together to rationalise treatment changes.

The case conferencing group agreed significantly more medical changes and the benefit persisted at 6 months but did disappear by 9 months.

It is likely that the extra costs were offset by savings and the paper supports the notion of regular case review between pharmacist and GP.

Periodic telephone counselling for polypharmacy improved compliance and reduced mortality. *Evidence-Based Medicine*, 2007; **12:** 22
The following paper is reviewed
Effectiveness of telephone counselling by a pharmacist in reducing mortality in patients receiving polypharmacy: randomised controlled trial
Wu JYF, Leung WYS, Chang S *et al.*
BMJ, 2006; **333:** 522

Telephone follow-up from a pharmacist to non-compliant patients saves lives according to this Hong Kong study. The patients were on five or more drugs and received periodic telephone counselling to reinforce the benefits of the medication, clarify treatment regimes and clear up any misconceptions.

Over the two years of this intervention there was a 40% reduction in death with the NNT being 16. Use of health resources was also reduced in this group showing the value and necessity of continuous support in order to change behaviour.

This was a robustly designed study with impressive results. It is not clear how much of the effect observed is due to taking the tablets as opposed to increased health awareness and improved continuity of care. The intervention nevertheless appears highly desirable.

OTC MEDICATION

Switching prescription drugs to over the counter
Cohen JP, Paquette C, Cairns C
BMJ, 2005; **330:** 39–41

Prescription drugs are usually considered for over the counter availability when they ease a non-chronic condition that is fairly easy to self-diagnose and has low potential for harm. But recent switches, such as simvastatin in May 2004, break this pattern.

What are the motives? This article suggests three possibilities, pharmaceutical firms' desire to extend their market, attempts to reduce NHS costs, and the self-care movement. Cost has caused omeprazole to jump over the counter in

Switzerland but that is unlikely to be the main motive for simvastatin in the UK as those at moderate risk of heart disease will still receive it on the NHS.

The number of drugs available this way will undoubtedly grow as pharmaceutical companies whose patents are expiring explore new markets.

ACCESSING CARE

The Challenge

The NHS Plan states that patients should be able to see a health professional within 24 hours and a GP within 48 hours. Yet primary care demand is higher than ever so how best do we balance daily appointment capacity with demand while also increasing satisfaction? At the same time, the style of care in the UK seems to be changing as requests for laboratory analysis went up by over 80% between 2000 and 2004, raising concerns that some are investigating inappropriately.

Advanced Access as proposed by the National Primary Care Collaborative aims to provide flexibility and reduce waiting times. Practices implementing the model have shown that telephone triage of requests for same-day appointments can reduce face-to-face consultations and follow-ups. However, concerns expressed about offering easier 'cosmetic' appointments for trivia at the expense of more appropriate review plans seem legitimate.

Many new models of care have leapt into the fray making first contact services an increasingly complex network marked by minimal evidence of safety or effectiveness.

Non-medical staff are increasingly being used to carry out assessments and treatment traditionally performed by doctors, despite lack of supporting evidence. Where evidence does exist, results are mixed. A direct access health advice line – NHS Direct – has nurse advisers using computerised decision support systems to advise callers. It is popular, safe and expensive.

Walk-in centres introduced in the NHS in 2000 are primarily nurse-led, have long opening hours and treat minor conditions with the intention of relieving the pressure on general practice and other providers of healthcare. Critics have worried about legitimising demand for minor illness and fragmenting care. There is minimal evidence of a benefit on waiting times and consultation rates and they seem to expensively duplicate rather than offer an alternative to the care provided by GPs. A lack of consensus on the core competencies needed by nurses working in walk-in centres and a lack of standardisation of induction, training or support does not help.

When patients do find their way to hospital, their average length of stay in the UK is more than twice that in the US, where strong financial incentives exist to facilitate early discharge and a greater use of intermediate care facilities.

There are many models of care setting out to use our resources better. These include GPwSI (GP with a special interest), joint consultations with specialists, virtual outreach (and shared care models. Most have been shown to be popular, improve treatment strategies and use investigation, referral and follow-up well.

What we know already:

- More patients who have planned appointments bookable in advance see their doctor of choice. Patients have been shown to have a good sense of when they value continuity over speed of access and use of combined appointment systems offer choice.
- Users of walk-in centres tend to be a more affluent group of working age but are a different population from conventional users of general practice.
- Both walk-in centres and NHS Direct improved access for the white middle class but may have increased health inequalities.

- In-house telephone triage by practice nurses is effective. During triage, practice nurses have the advantage of being able to access the medical record and provide a personal service based on previous knowledge of the patient. They can use their own competences more efficiently knowing there is always a GP nearby and this seems like the closest thing we have to an ideal triaging option.
- External management by NHS Direct is feasible but only at a higher cost. Most NHS Direct nurses have never worked in general practice. They are less likely to resolve the problem on the telephone and more likely to recommend a GP appointment. They take around 7 minutes longer to triage a patient using complex algorithms – two and a half times longer than a practice nurse.
- The sort of patients seen by GPs after introduction of a triage system have a higher number of presenting complaints and receive more consultations, prescriptions, and investigations. Appointment systems may have to be adjusted to ensure this particular 'distillation' of patients receive the time they appear to need from their GP.

Recent Papers

ADVANCED ACCESS

Impact of Advanced Access on access, workload, and continuity: controlled before-and-after and simulated-patient study
Salisbury C, Montgomery A, Simons L et al.
Br J Gen Pract, 2007; **57**: 608–614

This paper used anonymous telephone calls from simulated patients to test the hypothesis that Advanced Access appointment systems actually do lead to quicker appointments, as well as reducing workload and increasing continuity of care.

Overall there was indeed a slightly shorter wait in the 24 practices using the system. The NHS Plan 48 hour target was met in 71%, compared to 60% of the 24 control practices. Access to appointments increased at both groups of practices during the study period. There was no evidence of reductions in workload or increased continuity of care.

Does Advanced Access improve access to primary health care? Questionnaire survey of patients
Salisbury C, Goodall S, Montgomery A et al.
Br J Gen Pract, 2007; **57**: 615–621

Do the supposed advantages of Advanced Access really matter to patients? Or is it another triumph of targets over practical sense?

Questionnaires in 47 practices received replies on the subject from 74% – nearly 11 000 patients. While they confirmed that patients were generally seen more quickly, they also found they were less able to book in advance. Overall they were no more satisfied with the new system. Perhaps this was because most (70%) were consulting for a problem they had had for a few weeks.

The resounding message continues to be that patients need flexible systems with appointments that match their priorities

Preferences for access to the GP: a discrete choice experiment
Rubin G, Bate A, George A *et al*.
Br J Gen Pract, 2006; **56**: 743–748

How the targets of the NHS Plan compete with patients' desires for flexibility in choosing their timing and doctor is unclear.

This study of six practices in Sunderland found that the waiting time until an available appointment was only important for children and new health problems. Others would happily wait longer to see their own choice of doctor or choose their own time. This was particularly important for those who worked – they valued it six times more important than the waiting time. It was also of particular importance for those with a chronic illness, women and the elderly.

WALK-IN CENTRES

Impact of NHS walk-in centres on primary care access times: ecological study
Maheswaran R, Pearson T, Munro J *et al*.
BMJ, 2007; **334**: 838

This large study looked at the impact of having 32 walk-in centres within 3 km of 2500 general practices to promote shorter waiting times for GP appointments.

Over the 21 month study period up to the end of 2004, target waiting times improved markedly in the GP practices, but the proximity of the walk-in centre made no difference. Waiting times were longer in more socio-economically deprived areas and shorter in larger practices.

Only since 2006 have practices been blinded to the type of appointment requests made during research such as this. Prior to this, overestimations of the ease of access have been made as such claims benefit the practices' financial interests.

NHS walk-in centres
Salisbury C
BMJ, 2007; **334**: 808–809

This editorial acts as a nice summary of the position regarding walk-in centres. In an ideal world, they would reduce demand on GPs and allow speedier appointments. In reality, we may be catering for previously unmet demand and providing duplicate consultations.

The NHS 48 hour access target has questionable validity and research does not take into account the flexibility that general practice already offers to see patients in need, such as open surgeries and additional appointments for emergencies.

Walk-in centres are unlikely to have a meaningful impact on demand on general practice unless there is a massive expansion. Given their limited range of services and high cost per consultation this would be hard to justify. In fact, the additional service it offers could easily be incorporated into general practice.

Many countries use walk-in services but this may describe all sorts of different entities. When we finally realise how best to use each healthcare provider, we will know more about how to set up our services.

TELEPHONE TRIAGE

Safety of telephone triage in general practitioner cooperatives: do triage nurses correctly estimate urgency?
Giesen P, Ferwerda R, Tijssen R *et al*.
Qual Saf Health Care, 2007; **16:** 181–184

Nurses are increasingly being used to decrease GP workloads but the safety of their telephone-based triage decisions is underassessed.

Unlike the Danes who use doctors for telephone triage, the Netherlands and the UK uses nurses with a primary or secondary care background. This Dutch study used five standardised simulated patients to study decisions by nurses in four GP cooperatives totalling 352 contacts. The level of urgency attributed was compared with a gold standard.

- Correlation was found with the gold standard in about two-thirds.
- Sensitivity and positive predictive values were not high, meaning there was underestimation of urgent complaints in 19% of the contacts.
- Specificity and negative predictive values were high, indicating a high level of efficiency.
- Results showed no correlation with educational background.

The authors conclude that telephone triage by nurses is 'efficient but possibly not safe'.

This may sound harsh when we know that such a mechanism can substantially decrease the immediate workload of a GP. But we also know that some triage increases GP contact so we can say that at the very least it is operator-dependent.

Telephone triage is the most complex and vulnerable part of the out-of hours care process. It has not yet been proven safe. In an effort to improve safety, the Netherlands increasingly uses doctors to supervise a bank of nurses.

In a high quality model, safety trumps efficiency so are we dumbing down our care with these newer models? Can doctors prove they are any better at triage themselves? Perhaps the telephone is an intrinsically unsafe medium.

RATIONING

Rationing in the NHS
Klein R
BMJ, 2007; **334:** 1068–1069

This editorial returns in force to the debate on rationing. The days of rapid growth in the NHS budget are almost over and it is time to balance the books, claims the author.

Payments for targets achieved make the NHS a demand-generating machine for the first time in history. So how should competing demands jostle for position? The priority setting that follows is rationing.

A BMA discussion paper from May 2007 – *A rational way forward for the NHS in England* – calls for safeguarding the core values of the NHS against the incoherence of a constant wave of poorly integrated initiatives from government. The report calls for a separation of national politics from the everyday running of the

NHS. Parliament would determine the core services to be made available nationally and an independent board of NHS governors would be accountable for ensuring the constitution is delivered. Local health authorities could then provide additional services from their own budget and shape and deliver services based on local innovations.

Countries, however, that have tried to define core services have found that exclusions remain highly contestable and some excluded services have still slipped in by the back door. The very concept of a core service is too flexibly interpreted.

Primary care trusts have large unexplained variations in what they spend on particular services with large variances in their decision making. So when does local discretion become postcode prescribing? In addition, too strict legislation will stifle the local innovation that the BMA proposals are trying to encourage.

The danger as ever is too many systems conspiring to clog policy, logic and the practice of delivering health care with professional discretion.

OUT OF HOURS

Should general practitioners resume 24 hour responsibility for their patients? Yes
Jones R
BMJ, 2007; **335:** 696

This head to head argument revisits the 2004 issue of GPs relinquishing 24 hour responsibility for their patients.

Jones argues for rolling back the changes and points to advantages in GP training, benefits in quality and continuity of care, and suggests that patients would welcome back the old out-of-hours service and use it more appropriately than they did last time.

Our best-trained GPs focus on daytime care while patients who become ill at night are potentially seen by doctors with a shallower depth of experience. He notes that complaints to defence societies have risen sharply in relation to doctor–patient communication and diagnostic errors in the years since the changes.

Despite telling us that Scotland finds their out-of-hours services to be financially unsustainable, he claims that a reversion to the old ways is likely to be cost-effective. He continues to refer to the benefits for younger doctors 'more able to tolerate broken sleep' being attracted to this additional income. He barely seems to realise the self-imposed contradiction in his argument. He ends with a Barnum statement giving us his opinion that 24 hour responsibility would 'reap enormous benefits'.

Should general practitioners resume 24 hour responsibility for their patients? No
Herbert H
BMJ, 2007; **335:** 697

Herbert's response shakes Jones out of his time-warp and reminds us of the reasons the changes were made in the first place.

GPs are isolated and unsupported for their many daily decisions without the luxury of a hospital team to cross-cover. The new measures allowed doctors to avoid working all day and be on call at night before working another day in a system openly abused by some patients. Doctors can now avoid making life-threatening decisions, sidelining the sort of sleep deprivation that lorry drivers or airline pilots would not be asked to tolerate. The concept was for patient safety and a satisfactory work-life balance.

GPs are the solution to improving urgent care services rather than the problem. Designing services around clinical needs as opposed to government whim is the way to go. If newer models of care and services cause confusion that can hardly be their fault. Excellent models of primary care are already possible, such as those in place for terminal illness which anticipate problems, facilitate good communication, and allow for systematic care and follow up.

A role in advocacy of excellence in anticipatory care is the responsibility of modern general practice.

A qualitative study exploring variations in GPs' out-of-hours referrals to hospital
Calnan M, Payne S, Kemple T *et al*.
Br J Gen Pract, 2007; **57:** 706–713

This set of interviews set out to look at the reasons for the wide spread of referral rates among doctors.

High referrers were cautious and believed in admitting if in doubt. They expressed anxiety about the consequences of not admitting for both the patient and themselves.

Lower referrers were more confident about their decisions and more positive about alternatives to hospital admission. They felt able to resist pressures from family or carers and saw hospitals as places to be avoided, viewing their goal as preventing admission.

The authors call for more education at a level which builds confidence. This is surely timely as younger less experienced doctors may be more likely to be working in out-of-hours services.

NEWER MODELS

Effectiveness of paramedic practitioners in attending 999 calls from elderly people in the community: cluster randomised controlled trial
Mason S, Knowles E, Colwell B *et al*.
BMJ, 2007; **335:** 919

With demand for ambulances rising by as much as 8% per year and the statistic that half of their human deliveries to emergency departments require neither treatment nor referral, this well-powered randomised trial looked at the impact that an extended scope paramedic programme could have.

This model of care involves specially trained paramedics who have undergone a 3 week course and 45 days in supervised practice making home visits to elderly patients with minor illnesses. They responded to falls, burns and injuries, and among their skills was a degree of competence in neurological, cardiovascular, respiratory and joint examination. They could refer to GPs or emergency departments and request X-rays.

The survey had over 3000 responses from patients over 60 who had called 999. The most common presenting complaint was a fall. Within 28 days of the initial call, over 40% had required hospital admission and 5% had died, showing the group was high-risk but mortality was similar in the control group who received standard 999 service.

Attendances at the emergency department and hospital admissions in the following month were reduced and the service was popular with patients.

In an accompanying commentary (*BMJ*, 2007; **335:** 893–894), Woollard warns against generalising these findings and calls for more high quality studies before rapid costly expansion.

NURSE PRACTITIONERS

The Challenge

Rising demand and expectations have led to a shift of care to different health professionals, notably nurses. The trend towards advanced nursing practice is government-led and reflects international trends.

The role of nurse practitioner is as a co-practitioner in the primary care team, involving responsibility for assessment and treatment decisions.

Unfortunately, the term 'nurse practitioner' is often used vaguely and research in the area is not always relevant to general practice. The different abilities, amount of training, and degree of autonomy of nurse practitioners makes the role as a whole difficult to recommend with evidence. Generalisations regarding the value of the role sometimes extend beyond the conditions actually studied, which are often trivial illness and minor injury.

There have been successes but a recent expansion in nurse prescribing has caused widespread safety concerns.

What we know already:

- Nurses can successfully undertake much of the health promotion work of general practices and they have a leading role in chronic disease follow up.
- According to systematic review, nurses spend around 4 minutes longer than doctors per consultation and order more investigations with little difference in health outcomes. This could indicate a lack of diagnostic ability or a lack of time-efficient management.
- Employing a nurse practitioner skilled in chronic case management in a general practice failed to reduce workload for GPs in a controlled Dutch study. The change actually increased the GPs' consultations during surgery hours by around 5 per week.
- The standards of consultation required of GP registrars do not apply to nurses. Patient satisfaction is offered as an oft-quoted surrogate.
- Since May 2006, independent nurse prescribers in England have been able to 'prescribe any licensed medicine for any medical condition within their competence'.
- Nurse Independent Prescribers are professionally responsible for their own actions. However, employers may also be held vicariously responsible for the nurse's actions. Many GPs think nurses should be fully accountable for their own prescribing.

Recent Papers

Extended prescribing by UK nurses and pharmacists
Avery AJ, Pringle M
BMJ, 2005; **331:** 1154–1155

The Department of Health's announcement that nurse and pharmacist prescribers will be able to independently prescribe any licensed drug except controlled drugs was radical. It was the most far reaching development of its type anywhere in the world and stunned more than a few.

With a relative absence of evidence of either safety or benefit, the BMA has suggested that diagnostic skills just might be a valid part of safe prescribing, but this diplomatic article seems to get behind the propositions, reassuring itself that nurses will always act within their own areas of competence. There is no mention of the unknown incompetence that haunts some of us on a day-to-day basis. The authors admit it 'is impossible to draw clear conclusions on the safety and appropriateness of extended prescribing' and want to rely on clinical computer systems (as yet poorly developed) to provide the safety net. By the end of the article they seem to change their tune with the phrase 'thorough risk assessments should be done nationally and locally before prescribing is extended to new clinical areas.'

Developing nurse prescribing in the UK
Avery AJ, James V
BMJ, 2007; **335**: 316

Training for independent nurse prescribers involves 26 days of theory, 12 days of mentored practice and 5 assignments. Currently more than 8000 nurses have access to prescribing the full formulary that doctors use.

Some early analysis suggests that nurses prescribe within their areas of competence. However, detractors point to other research which draws attention to the lack of decision-making ability and pharmacological knowledge. In one recent analysis of 25 scenarios, only a minority of nurse prescribers were able to identify more than half the pharmacological problems relevant to each case and suggest a course of action.

Advocates suggest that in these cases they would have asked for help or, to use modern parlance, 'referred to a GP'.

While it is possible to dismiss criticism as concerned doctors worrying about having nurses on their traditional turf, there seem to be legitimate worries with this development.

The standalone training module was designed to allow rapid expansion among experienced nurse practitioners. With the next wave, it is time to build prescribing into a more comprehensive foundation of assessment, diagnosis, decision-making and audit. Expansion is likely to happen but there is much to be proven in terms of safety, effectiveness and the actual value of nurse prescribing.

Nurse practitioner and practice nurses' use of research information in clinical decision making: findings from an exploratory study
McCaughan D, Thompson C, Cullum C *et al.*
Fam Pract, 2005; **22**: 490–497

How do nurses deal with uncertainty? They ask a doctor. This qualitative study of information-seeking behaviour on a sample of 29 practice nurses and 4 nurse practitioners in the North of England showed that human sources of information were overwhelmingly preferred to books or the internet. The nurses involved, including the more independent role of nurse practitioner, rarely used evidence-based resources to seek answers to questions regarding diagnosis and treatment.

Epilepsy and supplementary nurse prescribing
Hosking PG
BMJ, 2006; **332**: 2

This editorial written by an epilepsy nurse specialist points out that we can do a lot more to prevent epilepsy-related deaths. Incentives can encourage GPs to conduct annual reviews and nurse specialists are known to improve patient management, reducing the need for contact with doctors.

However, she tells us that less than half of all epilepsy nurse specialists have postgraduate qualifications relevant to the responsibility of case management, casting doubt on titles such as 'specialist nurse'.

They propose that the correct level of education is a generic masters degree which can be adapted for epilepsy. This will provide the necessary familiarity with classification, differential diagnosis, pharmacology, neurophysiology, neuro-imaging, and psychosocial aspects of care. They would be able to advise GPs directly and be responsible for a caseload of around 1000 epileptics each.

Comparing the cost of nurse practitioners and GPs in primary care: modelling economic data from randomised trials
Hollinghurst S, Horrocks S, Anderson E *et al*.
Br J Gen Pract, 2006; **56**: 530–535

This cost analysis of two randomised controlled trials included costs of training and estimated the cost of nurse practitioner consultation (£30.35) as costing much the same as a salaried GP (£28.14). Confidence intervals overlapped. The costs were higher because of the time spent by GPs contributing to the nurses consultations and doing return visits.

They point out that proven abilities of nurse practitioners are very mixed and employment should depend more on the actual role fulfilled than a cost analysis like this.

INFORMATION TECHNOLOGY

The Challenge

The NHS Plan, NSFs and the NHS information strategy all promote use of electronic patient records, but incompatible systems and databases have made integration difficult and the UK somewhat lags behind similar countries in terms of IT.

The NHS information and technology programme is the largest civilian IT programme in the world and Connecting for Health is the agency responsible for delivering the programme. The main features are a new broadband networking service, electronic booking called Choose and Book, electronic transfer of prescriptions, and a nationally accessible summary of patients' records, called 'the spine'.

NHS HealthSpace (www.healthspace.nhs.uk) is a secure online personal health organiser available to all patients in England. Despite delays in progress it is set to become the world's first fully national system of electronic personal health records. Projected expenditure is over £12 billion and the programme has been dogged with concerns about maintaining patient confidentiality, resulting in a slow-down in implementation.

As yet we have little evidence on how to translate the potential of technology into daily care. For example, assessment of clinical gains from use of decision software and hardware is seriously lacking. A focus on gadgets must not avert our focus from the human element. Elderly and disabled people are most disenfranchised by new technologies such as online communication tools, leading to a worsening of health inequalities.

What we know already:

- Electronic medical records in general practice contain inaccuracies in 40% of their summaries.
- Over 90% of doctors use computers in clinical care and over 90% of prescriptions are now issued on computers.
- Computers have already increased safe prescribing by as much as 60% with legible, complete prescriptions.
- The software for detecting prescribing errors still seriously underperforms. Better system design that matches the patient record with external sources of data is needed to improve safety features.
- The internet comes with the appealing characteristics of 24 hour availability and privacy and the unappealing ones of poor quality sites and unscrupulous marketing.
- Health information is some of the most retrieved information on the internet. Patients use it to check the experiences of others, identify questions to ask the doctors and check their advice and treatment, but most research focuses on measures far removed from health outcomes making interpretation an art.
- Online learning for patients can produce objectively measured changes in behaviour and knowledge that are at least as good as learning 'live'.
- Patients value the unique environment provided by web-based disease management programmes, feeling an enhanced sense of security about their health, but they are disappointed at times when the programmes did not meet their expectations. Patients

---

used to doing all their banking at home may need to lower their expectations of what web-healthcare can deliver.

- Technologies may move too rapidly to make RCTs as useful as we need them to be, outpacing our ability to judge them.
- Paperless records compare very favourably with paper-based systems. They are more understandable, fully legible and contain more information in terms of diagnoses, advice, referral details and drug doses. Paperless doctors can recall more of the advice they gave to patients.
- Online advertising is a viable and cost-effective strategy to attract internet users to health promotion advice such as screening programmes.

Recent Papers

ELECTRONIC PATIENT RECORDS

Implementing the NHS information technology programme: qualitative study of progress in acute trusts
Hendy J, Fulop N, Reeves BC *et al.*
BMJ, 2007; **334:** 1360

Those involved with implementing changes in the NHS IT programme were interviewed over a two year period about the challenges they continue to face. Despite growing support for the overall aims there was frustration with delays and serious concerns with the following:

- local financial deficits and competing priorities
- delayed implementation of standardised systems risking loss of integration of the programme
- poor communication with local managers from Connecting For Health
- risk to patient safety with the ongoing delays
- discontent with the Choose and Book system

The authors warn of the need for suitable interim systems and realistic timetables to ensure long-term compatibility and value for money.

Potential of electronic personal health records
Pagliari C, Detmer D, Singleton P
BMJ, 2007; **335:** 330–333

HealthSpace (www.healthspace.nhs.uk) is a secure online personal health organiser available to all patients in England. It will allow access to the provider's electronic care records (summaries only at first), opening a gateway for interactive health care which will enhance continuity of care and efficiency. It facilitates the booking of appointments and reordering of prescriptions and could possibly be expanded to allow the seeking of direct professional advice by email as is done in parts of the US.

In the long run, it will ideally empower patients through shared decision making and increase safety by exposing diagnostic errors and mistakes in prescribing. Fragmentation will be reduced and continuity of care could benefit.

The system could expand to offering self-management support such as care plans, passive biofeedback and decision aids, but it may still be a considerable time before its full potential is reached. Without access to clinicians to interpret it, this may not all be beneficial.

Online access is being piloted in a limited number of practices in the first place due to ongoing anxieties surrounding confidentiality and security. Patients may ultimately have to decide whether they find the risk acceptable.

Professionals and patients need to be involved in the design, development and implementation of new IT systems to anticipate more problems.

Soft paternalism and the ethics of shared electronic patient records
Norheim OF
BMJ, 2006; **333**: 2–3

This paper discusses the ethics relating to the proposed network of integrated databases regarding patients records.

Rapid access to a single resource may improve quality of care but also makes patients vulnerable when records contain sensitive private information.

They note that the Royal College of General Practitioners strongly recommends an 'opt in' policy for citizens whereas Connecting For Health, the agency building the new electronic records service, wants an 'opt-out' policy.

Standard medical ethics suggests that where the path is unclear the public should be fully informed and only be included if they give explicit consent. This preserves freedom of choice, but as people are not always rational and may be too lazy to make a well-informed opinion, their health and welfare may suffer. On the other hand, automatic opt-in without the possibility to opt out promotes health and welfare at the cost of liberty

This article puts the case for 'soft paternalism', automatically opting people in unless they strongly disagree. This preserves freedom of choice and promotes health.

However, there are some caveats. The NHS must convincingly show that technical and legal safeguards are bulletproof and that the control of access is strict and transparent.

ᴇHEALTH

Email consultations in health care: 1 – scope and effectiveness. 2 – acceptability and safe application
Car J, Sheikh A
BMJ, 2004; **329**: 435–438, 439–442

Electronic communication has revolutionised the industries of banking and retail but what can it do for healthcare? Although little evidence currently exists on electronic models of care, patients want email access to doctors and this pair of papers considers its potential.

Advantages are:
- user-friendly, efficient and versatile in facilitating asynchronous communication

- increases patient choice and many would be prepared to pay for this service
- may be cost-effective, time-efficient and reduce need for face-to-face contacts
- addresses unmet need and delivers care to those who would not normally present
- plenty of scope for preventative health care and managing non-urgent conditions
- role in receiving straightforward test results or doing follow up checks
- useful for improving non-attendance rates with cheap reminders
- certain responses can be automated
- avoids face to face embarrassment of rescheduling appointments
- written record of important points to remember or clarify
- increased reporting of adverse events
- delivering information to many people simultaneously
- feedback from patient selfcare assignments particularly in chronic care
- surveys report greater honesty in electronic questionnaires than in person by an interviewer

Disadvantages are:
- potential for overwhelm due to increased communication burden
- satisfaction decreases markedly if replies take longer than 48 hours
- may widen social disparities of care
- loss of subtle emotive clues and patient-centredness
- inability to examine and risk of diagnostic errors
- lack of data security measures results in threats to confidentiality
- system must seamlessly integrate e-contacts with the usual medical record
- not currently recommended outside existing doctor–patient relationships

Guidance will be needed on organising the service with suitable standards and strategies that mitigate risk at all stages. Patients and doctors will need to understand the limitations and risks involved. Ideally, informed consent should be obtained.

THE INTERNET

Googling for a diagnosis – use of Google as a diagnostic aid: internet based study
Tang H, Ng JHK
BMJ, 2006; **333**: 1143–1145

Using one year's worth of case histories from one journal (*New Engl J Med*), this study looked at the accuracy of Google in coming up with the correct diagnosis.

Doctors chose the search words and opted for distinctive combinations of three to five terms. The three most prominent diagnoses that seemed to fit the signs and symptoms were selected and compared to the case record. If one of these was the right answer, the search was deemed a success. Google got it in 58% of cases.

Physicians have been estimated to carry 2 million facts in their heads in order to be a diagnostician. Google already accesses 3 billion articles.

Searches by patients may be less efficient than this figure but, at the very least, search engines can clearly be an additional tool to help doctors diagnose difficult cases with unique symptoms.

Diagnosis using search engines
Gardner M
BMJ, 2006; **333**: 1131

Although thousands of computer systems have been developed, most have made little impact. That said, they have not had the same speed, accessibility, simplicity and lack of cost as Google. No special equipment is required and no maintenance bills will come your way.

This editorial asks clinicians not to feel too discouraged. Although the press loved this story, we are reminded that doctors chose the search terms in the study above and that inferring a diagnosis also depended on the assessment of doctors.

However, developments in years to come will herald a much more powerful 'semantic web'. When future search engines can access data and resources that reside in databases other than HTML code, they will be increasingly important assets.

FUTURE OF GENERAL PRACTICE

The Challenge

The GMS contract, new in 2004, constituted the biggest change in primary care for decades. The UK general practice model has successfully demonstrated marked improvements in quality of care in many areas in recent years with financial incentives closely linked to the quality improvements. Further major structural review of the delivery of primary care is now well under way.

Recent requests for extended opening hours and a new initiative for 'polyclinics' have been announced. To many this may feel like déjà vu and this is despite evidence failing to consistently demonstrate associations between practice size and quality of care.

What we know already:

- Patients want a service that will be there when they need it which is free at the point of delivery.
- Although younger patients are willing to trade continuity for faster access, older ones particularly value continuity of care.
- The evidence shows that patients value 'humaneness' in their doctors above all other qualities. They want GPs who engage, take time, explain and have up-to-date skills, but change is coming at a speed which may override these subtle preferences.

Guidance

The future of general practice. A Statement by the Royal College of General Practitioners. **London: RCGP, September 2004** (www.rcgp.org.uk/PDF/Corp_future_of_general_practice.pdf)

Recent Papers

Gordon Brown's agenda for the NHS
Ham C
BMJ, 2008; **336:** 53–54

Reflecting on the sixtieth year of the NHS, the Prime Minister has indicated a broad direction for the future, although detail is markedly lacking at this stage. His agenda emphasises preventative care and screening although this editorial notes the many false dawns of the past on this issue.

Patients should receive help in managing their own conditions with an expansion of the lay-led Expert Patient Programme. Schools and employers will be encouraged to promote healthy lifestyles.

Primary care will have a part in accessing routine tests and GPs have been told to extend opening hours. He indicated that NHS foundation trusts would be allowed to provide primary care in the future adding that there were no 'no-go' areas for reform. The detail is expected when the NHS constitution is published.

Good general practitioners will continue to be essential
Lakhani M, Baker M
BMJ, 2006; **332:** 41–43

> These authors argue there will still be a need for care from a doctor with whom they have a relationship. Care will flow from a relationship-based model which commits to interpersonal care and becomes more necessary as health care becomes more complex. Patients will take part in planning health services and assessing quality as well as self-management of chronic illness.
>
> The unique skills of GPs are dealing with uncertainty and managing comorbidity. Cost-effective management of undifferentiated problems will be more important than ever. There will be more mediation with specialists and GPs will work within communities to develop partnerships to promote an agenda for health in schools and workplaces.
>
> A broader range of professionals will be based in primary care and providing a range of skills in an integrated fashion at a convenient location close to home will be crucial to match what the public requires. Virtually all problems including mental health will be dealt with in primary care, with short term referral to specialists as needed. Interfaces of care are dangerous for patients and primary care clinicians. Good clinicians will help prevent fragmentation of care using intelligent systems which ensure quality and accountability.

The magic roundabout
Lapsley P
BMJ, 2006; **332:** 43–44

> In 2015, unreasonable targets to be seen by a doctor within 2 days have been dropped due to effectively penalising working patients. Working out of hours has been made more attractive to GPs. Patients have finally been recognised to have responsibilities as well as rights in terms of leading healthy lifestyles, turning up for appointments and conforming with care plans. This seems to have started with the ban on smoking in public places.
>
> Health promotion messages have started to hit home and alternative health practices have been coordinated into NHS new age clinics which are well placed to provide practical advice on diet and fitness, as well as offering services such as acupuncture and chiropractic. Doctors and nurses are free to spend more time with patients who really are partners in their own health care.

General practice under pressure
Meldrum H
BMJ, 2006; **332:** 46–47

> A darker vision is that of GPs feeling undervalued due to eroded incomes and ongoing political interference.
>
> Charges have been introduced for many non-essential items including sickness certificates. Mobile video phones allow consultations with healthcare

professionals in their practice and, if investigations are needed, patients visit a mobile resource centre which feeds results back to the practice.

The clutches of the private sector are extending as Tesco Health takes over a failing NHS Direct. NHS facilities have found it difficult to compete with an aggressive cherry-picking private sector but a few larger practices (with many more salaried doctors) have succeeded in radically improving the number and quality of services offered.

MODERN TRENDS

Who needs health care—the well or the sick?
Heath I
BMJ, 2005; **330:** 954–956

This beautifully poetic article is well worth a read.

Dr Heath suggests there is a paradox that the more we concentrate on health at the expense of some of the other joys of living, the unhealthier we become. Rich countries are swept along in the 'excessive self confidence of preventative medicine' which could be tipping them towards a 'foundation of fear' and misery. Self-reporting of illness can be too low in poorer nations but is extremely high in the United States despite their health care never having been more advanced.

The measure of health care in rich countries seems to have become the simple prolongation of life. Swarms of protocols seem to express certainties where they do not exist and this may be a form of bullying. Bullying by doctors, by politicians and by multinationals who may have a lot to gain from the medicalisation of populations into the 'worried well'. We live in a time where more money is invested into research into the prevention of disease than into treatments. Money that could make a huge difference to poorer nations contributes towards relabelling risk factors as the latest illness.

As each generation looks back on the ignorance of the last, are we really sure we are doing more good than harm? Are we really addressing our patients' concerns? Or just doing everyone a favour by saying we can deliver life from its inherent thrill – uncertainty?

Competition in general practice
Marshall M, Wilson T
BMJ, 2005; **331:** 1196–1199

This is one of the articles under the issue banner 'The NHS Revolution' and looks at how competition might affect general practice. Alternative models of primary care have already arrived in communities that have failed to replace retiring GPs and challenged the priority of continuity of care which has been so successful in minimising competitive forces at the expense of patient choice.

General practice performs well in term of equity (although some inequalities remain), efficiency (where it is one of the most cost-effective healthcare systems in the developed world, with its emphasis on dealing with uncertainty and rationing expensive services), and quality (where clinical governance is starting to bear fruit).

But other models could be used:

- Commercial takeover, e.g. by a high street retailer or pharmaceutical company
- Mergers of existing practices allowing a common executive team
- Hospital-based services with primary care clinics closely linked to hospitals
- Population-specific services in which a provider might deliver all services aimed at a specific age group, e.g. teenagers
- Condition-specific services – where independent providers might deliver hypertension clinics or investigative facilities

The trade off in personal care might suit those who want technically efficient, accessible care. But fragmentation might lead to exacerbation of inequalities and reduce care for the growing number of people with comorbidities. And if general practice has been as cost-effective as it is claimed, new entrants in the market may be unable to compete with current providers.

Either way, the monopoly is disappearing and the article opines that positive things will come of integrated measures such as takeovers and mergers. Negative effects are more likely with different packages of care coming from different directions such as population-specific and condition-specific approaches.

PRACTICE SIZE

The future of singlehanded general practices
Majeed A
BMJ, 2005; **330**: 1460–1461

This editorial is a good summary of the position regarding single-handed practices.

Between 2003 and 2004 the proportion of such practices in the UK fell to 6% with a larger fall over that one year than in the preceding nine years. Yet the value of such doctors in communities, especially rural and inner city practices, has been unquestionable. Although they have the shadow of Harold Shipman leering over them, the balance of evidence for general practices does not insist that bigger is better. Government recommendations to do something about the clinical isolation of single-handed practitioners flies in the face of a well-liked service that offers patients a choice (at a time when choice is quite a popular idea) and has been found by patients to be more accessible and deliver higher rates of satisfaction than larger practices.

Doctors may well like the flexibility of working in a large practice to allow time for family or other interests as well as the opportunity to work with more support staff. But for those that might choose single-handed practice, perhaps the market rather than the government should decide their fate. Good comparative information on measures of quality of care will identify those underperforming. Perhaps in the future these data will even be published so patients can vote with their feet. Single-handed practices can then die a fair and equitable death. But who would bet against them flourishing? Nearly half the family practitioners in the US are single-handed.

Determinants of primary medical care quality measured under the new UK contract: cross sectional study
Sutton M, McLean G
BMJ, 2006; **332:** 389–390

This study in 60 Scottish general practices found that higher quality scores were obtained in deprived areas (contrary to early concerns that the new contract would increase health inequalities) and where the teams of doctors and practice nurses were larger. Practices with fewer than four full time clinicians had lower recorded quality.

Factors not statistically associated with quality were accreditation, training status and age of the GP. This implies that the size and the composition of the clinical team are the most important determinants of the quality of primary medical care. We should focus on this structure when looking to the future.

CHILDREN

Primary care for children in the 21st century
Hall D, Sowden D
BMJ, 2005; **330:** 430–431

This editorial opens with a pat on the back for the model of general practice and then goes on to say how inadequate it will be in treating the children of the 21st century. It proposes that the lack of 24 hour care will mean more and more concerned parents will bypass primary care in favour of a trip to the hospital.

It suggests that GPs do not have a major role in managing chronic disorders in children and while the preventative care may be fine, this can easily be taken over by health visitors and other non-medical staff.

Teenagers need special attention and, despite some practices making an effort to make things more accessible in sensitive areas such as sexual health, clinics not attached to 'the doctor's' seem to be more popular with adolescents.

We are told that tomorrow's parents will expect their doctor to have 'confirmed competencies in acute and non-urgent children's care particularly psychological disorders and chronic disease'. It proposes the abandoning of the concept of the whole family doctor in favour of a new generation of general paediatricians who can work in the community as well as in hospitals.

It is written by a professor of community paediatrics.

DOCTORS IN PRACTICE

The Challenge

Complex interactions occur in general practice and GPs are at risk of high levels of stress and burnout. Doctors may carry grievances in relation to ever-increasing patient demand and a growing perception of a general lack of respect for the medical profession. They have a tendency to deny personal illness, to self-prescribe and have a high suicide rate.

Larger partnerships can reduce professional isolation and provide the opportunity for a supportive environment. However, personal morale and ability to cope with workload depends on perceptions of fairness in allocation of work and remuneration – topics often too emotive to discuss.

Managers are under increasing pressure to reach new targets and achieve major structural reform. They look at allocating resources to populations and the need for public accountability. Doctors tend to have different values. They focus on patients, desire professional autonomy and work towards evidence-based practice while yearning for a bygone age when managers knew their place. They tend not to like to give up professional autonomy to managers and management styles that annoy them may adversely affect quality of care.

Two distinct styles of manager are the directive authoritarian who sees doctors as obstacles, and the more appealing facilitative manager who pays attention to complex collaborations valuing mutual respect and nurturing the ability to live with different points of view.

The GP registrar joins this complex ecosystem with sometimes explosive results.

What we know already:

- Patients are best served by an ongoing tension between doctors and managers.
- Despite some junior doctors feeling isolated, those exposed to general practice at an early stage after graduation benefit from enhanced communication skills, patient-centred consulting, dealing with diagnostic uncertainty and developing understanding of doctor–patient relationships in the community.
- Twelve months registrar training may not adequately prepare doctors for general practice with many feeling that the year is too pressured and too focussed on examinations.
- A major reason for new GPs to express regret at joining a practice is the stress from the personalities of the partnership.
- Qualitative evidence has shown that training can occasionally be patchy in quality with some registrars frightened of their trainer and worried their form would not be signed, and some areas of training totally absent despite being signed off.
- Pilots which extend registrar training to 18 months have not convincingly resolved issues of feeling adequately prepared for independent practice if this is even possible. An extension of vocational training to a total of 5 years in line with other specialities has been proposed.

Recent Papers

JOB SATISFACTION

Selecting and supporting contented doctors
Peile E, Carter Y
BMJ, 2005; **330**: 269–270

Unhappy doctors underperform and can drag their colleagues down with them according to this editorial.

However, much of the perception of the stress in their lives can be directly attributed to their own personality, according to research on over 1600 medical graduates followed up 12 years after they had entered medical school. The trait of neuroticism, for example, predicts a disordered approach to work and perceptions of high workload and stress. Perhaps if we cannot socially engineer to fill medical schools with easy going contended candidates (after all where are we to get our supply of academics from?), we should use this psychological profiling to identify those in need of help. A process of mentoring and appraisal with the chief aim of supporting doctors and students can detect unhappiness early and do something to effect change.

PRACTICE RELATIONSHIPS

General practitioners' perceptions of sharing workload in group practices: qualitative study
Branson R, Armstrong D
BMJ, 2004; **329**: 381

Hats off to the authors! This paper looks at how GP partners get on with each other. Not generally without resentments and resignations of one kind or the other, it seems.

All the 18 GPs who agreed to be interviewed recognised the problems of inequitable distribution of workload. The most common cause of tension was between 'fast consulters', who felt they inherited extra visits, appointments and more repeat prescriptions, and 'slow consulters' who saw themselves as providing a higher quality service with more stress resulting from attending to psychosocial issues.

Doctors were irritated when covering a fast consulter's clinic made them realise that patients were being reviewed for trivial reasons.

Perceived inequality is a major source of resentment and stress in general practice but erosion of trust is shared with many areas of modern society. Interestingly, legitimate data fails to back up perceptions of being a harder worker with actual facts. The conclusion is that workload is not as misallocated as presumed.

Small practices needing more flexibility between colleagues in order to provide a full service relied on mutual trust to manage this hurdle. Larger practices had more rigid systems that allowed them to predict workload. Some even allocated points linked to financial rewards, but fairness still depended on who designed the system.

Practice meetings could be useful to air grievances but a lot of lengthy meetings became self-defeating and increased stress levels.

Ultimately, solutions to the problem depended on a cyclical acceptance of periods of contentment and resentment or, like any other marriage, divorce.

I like the comment in the rapid responses: "[In the complex work of general practice] if you don't think you are working harder than your partners then you're not working hard enough".

THE PHARMACEUTICAL INDUSTRY

The Challenge

Doctors need to use the products the pharmaceutical industry comes up with and it is reasonable that the industry should promote these products.

The pharmaceutical industry funds trials at all stages of a product's life cycle. But the questions asked in those trials are designed to get drugs registered as quickly as possible with the least restrictive indications. The best questions may therefore not be asked and because of ethical constraints in future trials they become unanswerable.

Trials can be carefully designed to show 'equivalence' or 'non-inferiority'. Trials powered to detect superiority would be a disaster for the new product if the drug did not win the head-to-head race. If in doubt, use your competitor's drug in the wrong dose. Keep the dose nice and high so you can show your drug has fewer toxic effects, or nice and low so you can say yours is more effective. If it all goes wrong of course, you can bury the results in a drawer labelled 'unpublished'. Add in a hideously complex economic evaluation paper and the brain of the average journal editor could be spinning, never mind that of the poor pressured GP trying to divine the truth. There is potential for huge conflicts of interest and corruption charges have been brought in high profile cases in Italy.

Most medical journals have a substantial income from drug companies who crave favourable editorial coverage in credible journals above all things. For their part, doctors like to get journals for free even if they have lots of adverts in. Free publications work hard to increase their attractiveness to readers and therefore increase their advertising revenue.

Drug companies are not allowed to advertise to patients but that's not a problem because even patients' organisations are at it! Patients' organisations welcome opportunities (i.e. money) for expansion and publicity, and pharmaceutical companies are rich, whereas patients' organisations are poor.

The inequality raises serious questions. Drug companies might persuade patients to lobby for them against restrictive health service policies. This has massive potential to pervert real agendas and has been exploited in various sneaky ways in the US.

What we know already:

- Contact with pharmaceutical representatives increases prescribing costs.
- Requests from patients for specific medications increases their prescribing.
- The Association of the British Pharmaceutical Industry (ABPI) have a national Code of Practice that prohibits all but the most modest hospitality towards doctors. The going rate is £6 per gift and it has to be work-relevant.
- Studies have shown that references cited in drug advertising can be impossible to track down and independent review of the evidence they quote often leads to different conclusions than those claimed. The high quality of the work, however, is not in question.
- Characteristics of GPs who have contact with drug reps are greater willingness to prescribe new drugs, increased likelihood of agreeing to a request for a drug not clinically indicated and reluctance to end consultations with advice alone.

- The Department of Health's drive to persuade doctors to prescribe statins generically (saving an estimated £84 million a year) is being legally challenged by ABPI who are trying to insist that patients provide informed consent.

Recent Papers

The influence of big pharma
Ferner RE
BMJ, 2005; **330:** 855–856

A government report on '*The influence of the pharmaceutical industry*' from April 2005 paints a picture of an industry that buys influence over doctors, charities, patient groups, journalists and politicians, and whose regulation is at worst weak and at best ambiguous. Half of all postgraduate medical education, and a great deal of nurse education, is funded by the pharmaceutical companies. They finance 90% of drug trials but come up with few innovative products while publishing positive results in a variety of guises and dismissing negatives results as flawed.

Advertising associates their brands with emotional attributes to appeal to doctors as they push their promotions as powerfully as they can.

The report suggests new limits on marketing and prescribing during 'probationary periods' for new drugs, with formal trials of efficacy performed within the NHS to improve pharmacovigilance.

Influence of pharmaceutical funding on the conclusions of meta-analyses
Epstein RA
BMJ, 2007; **335:** 1167
and
Financial ties and concordance between results and conclusions in meta-analyses: retrospective cohort study
Yank V, Rennie D, Bero LA
BMJ, 2007; **335:** 1202–1205

Yank's study looked at meta-analyses relating to antihypertensive drugs and found that we should question the interpretation of results in such studies. The conclusions of meta-analyses which are sponsored by drug companies enjoyed more positive spin than those that were not. The effect was particularly marked when the sponsor was a single company. That the bias remained unspotted and was published also exposes a failure of editorial and peer review.

The effect disappeared completely when funding was from non-profit institutions and these meta-analyses showed excellent concordance between results and conclusions.

Clearly some control is being exerted even though the actual areas of bias may be well-disguised. It has therefore been suggested that drug companies should have a more restricted role in financing and preparing such research. As they are responsible for so much funding, however, there are fears the research may dry up. Nobody is questioning the quality of the research, just the interpretation.

The editorial by Epstein therefore argues that we should continue with the higher number of studies with the inherent risk of bias rather than have no studies at all. Then we can safeguard by getting other investigators to double-check the same data and see if they agree with the conclusions. Editorial comment perhaps published elsewhere could then flesh out a fuller perspective of what the data are really saying. Authors would then be subtly cajoled into softening their basic claims.

The Pharmaceutical Price Regulation Scheme
Collier J
BMJ, 2007; **334:** 435–436

The Pharmaceutical Price Regulation Scheme (formerly the Voluntary Price Regulation Scheme) has been running since 1956. It is a voluntary arrangement between the Department of Health and individual drug companies and it determines the prices companies can charge the NHS for their drugs.

In February 2007, the Office of Fair Trading proclaimed that it was no longer fit for purpose. With a concurrent agenda to obtain drugs at reasonable prices as well as sponsor the well-being of UK companies there is too much conflict.

The pharmaceutical industry alone determines the price it considers to be the value and high prices at launch are guaranteed.

An independent commission is now proposed to determine the new value and involving NICE will streamline rapid access to early official endorsement immediately after launch. Until now the drug companies have shared the risk of drug development with the NHS who could provide reimbursement if things went wrong. Under the changes proposed they would now be on their own.

Who pays for the pizza? Redefining the relationships between doctors and drug companies.
1. Entanglement 2. Disentanglement
Moynihan R
BMJ, 2003; **326:** 1189–1192, 1193–1196

This pair of papers is based on the American system but looks at how doctors and drug companies are 'twisted together like the snake and the staff'. There is a new urgency to address this area in the face of rising pharmaceutical costs.

- In the US about 90% of doctors see drug reps. They receive gifts and attend events which highlight the sponsor's drug.
- Most deny their influence despite evidence to the contrary.
- Entanglement is widespread and undermines rational prescribing strategies.
- Medical journals rely on drug company-funded trials, advertisements, company-purchased reprints and ad-laden supplements.
- The impact is to fundamentally distort the evidence base of healthcare.
- 'Food, flattery and friendship are all powerful tools of persuasion'.
- Increasing access to young medics means that a culture of gift-giving could breed a long-term sense of entitlement and indebtedness.
- Young doctors unrealistically believe they are immune to promotional influences.

- Calls for disentanglement are being made by medical reform groups (such as www.nofreelunch.org).
- The 'systematic bias' in sponsored research comes not from bad science but the fact that the questions asked in the first place are in the interests of the sponsors not the patients.
- Reporting all trials rather than burying important negative findings should be job number one.
- The analogy that we would not tolerate judges taking money from those they judge may be a realistic one.

The debate seems to have started now that the American healthcare system is at a crisis point. There may still be some valid points for the UK system.

Direct to consumer advertising
Mansfield PR, Mintzes B, Richards D *et al*.
BMJ, 2005; **330:** 5–6

With New Zealand introducing a ban in 2005, the United States is left as the only industrialised country allowing full direct-to-consumer advertising of prescription medicines.

Generally, nations feel that there is no net benefit for their communities from minimising risk information and exaggerating benefits with advertising gloss. It increases prescriber workloads and expenditure for the larger employers that provide healthcare benefits.

Advertising is most profitable for new drugs where long-term health effects are unknown. It may increase knowledge but not in a balanced way as the idea is to persuade rather than inform. It also provides a potential conflict for doctors striving to be both patient-centred and evidence-based.

How conducting a clinical trial affects physicians' guideline adherence and drug preferences
Andersen M, Kragstrup J, Søndergaard J *et al*.
JAMA, 2006; **295:** 2759–2764

This Danish study in 10 general practices shows how a pharmaceutical company-sponsored clinical trial can influence doctors to prescribe their drugs. Over 5000 asthma patients were compared to 60 000 control patients from 165 practices.

There was no influence on adherence to guidelines but the sponsor's share of the asthma drugs prescribed rose by a healthy 6.7% over the 2 years of the trial. This could be attributed to a higher preference for the company's drugs but we know pharmaceutical companies use various means to influence doctors. GPs in this trial were paid around £440 for each recruit. The trial compared two different dosage regimens and was never published. 'Seeding trials' were first described in 1994 and pay doctors for trials of dubious virtue while the hidden agenda is really to influence physician and patient behaviour.

Should patient groups accept money from drug companies? No
Mintzes B
BMJ, 2007; **334**: 935

In this head to head feature Mintzes presents a strong argument.

Estimates indicate that roughly half of UK and European patient groups accept industry funding. Patients' groups provide important information and in the current climate have increasing influence, but how can they be impartial if funded by companies that sell products to treat those illnesses?

Big pharma may look at this as a good channel for promotion through a seemingly neutral third party with increasing clout and the confusion between patient and sponsor's interest provides a nice smokescreen. The article gives several examples of industry using these platforms to help underplay risks and talk up new treatments.

Mike Rawlins, the chair of NICE, warns that in the long term the immense damage to the patient groups will undermine confidence in their neutrality. This is particularly important as their representation on so many advisory and legislative committees grows.

Should patient groups accept money from drug companies? Yes
Kent A
BMJ, 2007; **334**: 934

Kent argues that that is all very well but he would rather have the money.

The reduction in the potential voice of the patient groups would be too much to bear. He finds nothing wrong with collaboration if there are mutual interests, providing that the source of the funding is acknowledged.

The 'feeling' of the person accepting the cash is his benchmark for accepting or refusing the investment. As a few sentences later he describes walking away from a funder to be 'painful', it seems that the feeling needs to be quite acute to turn down the money.

He mentions some questions of conscience that some may choose to ask. Was the idea their own or did a third party request it? Do they retain control over the output? This simplistic approach shows no appreciation of the subtle and admirable power of the big guys. "Patient groups are not naïve" he reassures us, "they are quite capable of spotting the strings that may be attached to funding".

Kent is at least honest. He really wants the money and to him the end justifies the means. "If drug company money makes possible [effective advocates], bring it on. Ideological purity.... should be rejected as a cop-out".

His words not mine. Oh dear!

CLINICAL GOVERNANCE

The Challenge

Many approaches have been tried such as audit, guidelines in the form of national service frameworks, disease management programmes, public reporting, and accreditation and revalidation. But, despite considerable efforts to improve the quality and safety of health care through concepts of clinical governance, there are of course still huge challenges.

Reticence to change, complex organisational structures and dysfunctional financial incentives have made real improvements painfully slow at times.

Successful implementation of changes requires a profound understanding of how decisions are made. Quality research on where we need to improve is not yet fully developed.

An expanding role for NICE, first introduced in the NHS Plan of 1998, seems inevitable. Currently it aims to promote evidence-based medicine, improve standards of care, and reduce inequalities in access to innovative treatments. It dovetails scientific evidence with what is good for society (social value judgements), assessing costs as well as clinical effectiveness in order to create guidelines for the NHS.

NICE prefers to use the QALY – the cost per quality adjusted life year – but if quality of life data are not available, alternatives such as the cost per life year gained are used. It avoids an absolute threshold and claims not to consider affordability. If it decides something is cost-effective then they consider deeming it unaffordable to be a matter for the government. To facilitate social value judgements, NICE has formed a Citizen's Council to ensure these values resonate broadly with the public.

Some argue that the real issue is not whether to ration but how. They suggest that NICE must expand into fully informed rationing for the NHS giving it a real budget to fund all its advice.

What we know already:

- Many clinicians feel that the 'cookbook' approach promoted by prescriptive guidelines can undervalue and undermine clinical experience.
- A study of 338 recommendations from nine guidelines for management of cardiovascular risk found that fewer than one-third were supported by high quality evidence.
- Research shows that doctors rarely tend to access explicit guidelines. They tend to use 'mindlines', referring to tacit internal guidelines which are perhaps 'evidence-informed' rather than 'evidence-based'.
- GPs top up their personal experience with shortcuts to evidence such as brief reading of trusted sources as well as listening to colleagues and patients. They also value interactions with respected opinion leaders.
- Guidelines are more likely to be followed by GPs if they are clear, applicable to daily practice, avoid complex decision trees, require no new skills, and are supported by evidence. The punchier the better but brevity alone may not be enough to make them more likely to be implemented.
- Increasing awareness of variable quality in primary care led to the introduction in April 2004 of quality and outcomes frameworks which match quality indicators with financial incentives.

- Published data alone cannot be relied upon to recommend specific drugs. Bias such as multiple publication of results, selective publication (with positive effects more likely to make it into print) and selective reporting by, for example, failing to report intention to treat has too much influence.
- Patterns of implementation of NICE guidelines have been mixed and in its present form NICE fails to stimulate rapid universal implementation of evidence.

Recent Papers

MEASURING QUALITY

Measuring performance and missing the point?
Heath I, Hippisley-Cox J, Smeeth L
BMJ, 2007; **335**: 1075–1076

Since April 2004 the performance of GPs, and thereby their remuneration, has been measured using a limited number of easily measurable clinical processes, an initiative unique in the world and under scrutiny.

The chosen activities are easy to measure but three-quarters of the population have none of the diseases under scrutiny. In addition none of the parameters estimate clinically tangible outcomes. These are much harder to measure, especially at the level of individual practices.

Improvements such as those in diabetic control have shown successes, and innovations such as computer prompting have been praised, but are we in danger of missing the point? Although the quality and outcomes frameworks are largely evidence-based, their blanket approach fails to see the individuality in patients or recognise variables which may put them out of sync with the groups from the original research.

Evidence-based medicine was never intended to be a substitute for clinical judgment and this inflexibility stifles innovation. The emphasis away from grappling with the inherent uncertainty of specific symptoms and patient preferences steers us away from fundamental decisions for appropriate treatments.

The focus on points-scoring reduces the responsibility of doctors to think and some groups of patients will be systematically harmed by the new approach. The authors offer the example of the dangers of over-treating hypertension in the elderly when no allowance is made for age and frailty.

'Reductive linear reasoning' views the body as a machine when it should more usefully be regarded as a complex adaptive system, making much more sense of clinical experience.

Socio-economic issues mean that such measures can even exacerbate inequalities in deprived areas and create the illusion that such issues are an area for the NHS alone.

Future of quality measurement
Lester H, Roland M
BMJ, 2007; **335**: 1130–1131

Use of quality measures is controversial but this paper argues that while it has been beneficial it cannot remain static.

Rather than get swamped with more and more indicators, they suggest a rotation of different measures to improve a wider range of conditions, although they advise a careful pilot study to spot any unintended consequences.

A revision and expansion of the quality and outcomes frameworks in 2006 put GPs firmly into new territory by using standardised questionnaires for depression and more active management of chronic kidney disease. The authors warn that changes such as these should be piloted carefully for at least 12 months to identify professional and educational concerns.

They also warn that in the quest to meet our surrogate targets, there is an urgency to avoid creating a generation of doctors who are losing grasp of the less definable aspects of care. This would devalue the quality of interpersonal care and undermine the core complexity of general practice.

Use of process measures to monitor the quality of clinical practice
Lilford RJ, Brown CA, Nicholl J
BMJ, 2007; **335**: 648–650

This analysis also supports the use of process measures as the best tool for judging and rewarding quality. They warn that outcomes actually have a poor relation with quality because they are affected by factors other than quality of care, producing what the authors call a 'low signal to noise ratio'.

For example, systematic review has shown poor correlation between quality of practice and hospital mortality. Hence mortality is neither a sensitive nor specific test for quality. It is a fallacy that statistical adjustments of risk will solve such a problem. For example, such statistics will not factor in the existence of a local hospice which eases the general hospital's mortality rates.

Some of these data can be used for sanction or judgment – perhaps suspension of a doctor – rather than in the spirit of continuous improvement. In these cases the authors warn that strong correlations with quality rather than just statistical associations are required. Outcomes being generally a poor measure of quality, there is higher burden of proof if the data are used to brand someone as 'bad'.

The value of an actual outcome they argue is simply as a research tool. Observable changes in outcomes would be an indication for further investigations of processes. Process, they argue, encourages a more universal improvement.

Process rules!

Quality failures in the NHS
Ham C
BMJ, 2008; **336**: 340–341

In 2008, the Healthcare Commission produced *Learning from Investigations*, a report echoing many of the recommendations from *An Organisation with a*

Memory (Dept of Health 2000). Depressingly familiar themes of weak leadership, conflicting targets, lack of teamwork and poor standards of ward care recurred.

Why can we not learn from the mistakes of the past?

First, it's the sheer size of the NHS and the absence of well-developed systems. The lack of direction and the lack of a safety culture do not help, and continuous restructuring is counterproductive to quality.

A nuanced approach that turns the NHS from a 'doing organisation' to a 'learning organisation' with continuity of leadership is proposed here, somewhat vaguely. Would the airlines and nuclear power industries accept similar levels of safety to the NHS?

NICE

NICE's cost effectiveness threshold
Appleby J, Devlin N, Parkin D
BMJ, 2007; **335**: 358–359

NICE's judgements on cost-effectiveness are the subject of this editorial. The value of £20 000–£30 000 per QALY is unchanged since inception and has no basis in evidence. It is probably far too generous and means that NICE may have diverted resources away from other services and reduced the efficiency of the NHS.

The average primary care trust spends £12 000 per QALY in circulatory disease and around £19 000 in cancer, but analysis suggests that NICE may upgrade that when it suits them to around £45 000.

Two solutions have been proposed. Either set the value of a QALY and select NHS care below that value. Or, decide how much to spend on the NHS budget and let the value of a QALY emerge from the purchasers. This risks inconsistent decision-making based on dubious and variable valuations of health gain.

Any threshold is always going to be a moving target with many economic considerations beyond the control of NICE. The economists writing this editorial therefore propose an independent threshold committee that sets the value that NICE, primary care trusts and other purchasers are required to adopt. This will inject efficiency and fairness back into the NHS.

Parliamentary review asks NICE to do better still
Collier J
BMJ, 2008; **336**: 56–57

In January 2008, the House of Commons Health Select Committee published its second inquiry into the work of NICE. This was written six years after the first in a changing landscape and is chock full of hard-hitting detail and potential consequences. They made the following recommendations.
- More communication with stakeholders – a clarification of their role as a rationing body.
- Some advice should be compulsory and re-designated as NICE Directives, leaving other advice to be referred to as guidance or guidelines.

- An independent body should set the threshold for clinical effectiveness. The customary level of less than £30 000 per QALY was noted to have no basis in hard science, does not factor in costs of carers, and was actually chosen by NICE itself.
- NICE should appraise all new drugs with 'rough and ready' advice available at launch. Currently we are waiting up to a year for an expensive new drug to be appraised that might only be of use in secondary care.
- NICE should have access to the same high quality data that the UK drug licensing authority does. Reliable decisions are sabotaged by drug company data where weakness and bias may be well disguised.
- They should begin evaluating older possibly cost-ineffective treatments to allow 'disinvestment' in drugs not fit for purpose.

INPUT FROM PATIENTS

Can patients assess the quality of health care?
Coulter A
BMJ, 2006; **333:** 1–2

Coulter reflects on a paper in the same issue (Rao *et al. BMJ*, 2006; **333:** 19) that showed no correlation between patients' evaluations of the quality of technical care by a GP, compared with evidence-based indicators. The authors conclude that patients cannot reliably assess technical aspects of care but this editorial says this is a generalisation too far.

The public tends to value excellent communication skills and sound up to date technical skills as equally important, and together these are the two most importance factors in having confidence in their doctor.

Questionnaires continue to be popular tools for practice accreditation and clinical governance, appraisal and revalidation. The General Practice Assessment Survey used in Rao's paper has now been replaced with the General Practice Assessment Questionnaire which has no such assessment of technical skill (www.gpaq.info).

The authors comment that it is difficult enough for doctors to rate the technical skills of other doctors, so it is nigh on impossible for patients with no training.

ASSESSING EVIDENCE

How quickly do systematic reviews go out of date? A survival analysis
Shojania KG, Sampson M, Ansari MT *et al.*
Ann Intern Med, 2007; **147:** 224–233

Systematic reviews may only have a short shelf life according to this sample of 100 such reviews. About a quarter need an update within 2 years and 15% within a year. Over half needed an update within a median time of 3 years. The median overall for the sample was 5.5 years before they were out of date.

Although the studies chosen were directly relevant to clinical care they were not necessarily generalisable to all such reviews. Nevertheless, speedier publication is called for as 7% were out of date by the time they were published.

HEALTH INEQUALITIES

The Challenge

The socio-economic classification we now use is based on current employment and has seven main classes based on the responsibility in the occupation, and an eighth class for the long-term unemployed. Reducing health inequalities between socio-economic groups is a government priority but the new general medical services contract takes no account of deprivation or ethnicity on target levels.

In 2007 the Government committed to the most comprehensive strategy so far to improve access to care and life expectancy in the areas with the worst health and deprivation. However, mortality data are the only measurement of population health, and problems of homelessness, poverty, ethnic differences and socio-economic deprivation pose other serious health risks. Lung function, for example, is an important indicator of general health. Being in a manual occupational social class, having no educational qualifications and living in a deprived area all separately predict reduced lung function, even after controlling for smoking. These factors may exert their influence through poor diet, lack of exercise, poor housing that increases respiratory infections, or environmental tobacco smoke.

What we know already:

- The north – south divide in social class inequalities is real but it is a more of a north west – south east divide. There are considerable inequalities depending on region (with the south east coming off best).
- Within each region of Britain, there are large inequalities of health related to social class. Those in class 7 have rates of poor self-rated health more than double those of class 1. Scores are worse in women than in men in each region and class.
- Scotland and London have the widest health divides, adding to the debate on how to allocate resources to tackle the divide.
- Over the past decade, the UK ethnic minority population has grown by 53% and now comprises 8% of the total population with South Asians, the largest group, now accounting for 50% of ethnic minority groups.
- Inhibited access to general practice means homeless people often access healthcare inappropriately through A&E.
- A Danish study found that homeless people, particularly young women staying in hostels, were four times more likely to die early than the general population.
- Studies have shown the incidence of heart failure increasing by 44% between the most affluent and most deprived socio-economic strata. The most deprived patients were 23% less likely to see their GP for follow up. Those with closer follow up did better.
- People in areas of high deprivation or with large ethnic minorities are less likely to have their diabetes care recorded thoroughly. Practices in deprived areas need to work harder to achieve recommended standards.
- Lower socio-economic groups are under-represented in medical schools but academically able 14–16 year olds in these groups are markedly less likely to want to be a doctor. They underestimate their chances of success, allow cost worries to affect their choices, and are

not keen on what they perceived as prohibitive personal sacrifice. Pupils from less deprived backgrounds are more attracted by the challenge of medicine and potential for achievement and fulfillment.

Guidance

Tackling health inequalities: 2004–06 data and policy update for the 2010 national target. www.dh.gov.uk/healthinequalities, December 2007.
The report provides an update on progress to meet the health inequalities national target and reduce the gap, as measured by infant mortality and life expectancy, by 10% by 2010.

Recent Papers

ETHNICITY

Perceptions and experiences of taking oral hypoglycaemic agents among people of Pakistani and Indian origin: qualitative study
Lawton J, Ahmad N, Hallowell N et al.
BMJ, 2005; **330:** 1247

Interviews with British Pakistani and Indian diabetics illustrated that ambivalent attitudes towards oral hypoglycaemics exist. Many perceive such medication as necessary but also harmful which backs up the particularly poor adherence to medication and poor glycaemic control noticed in this group.

Most trusted their doctors' expertise, appreciating the NHS delivery of prescriptions free of financial incentive for the doctor, and considered the medicines available in Britain to be better than those available in the Indian subcontinent. Their beliefs about Western medicines, however, may lead them to self-regulate their doses in ways that seem rational to them but go against medical advice.

The authors make recommendations to tackle these observations by having a high index of suspicion that patients will self-regulate, asking about it in a non-judgmental way, asking the patient what they think each medication is doing for them and, in particular, if they make dietary changes (which may be counter to their diabetes recommendations) as a result of taking the medications.

Excess coronary heart disease in South Asians in the United Kingdom
Kuppuswamy VC, Gupta S
BMJ, 2005; **330:** 1223–1224

This editorial suggests that inequalities are indeed widening, with death rates in South Asians from Bangladesh, Pakistan and India (in order of how badly they fare in coronary mortality statistics) declining at a slower rate than the 'indigenous' population.

They theorise that the increased prevalence of the metabolic syndrome and diabetes in second and third generation Asians is the most compelling aetiology.

Lack of exercise, unhealthy diets and a reduced likelihood of receiving statins as well as failure to take up cardiac rehabilitation all add to the mix.

The authors argue that the usual methods for risk stratification, such as Framingham data, underestimate risk in this ethnic group and that treatment ranges may need to be redefined. They also point to possible linguistic and cultural barriers and the need for more patient education, a higher index of suspicion among doctors and perhaps 'well Asian' clinics to provide some intensive primary care.

Religious beliefs about causes and treatment of epilepsy
Ismail H, Wright J, Rhodes P *et al.*
Br J Gen Pract, 2005; **55**: 26–31

A study of the use of healers and complementary therapies by South Asian epileptics in Yorkshire revealed that over half of responders attributed their illness to fate, the will of God, or as punishment for the sins of a previous life. There was a network of healers who were seen as providing a parallel and complementary system of care.

Although families of Asians encouraged them to turn to these traditional religiospiritual treatments in desperation for a cure, many were sceptical about their effectiveness. It is important doctors are aware of these belief systems and consider if there are conflicts with Western health care.

Trends in opioid prescribing by race/ethnicity for patients seeking care in US emergency departments
Pletcher MJ, Kertesz SG, Kohn MA *et al.*
JAMA, 2008; **299**: 70–78

Some 23% of pain-related visits in 1993 were treated with opioids, rising to 37% in 2005. But although ambitions for higher prescription of pain relief have been met in US emergency departments, an ethnic divide still exists.

A study covering 13 years found that white people in pain consistently received more opiates (31%) than other ethnic groups such as black (23%), Hispanic (24%), or Asian/other patients (28%). The severity of pain was adjusted for but still the worse the pain was, the more marked the difference. The differences did not diminish over time. In 2005, 40% of white people received opiates compared to 32% for all other people.

Should Muslims have faith based health services?
Sheikh A
BMJ, 2007; **334**: 74

Muslims have some of the worst overall health in Britain. Sheikh blames "general failure among academics, policymakers, and clinicians" to appreciate and tackle this problem. Faith-centred healthcare initiatives are needed but his agenda is a longer term goal of aiming to get everyone to understand religious identity.

The author tells us that for many British Muslims religion defines them much more than ethnicity. He tells us of the "evil" institutionalised racism affecting all British public services.

For historical reasons, Muslims are predominantly congregated in the inner-city areas with high unemployment, poverty and poor educational records, and may be twice as likely as the general population to self-report poor health and disability

Sheikh calls for a better picture of the health profiles of Muslims and specific measures such as:

- male circumcision available on request on the NHS to avoid use of the poorly regulated private sector
- a choice of gender of clinician
- better access to prayer and ablution facilities
- Muslim 'chaplains' for spiritual care
- a service to avoid ingestion of porcine and alcohol-derived drugs
- GPs to offer consultations before Ramadan and the Hajj pilgrimage to inform their patients how to modify their treatment regimes
- Muslim representation on the boards of government, NHS trusts and charities

---

Should Muslims have faith based health services?
Esmail A
BMJ, 2007; **334:** 75

Esmail, an anti-racism campaigner and professor of primary care, reminds us that there are many complex components to human identity. Fostering a single identity has led to persecution and violence throughout history. The emergence of Islamophobia has encouraged many to assert their singular identity and this can progress to requests for treatment as a special case.

Faith does matter to some in healthcare settings and doctors should be sensitive to these needs. Access to chaplains for different faiths may be important as is the provision of halal or kosher food.

A list of accredited surgeons for circumcision seems sensible but that is no reason to divert NHS resources to these operations. Meeting every demand is impractical and some preferences such as female circumcision would be unethical.

Neither is religious identity homogenous. Different sects may have different needs for faith-based services. He advises respect and tolerance for the patient as an individual without having to subscribe to special treatment which would risk stigmatisation and stereotyping everyone who shares similar needs and belief systems.

ETHICS

The Challenge

Decisions to withhold or withdraw treatment are among the most difficult that health professionals face, and debate on legalisation is growing in many countries.

Both voluntary active euthanasia and physician-assisted suicide have been openly practised in the Netherlands for more than 25 years and formally legalised since 2002. A more restricted position involving physician-assisted suicide only was legalised in Oregon in 1997. In this model, patient control is enabled by limiting the doctor's role to assessment and prescribing, but with the patient self-administering the fatal drugs.

It helps when patients express their preferences in advance. Advance decisions (previously known as advance statements) may be as simple as a record of a conversation or a note that conveys a sense of the individual's wishes, but to be legally binding must fit certain criteria. Advance directives (living wills) are clear instructions refusing a medical intervention and are to be referred to in the event that the patient becomes incapable of expressing them. They are made voluntarily by a competent and informed adult, and if unambiguous are likely to have legal force but are not bound by statutory law.

What we know already:

- Evidence suggests that doctors have difficulty balancing subjective impressions of a quality of life worth preserving with a patient's expressed desire for autonomy and the right to have treatment withdrawn. This implies that anyone with an advance directive cannot assume that any particular outcome will result from its implementation.
- Supporters claim euthanasia is a continuation of palliative care and that doctors must respect patients' autonomy.
- Evidence suggests we lack sufficient training in palliative care at the end of life. Tackling this might be a good place to start before clarifying a place for euthanasia.
- In May 2006, *The Assisted Dying for the Terminally Ill* Bill which had aimed to legalise physician-assisted suicide in the UK was thrown out of the House Of Lords.
- The Royal College of Physicians and the Royal College of General Practitioners also opposed the bill. The BMA maintained its neutral stance.
- In June 2006, voting from BMA members made clear that the majority oppose such legislation. Therefore the BMA has dropped its neutral stance and its current position is to oppose all forms of assisted dying.

Guidance

Assisted dying – a summary of the BMA's position. www.bma.org.uk, June 2006.

Withholding and withdrawing life-prolonging treatments: good practice in decision-making. *GMC*, August 2006.

Recent Papers

ADVANCE DECISIONS

Controlling death: the false promise of advance directives
Perkins HS
Ann Intern Med, 2007; **147**: 51–57

Advance directives have actually delivered very little. Complexities, ambiguities of interpretation and the strong will of third parties can derail even the most thorough directives. Most patients do not complete them. If they do, most do not keep them updated. Proxies often do not know the patient's wishes in enough detail to make them effective.

It may be that expectations of advance directives are simply unrealistic and that their very concept is fundamentally flawed. They suppose more control over the future than is possible.

Until we come up with something better, Perkins emphasises that emotional preparation for patients and families in crises is a much more important priority.

Advance decisions and proxy decision-making in medical treatment and research
Guidance from the BMA's Medical Ethics Department. June 2007 (www.bma.org.uk)

The BMA's latest advice is for people in England and Wales to consider appointing a relative or friend to make decisions for them in the event of losing mental capacity.

Since October 2007, a lasting power of attorney can be drawn up and the proxy can make treatment decisions on their behalf. Healthcare teams ensure certain safeguards are met before consenting to or refusing life-prolonging treatment. The document should have sufficient scope and be registered with the Public Guardianship Office. Disagreements go to the Court of Protection.

The guidance reminds doctors that an obligation to extend life does not need to extend to treatments not thought to be clinically indicated, although obtaining a second opinion is wise.

EUTHANASIA

Legalised euthanasia will violate the rights of vulnerable patients
George RJD, Finlay IG, Jeffrey D
BMJ, 2005; **331**: 684–685

This paper fails to see a distinction between legalised euthanasia and therapeutic killing. This 'insoluble ethical conflict' may mean that the voice of the vulnerable and incapable is drowned out, making coercion and the inference of a 'duty to die' a real risk. In Oregon requests for physician-assisted suicide because of 'being a burden' have increased as people shop around for compliant doctors. Can we afford the moral cost to society?

And this at a time when research consistently shows that GPs, each dealing with fewer than five dying patients per year, could do a lot better with the palliative care they deliver.

Physician assisted death in vulnerable populations
Quill TE
BMJ, 2007; **335**: 625–626

This editorial addresses concerns put forward about the consequences of legalising physician-assisted death.

It reassures us that since legalisation in Oregon, which is amongst the nation's leaders in end of life care, there has been no significant change in the frequency of its use. More than 85% were enrolled in hospice programmes. Similar stability has been seen in Holland. There was no evidence to suggest that the burden of this practice would fall disproportionately on the deprived and vulnerable. There was no increased incidence in populations with low socio-economic status, minors, ethnic minorities, or those with physical disabilities. Research which attempted to uncover the secret practice of assisted dying in the US estimated significantly higher rates than in Oregon after legalisation.

All this suggests that legalisation with regulation and appropriate safeguards protects rather than facilitates the practice. There was no clear evidence that the legalisation has created a slippery slope, rather that objectivity and honesty towards all aspects of care of the dying helps us deliberate with patients and families in an open and accountable environment.

Role of non-governmental organisations in physician assisted suicide
Ziegler SJ, Bosshard G
BMJ, 2007; **334**: 295–298

This article tells us how non-government organisations can help to limit the role of doctors in facilitating suicides. In Switzerland and Oregon a large majority make use of organisations (92% and 75% respectively) whose volunteers offer knowledge and unrushed advice ensuring openness and dignity.

These 'right to die' organisations could help to solve the ethical problems doctors face by sharing responsibility. But the authors warn that involving organisations can bring other problems and ultimately the doctor must decide whether involvement at any level is actually a violation of his professional integrity.

CONSCIENCE

Should you tell patients about beneficial treatments that they cannot have? Yes
Marcus R
BMJ, 2007; **334**: 826
and
Should you tell patients about beneficial treatments that they cannot have? No
Firth J
BMJ, 2007; **334**: 827

This head-to-head debate looks at the moral obligations when coming face-to-face with the financial limitations of the healthcare system in which you are working.

Firth uses the example of prescribing erythropoietin for a fatigued kidney patient who is not yet on dialysis. With no budget for this and with the patient unaware of its existence, he feels that telling him about this unattainable possibility is 'bad medicine'. Although this could be looked at as failing to respect patient autonomy, the harm caused would not be justifiable.

Marcus argues that not acting in the patient's best interests is a betrayal of trust. He notes that a virtual state monopoly for healthcare in the UK challenges doctors with a dual loyalty to patients and employer. Even so, patients have a right to know of treatments that may help them even though no healthcare system can fund everything.

A doctor cannot be the passive tool of the state and not inform a patient of all his options. Who are we to know that the patient might not have the resources to afford the treatment privately or feel empowered enough to start to lobby government or community groups. Although it may be harmful to tantalise, keeping the poor in deliberate ignorance could be seen as a failure of duty of care.

Religion, conscience, and controversial clinical practices
Curlin FA, Lawrence RE, Chin MH *et al*.
N Engl J Med, 2007; **356**: 593–600

Over 1100 US physicians participated in this study. When asked, the majority did feel that they were obliged to inform patients about all possible treatments and offer referral to another physician if they themselves had moral objections to the treatments in question. Offering terminations and providing contraception for minors were two such examples.

However, 62% found it acceptable to tell patients of their own personal objections and 8% felt they had no obligation to tell patients of such treatments in the first place or to refer to a doctor more willing to treat them (18%). Religiously inclined doctors were the worst offenders and men were worse than women.

If representative, the number of people in America potentially prevented from accessing effective and legal treatments could reach 100 million.

CONSENT

Gillick or Fraser? A plea for consistency over competence in children
Wheeler R
BMJ, 2006; **332**: 807

This article emphasises the difference between the terms 'Gillick competence' and 'Fraser guidelines'. Synonymy has been encouraged following an urban myth that Mrs Gillick did not want to associate her name with the ruling.

Adulthood is reached at 18 years in the UK and, to a limited extent, 16 and 17 year old children can make medical decisions independent of their parents.

The Gillick test for competence in those under 18 dates from 1983 and requires the child to demonstrate sufficient maturity and intelligence to understand and appraise the nature and implications of the proposed treatment (age alone is recognised as an unreliable predictor of this capacity).

Lord Fraser was one of the Law Lords in the Gillick judgement and specifically addresses the dilemma of contraceptive advice without parental knowledge. To protect the welfare of these girls he emphasised the desirability of parental involvement and understanding the risks for unprotected sex. So Gillick is a general assessment of competence. Fraser fuses this with the specific provision of contraceptive advice.

Remembering this will protect the concept of Gillick competence as the central doctrine with which to judge capacity in children.

ALCOHOL

The Challenge

Alcohol is associated with a huge range of dose-related adverse consequences ranging from acute poisoning, cancer, and death on the roads, to anti-social behaviour and domestic violence.

There is a high prevalence of alcohol problems in those who commit suicide but most problem drinkers are unknown to their GPs. Screening instruments high in specificity and sensitivity seem to be needed, but using these tools liberally can disturb rapport and hijack the consultation – one GP likened it to having to do a rectal examination on everyone who walked in.

Costs to the British economy come in at an estimated £30 billion a year and mean that strategies to control alcohol consumption at a national and international level become essential.

Binge drinking has become commonplace and is a particularly harmful pattern of drinking. Direct and indirect costs to the UK are substantial.

Frequency of heavy drinking in pregnant women is associated with the occurrence of a range of completely preventable mental and physical birth defects collectively known as Fetal Alcohol Spectrum Disorders.

What we know already:

- The UK Government Guidelines define sensible drinking as a maximum of 3–4 units a day (28 units per week) for men and 2–3 units a day (21 units per week) for women.
- A report from the RCGP and the Royal Colleges of Physicians and Psychiatrists recommends no more than 21 units per week and 14 units per week for men and women respectively.
- In October 2007, the World Cancer Research Fund panel advised that men should drink no more than two units of alcohol a day and women no more than one unit a day.
- Scoring 2 or more on the CAGE questionnaire has a sensitivity of 71% and specificity was 90% for diagnosis of alcohol abuse and dependence, putting limits on its practical value. The score may be better treated like a graded measure rather than simply positive or negative.
- Meta-analysis has suggested that screening routinely in GP consultations and providing brief interventions to reduce excessive drinking may be cost-effective in ideal research conditions. It seems, however, to be of very little practical use when its effects are reviewed after a year. This makes universal screening questionable as a case finding approach. The rapport of a good consultation might be a better tool.
- Laboratory tests such as GGT and MCV are poor at identifying problem drinkers.
- The BMA has called for legislation to compel manufacturers of alcoholic drinks to clearly label their products with the number of units of alcohol. All alcoholic drink labels should contain this information alongside government recommended drinking limits by the end of 2008.
- A unit contains 8 g (1 cl) of pure alcohol and is often defined as a half a pint of beer or a small glass of wine. But that is inaccurate. A 125ml glass of wine with 12% alcohol content, for example, actually contains 1.5 units and standards vary around the world.

LIFESTYLE

- The benefits of light to moderate drinking on cardiovascular outcomes have been proven even after MI, but men drinking over 35 units a week double their risk of stroke, mainly haemorrhagic.

Guidance

Alcohol misuse: tackling the UK epidemic. *BMA*, February 2008 (www.bma.org.uk).

Recent Papers

SCREENING

Opportunistic screening for alcohol use disorders in primary care: comparative study
Coulton S, Drummond C, James D *et al*.
BMJ, 2006; **332**: 511–517

In this study of nearly 200 males, the Alcohol Use Disorders Identification Test (AUDIT) – a 10 item questionnaire – proved more efficient than levels of GGT, MCV and AST at correlating with alcohol consumption when used for opportunistic screening in six Welsh primary care practices. It had a higher sensitivity, specificity and positive predictive value than the biochemical markers for hazardous consumption, including binging as well as alcohol dependence. It was also cost-efficient at around £1.70 per patient.

Some 25% of attendees screened positive, showing the scale of the hidden problem.

TREATMENT

British drinking: a suitable case for treatment?
Hall W
BMJ, 2005; **331**: 527–528

Britain has one of the highest rates of alcohol dependence in the European Union and the usual approaches of public education and measures to improve policing do not seem to be making much headway.

Australians, on the other hand, have imposed lower taxes on weaker beer and low alcohol beer now accounts for 40% of beer consumed. Random breath testing on a large scale (and lower driving limits for alcohol) have gained public support following reductions in deaths and serious injuries.

Regarding treatment, the time may now be right for investment in two relatively brief psychosocial interventions – motivational enhancement treatment and social network therapy – allowing the UK government to make headway on their targets for alcohol related disease.

Effectiveness of treatment for alcohol problems: findings of the randomised UK alcohol treatment trial (UKATT)
and
Cost effectiveness of treatment for alcohol problems: findings of the randomised UK alcohol treatment trial (UKATT)
UKATT Research Team
BMJ, 2005; **331**: 541–544, 544–548

> These two papers compared the effectiveness of social behaviour and network therapy (up to eight 50-minute sessions) – a new treatment for alcohol problems aimed at building social networks to support changes in behaviour – with the proven track record of motivational enhancement therapy (three 50-minute sessions).
>
> No previous British randomised trial of non-pharmacological treatments for alcohol problems had had the statistical power to reliably detect effectiveness.
>
> This randomised trial followed over 600 outpatients for a year and showed that both interventions showed similar and substantial reductions in alcohol consumption and dependence as well as improvements in mental health. Both therapies saved about five times as much in terms of GP/hospital resources, social consequences and legal services as they cost.
>
> The two therapies were equally cost-effective despite the average cost of social behaviour and network therapy being £221 and that of motivational enhancement therapy being £129.

Brief interventions including information sessions, motivational interviews, and cognitive behavioural therapy reduce excessive alcohol consumption in primary care. *Evidence-Based Medicine,* 2007; **12**: 179
The following report is reviewed
Effectiveness of brief alcohol interventions in primary care populations
Kaner EF, Beyer F, Dickinson HO, *et al.*
Cochrane Database Syst Rev, 2007

> Brief interventions involving education, CBT, motivational interviews or action plans do reduce alcohol consumption, at least in men, according to this meta-analysis of 21 randomised trials. They also produced fewer heavy and binge drinkers than the control group. The data were relevant to primary care but very sparingly exploited in practice. Limitations of time, attitudes and resources mean we generally fail to deliver these treatments.

PREGNANCY

Is it all right for women to drink small amounts of alcohol in pregnancy? No
Nathanson V, Jayesinghe N, Roycroft G
BMJ, 2007; **335**: 857

> Abstention from alcohol in pregnant women and women trying to conceive is the latest government advice. It echoes that of the BMA, the Royal College of Obstetricians and Gynaecologists, the surgeon general of the US and WHO. Canada, France, New Zealand and Australia concur.

LIFESTYLE

The teratogenic damage from heavy consumption is well documented but there is no consensus on the effect of low to moderate drinking on pregnancy. Data are incomplete and the contribution of confounding factors is unknown. All this means there is no clear threshold of safety.

Possibilities exist that low to moderate drinking at two to five units per week may delay development of the nervous system permanently.

Confusion in the UK as to the actual quality of a 'unit' of alcohol persists, meaning intake is difficult to estimate. In addition many women in early pregnancy will not yet know they are pregnant and will drink as though they are not.

The only safe message is abstention for this group.

Is it all right for women to drink small amounts of alcohol in pregnancy? Yes
O'Brien P
BMJ, 2007; **335**: 856

The flipside of the argument is an equally articulate response. The Department of Health and BMA has changed from condoning 'one to two units of alcohol once or twice a week', but the change is not in the light of new evidence. So what is going on?

Mainly, confusion. People have never really understood what a unit of alcohol looks like and probably would not know how to pour one for themselves.

NICE's draft advice in September 2007 was that pregnant women should limit their alcohol intake to one standard drink (1.5 UK units) per day and avoid altogether in the first trimester. Although probably trying to keep things simple, with the conflicting advice out there, it seems to confuse. (NB In March 2008 it brought its guidance into line with the Department of Health and recommended abstention during pregnancy.)

In addition, the BMA fears an increase in fetal alcohol disorders will be a consequence of the rise in binge drinking young women and so is trying to put the brakes on that.

This author also quotes the Royal College of Obstetricians and Gynaecologists who found no evidence of harm at low levels, but omits their advice which comes down on the side of abstention. No evidence of harm, however, does not mean evidence of no harm. The author does not deny this but instead of playing safe in the interests of the baby, O'Brien thinks the autonomy of the mother comes first and that medics should keep their 'value judgments' to themselves. She feels that those we advise will turn against us for our paternalism.

This hard line will also worsen fear and embarrassment in mothers who continue to drink, and may worry those who previously drank at the limits that were previously decreed safe. Even with the previous advice, half of women avoid alcohol anyway. This appears to be enough for O'Brien. Is it enough for you?

DRIVING

Alcohol dependence and driving: a survey of patients' knowledge of DVLA regulations and possible clinical implications
Culshaw M
Psychiatric Bulletin, 2005: **29**: 90–93

A Glasgow survey of 58 patients with alcohol dependence showed that most heavy drinkers with a licence continue to drive, unaware that there are any restrictions from the DVLA. Only 14% said that a health professional had discussed the regulations with them – of these, four were GPs, one was a nurse, and one a psychiatrist. Doctors have a duty to inform the DVLA if they are aware such a patient continues to drive but are either unaware of this, avoid the issue, or worry about breaches of confidentiality and the effect on the doctor–patient relationship.

CLINICAL ISSUES

LIFESTYLE

DIET

The Challenge

The burden of health due to poor diet has been estimated as similar to that caused by smoking in terms of mortality and morbidity.

We know that some diets which rely on plant foods and unsaturated lipids have been shown to reduce cardiovascular end-points, cancers and overall mortality. The Mediterranean diet is one such approach. It is characterised by a high intake of vegetables, legumes, fruits, and cereals, a moderate to high intake of fish, a low intake of saturated fats, but a high intake of unsaturated fats, particularly olive oil, a low intake of dairy products and meat, and a modest intake of alcohol, mostly as wine.

An Indo-Mediterranean diet in which green leafy vegetables, mustard or soybean oils, certain nuts and whole grains replace fish, rapeseed and olive oils, also reduces risk of cardiac death by up to half – at least in Indian men.

Functional foods also known as 'nutraceuticals' or 'designer foods' are foods modified with supplements that claim to improve wellbeing or health. Probiotics – live micro-organisms which may confer a health benefit on the host – are one such trend. There is increasing evidence that they are beneficial in a range of gastrointestinal conditions. They include *Streptococcus thermophilus*, *Enterococcus* species, *Saccharomyces* species, and various species of lactobacilli and bifidobacteria.

Functional foods also make a lot of soft claims implying health benefits without naming a disease, and quackery is rife. They are intended for use as part of a healthy lifestyle but risk medicalising our daily intake with unproven claims. While safety is well regulated, health claims are not. They are highly profitable and aggressively marketed directly to consumers who cannot assess these claims.

What we know already:

- Total fruit and vegetable intake is inversely associated with risk of cardiovascular disease – at least five 'servings' a day are recommended. A once-daily serving of a green leafy vegetable has been shown to claim most of this benefit by cutting cardiovascular disease by over 10%.
- There are some beneficial ingredients in functional foods – sorbitol in chewing gum (which reduces dental caries), plant stanols and sterols (which lower LDL) and probiotic bacteria.
- There are also unproven candidates such as phytoestrogens for breast cancer and many herbal remedies are under review for benefit and more importantly for harm.
- Most studies have confirmed an inverse association between fish consumption and coronary heart disease and ischaemic stroke. Two to three servings of fish per week should provide sufficient omega 3 fatty acids to be of benefit.
- Studies that showed no such association were in populations with an already moderate fish intake, perhaps indicating a ceiling of benefit.
- EPIC found that eating more than 160 g of red meat per day means a 35% higher chance of developing bowel cancer than those who eat less than 20 g per day.

- Those who eat the most red meat are twice as likely to develop rheumatoid arthritis as people who eat half their amounts.
- Dietary magnesium (from whole grains, nuts, and green leafy vegetables) appears to protect against diabetes and heart disease.
- The Atkins diet books have sold more than 45 million copies over 40 years.

Recent Papers

GENERAL

Diet and the risk of cancer
Key T
BMJ, 2007; **335**: 897

This editorial describes the position taken by the second report from the World Cancer Research Fund into the effect of diet on cancer.

Alcohol consumption has increased globally in recent decades, increasing the risk for cancers of the mouth, pharynx, larynx, oesophagus, colorectum, and breast, and also leading to cirrhosis, which predisposes to liver cancer.

Obesity increases the risk of cancer of the oesophagus, colorectum, pancreas, breast, endometrium, and kidney. Mean BMI in adults in the UK is much too high at around 27 and enormous efforts will be needed to reverse this trend.

The role of fruit and vegetables, however, is less well understood. There may be protective effects against some cancers but there is no rock solid evidence for any one cancer. They still go with the advice to eat at least 5 portions a day, but caution about the implications for agriculture if people actually followed this advice. Financial costs are also important as this is expensive for people. Fruit and vegetables are low in energy and protein so may be taken in supplement to someone's normal diet. It may be better to push beans and cereals which contain energy and protein and so might substitute for meat. They confirm that red and processed meat convincingly causes colorectal cancer in a dose-responsive way – with those eating the most having a 30% higher risk than those eating the least. Men in the UK eat three times the recommended maximum amount of 300 g per week.

Fruit and vegetable consumption and stroke: meta-analysis of cohort studies
He F, Nowson C, MacGregor G
Lancet, 2006; **367**: 320–326

This meta-analysis totalled 250 000 subjects with nearly 5000 stroke events and showed that eating more than five servings of fruit and vegetables per day can cut the risk of stroke by as much as 26%. Three to five servings managed a reduction of 11%.

It is probably the combination of nutrients that does the trick. A portion might be a medium-sized apple, a cup of raw salad greens, half a cup of cut-up vegeta-

LIFESTYLE

bles, half a cup of cooked beans or peas, or three-quarters of a cup of 100% fruit or vegetable juice.

SALT

Long term effects of dietary sodium reduction on cardiovascular disease outcomes: observational follow-up of the trials of hypertension prevention (TOHP)
Cook NR, Cutler JA, Obarzanek E *et al.*
BMJ, 2007; **334**: 885

This landmark paper followed up cardiovascular outcomes in prehypertensive participants of two randomised lifestyle intervention trials – the trials of hypertension prevention phase I (TOHP I) and phase II (TOHP II).

Nearly 3000 patients were randomised to a sodium reduction intervention amounting to reductions of 2 to 2.6 grams per day.

After adjusting for other variables of cardiac risk, the risk of a cardiovascular event was 25–30% lower among those in the intervention group. They had cut their salt intake for at least 18 months and the effects persisted for an impressive 10–15 years after the original trial. This is pretty incredible considering the general tendency for behavioural interventions to attenuate over time. The study seems to have verified once and for all the dangers of salt intake.

Salt and cardiovascular disease
Cappuccio FP
BMJ, 2007; **334**: 859–860

Trials have shown that salt intake predicts cardiovascular events and that reduction improves hypertensive levels with no apparent threshold. The effect is also independent of age, sex, ethnic origin, baseline blood pressure, and body mass. Cook *et al.*'s study (*above*) strengthens further the case for salt limitation, but few countries have policies for this.

In the UK we are still far from our recommended target of 6 g per day. Most of the salt in our diet is derived from bread and processed food and the salt industry has been less than helpful in voluntary codes to reduce its profits. Therefore, it will be necessary and justified to legislate.

Advising patients in a primary care setting to eat less salt is pretty ineffective too. Cappuccio suggests a 24 hour urine collection will help us estimate our salt intake and make us aware how much we can reduce our cardiovascular risk. It is cheaper than testing cholesterol and could be part of the UK's National Service Framework.

FUNCTIONAL FOODS

Functional foods: the case for closer evaluation
de Jong N, Klungel OH, Verhagen H *et al.*
BMJ, 2007; **334**: 1037–1039

The EU is developing more detailed regulation and directives for functional foods but they mainly focus on safety and acceptable nutritional claims backed up by good nutritional science. They seem to be off the hook in having to prove their health claims, however, and their main appeal may be to anxious consumers.

There are some problems with their rush to the lifestyle marketplace:
- the evidence of harmlessness only comes from around 6 years of exposure
- it is unknown how usage affects compliance with prescribed medication
- once on the market, there are very limited data on the impact on the community and post-launch monitoring needs to be initiated
- if they have a benefit on public health, the government can incorporate them into national advice; if not, re-evaluation should be required

Functional foods
Lang T
BMJ, 2007; **334**: 1015–1016

Proponents argue that functional foods are a way of improving dietary intake through consumer choice. Fortified breakfast cereals and probiotic yoghurts are two of the largest markets and global sales are ballooning.

Sceptics argue that they represent a corporately driven exploitation of a niche market, affordable and appealing only to the worried well, and which is an extra burden on the finances of the poor.

Claims of performance enhancement and mental improvement are surely begging for post-marketing evidence, but until then it may just be another confounding factor for nutritionists to unravel.

DIET REGIMES

Comparison of the Atkins, Zone, Ornish, and LEARN diets for change in weight and related risk factors among overweight premenopausal women. The A TO Z Weight Loss Study: a randomized trial
Gardner CD, Kiazand A, Alhassan S *et al.*
JAMA, 2007; **297**: 969–977

Women under 50 years and with a BMI from 27 to 50 were randomised to one of four diets:
- Atkins (low in carbohydrate and high in fats and protein)
- Zone (low in carbohydrate, macronutrient balance)
- LEARN (lifestyle, exercise, attitudes, relationships, and nutrition)
- Ornish (very high in carbohydrate and very low in fat)

They attended classes led by a registered dietician once a week for 8 weeks and data were collected at 2, 6, and 12 months.

LIFESTYLE

- Women on the Atkins diet for 12 months lost an average of 4.7 kg more weight than women following the three other diets.
- There were no adverse metabolic effects in terms of lipid profiles or other cardiovascular risk factors, and systolic blood pressure came down significantly during the year.
- The other three diets worked about as well as each other with an average loss of 1.6–2.6 kg on average.
- The difference between Atkins and the others was significant after only two months and peaked at six months.

These results are reassuring that in the short term Atkins is unlikely to harm. Weight loss for these diets is still relatively modest, however, at around 5% of body weight.

The BBC diet trials
Arterburn D
BMJ, 2006; **332**: 1284–1285
and
Randomised controlled trial of four commercial weight loss programmes in the UK: initial findings from the BBC 'diet trials'
Truby H, Baic S, deLooy A *et al.*
BMJ, 2006; **332**: 1309–1314

The BBC diet trials were an attempt to compare the effects of four commercially available diets – Dr Atkins' new diet revolution ('the Atkins' – a low carbohydrate diet), Slim-Fast plan (meal substitution), Weight Watchers pure points programme (energy control), and Rosemary Conley's Eat Yourself Slim diet and fitness plan.

- Compared to a control group, there was little to choose between them – all produced weight loss of around 6% (6 kg) at 6 months
- Atkins produced faster weight loss in the first four weeks but was no more effective by the end. It did not adversely affect cholesterol and was the cheapest option. The Atkins book costs £8, 24 weeks of Rosemary Conley classes were £140, Weight Watchers classes cost £170, and twice daily Slim-Fast meal replacements cost £240
- Dropout rates were slightly higher for Slim-Fast and Atkins – the programmes which had less ongoing support

The BBC picked up the tab for the first 6 months but after that persistence with the diets was low and long-term inferences become impossible.

MEDITERRANEAN DIETS

Modified Mediterranean diet and survival: EPIC-elderly prospective cohort study
Trichopoulou A, Orfanos P, Norat T, *et al.*
BMJ, 2005; **330**: 991

EPIC – the European Prospective Investigation into Cancer and Nutrition study – is a very large prospective study reaching 9 European countries and 478 000 men and women from many European countries. It investigates the role of biological, dietary, lifestyle and environmental factors in cancer and other chronic diseases. It is coordinated by the International Agency for Research on Cancer and is the largest available database for investigating the role of diet in health.

This part of EPIC studied 75 000 men and women from 9 countries, aged over 60 and free of serious disease at enrolment. They aimed to see if the advantages for cardiovascular end points with the Mediterranean diet translated into years of longer life. They did better than they expected.

The diet was modified to make it more Euro-friendly by including polyunsaturates (much commoner in non-Mediterranean countries) in with the measure of the monounsaturated lipids so common in the olive oils of Greece and Spain.

A scoring system out of 10 was invented to measure adherence to the diet which may be a little arbitrary and discriminatory. However, the results were still impressive.

- There was significantly longer life expectancy in the healthy elderly cohort.
- A 2 point increase in the score corresponded to an 8% reduction in mortality and a 4 point increase led to a 14% reduction.
- A healthy 60 year old adhering to the diet can expect to live a year longer than one who does not adhere well.
- They conclude polyunsaturates are an acceptable substitute for monounsaturates.
- The benefits were strongest in Greece and Spain where they have the true Mediterranean diet.

Effects of a Mediterranean-style diet on cardiovascular risk factors
Estruch R, Martínez-González MA, Corella D *et al.*
Ann Intern Med, 2006; **145**: 1–11

This Spanish study found that the impact of the Mediterranean diet can be quick. They randomised 772 patients with a high risk of cardiovascular disease to a low fat diet or one of two Mediterranean diets – one provided free virgin olive oil and one provided free nuts.

Short term benefit on surrogate markers of cardiac disease were illustrated within 3 months. The Mediterranean diet improved plasma lipid profiles and CRP more than a low fat diet, reduced systolic blood pressure by 6 mmHg (oil) and 7 mmHg (nuts) and reduced serum glucose by 0.4 mmol/l and 0.3 mmol/l, respectively.

PROBIOTICS

Use of probiotic *Lactobacillus* preparation to prevent diarrhoea associated with antibiotics: randomised double blind placebo controlled trial
Hickson M, D'Souza AL, Muthu N *et al.*
BMJ, 2007; **335**: 80

A randomised double-blind study was used to assess a probiotic yoghurt drink containing *Lactobacillus* to see if it prevented diarrhoea associated with prescribing a course of antibiotics, and if it reduced diarrhoea caused by *Clostridium difficile.*

LIFESTYLE

Some 135 hospital patients with a mean age of 74 years were randomised to a twice-daily probiotic drink containing *Lactobacillus casei, L. bulgaricus,* and *Streptococcus thermophilus,* during a course of antibiotics and for 1 week afterwards.

- Diarrhoea following antibiotics was prevented by the probiotics with an absolute risk reduction of around 20% and the number needed to treat was 5.
- No one in the probiotic group had diarrhoea caused by *C. difficile* compared to 17% of the milkshake-drinking control group – an absolute risk reduction of 17% and with an NNT of 6.
- The cost to prevent one case of diarrhoea was £50 and to prevent one case of *C. difficile was* £60.
- There were no adverse events and the drink was well accepted.

The authors conclude that this paper adds to the young research base with a high quality approach. It shows the potential of probiotics to reduce the incidence of antibiotic-associated diarrhoea and *C. difficile*-associated diarrhea, and to decrease morbidity, healthcare costs, and mortality if used routinely in patients aged over 50.

DRUG MISUSE

The Challenge

Some 3.2 million people in Britain smoke cannabis, but associations with psychotic illnesses are increasingly confirmed. Most users are in their twenties and males outweigh females by 3:1. Adolescents are increasingly using it, with 40% of young people having tried it at least once.

Cannabis was reclassified from a Class B to a Class C drug across the UK in January 2004. As a controlled drug, production, supply and possession remain illegal, only the penalties have changed. Despite pressure and fears over psychosis, the Home Secretary refused in January 2006 to reclassify cannabis as a Class B drug. Stronger evidence in 2007 has led to requests to the Advisory Council on the Misuse of Drugs for clarification on the issue once again.

When the evidence is finally in, all the indications are that the effects of smoking cannabis will be at least as bad as those of smoking tobacco except at a younger age.

Drug misuse is an increasing problem that not only impairs the physical and mental health of people who misuse drugs, but also negatively affects their families and wider society (for example, in its association with crime).

All doctors will see drug users for a variety of medical and social problems, but recently expanded drug services in the UK involve GPs to a considerable degree. GPs care for at least one-third of the opiate misusers in treatment. Many clinicians, however, remain pessimistic about engaging drug users in treatment.

What we know already:

- Between 1993 and 1998 psychotic illness related to drug misuse increased by 50%. The average age of these cases decreased from 38 years to 34 years.
- Most users of cannabis also smoke tobacco, but cannabis cigarettes deposit four times as much tar on the respiratory tract as an unfiltered cigarette of the same weight.
- Both cannabis and tobacco smoking lead to inhalation of 4000 largely identical chemicals.
- Smoking cannabis is known to entail a two-thirds larger puff volume, a one-third larger inhaled volume, a fourfold longer time holding the breath, and a fivefold increase in carboxyhaemaglobin.
- The main active constituent in cannabis is THC (tetrahydrocannabinol) which has increased in concentration tenfold in the last 20 years in Britain, but is still only half the strength of that smoked in Holland.
- Between the mid-eighties and mid-nineties there was a fourfold increase in those testing positive for cannabis after fatal road accidents; it is an offence involving the same penalties as for alcohol, but legal limits are not defined, public awareness is low, and good testing devices are needed.
- Amongst drug misusers, heroin is the most used drug followed by methadone then cannabis and amphetamines.
- Methadone maintenance in a primary care setting can be effective in reducing crime and HIV risk-taking behaviour while improving physical and psychological well-being.

LIFESTYLE

- Contingency management programmes have been set up which involve incentives such as shopping vouchers to reward engagement with services and reduce illicit drug use. These are effective and are supported by NICE to encourage harm reduction such as rewarding attendance for hepatitis and HIV testing.
- Prescription of heroin to misusers is controversial. Although legitimate in the UK since 1926 (and known as 'the British system' abroad) it has been used in a limited way to stop destructive patterns of behaviour. Critics point to the further addiction and enslavement of suffering addicts.

Guidance

Drug Misuse and Dependence – Guidelines on Clinical Management. *Dept of Health,* September 2007 (www.smmgp.org.uk).
This is a comprehensive document incorporating NICE guidance on detoxification, maintenance therapy and psychosocial interventions for opiate uses.

Interventions to reduce substance misuse among vulnerable young people. *NICE,* 2007 (www.nice.org.uk/PHI004).

Guidance for working with cocaine and crack users in primary care. *RCGP,* Sept 2004.
This is a detailed document looking at issues related to primary and shared care for different types of user communities.

Recent Papers

CANNABIS

Prospective cohort study of cannabis use, predisposition for psychosis, and psychotic symptoms in young people
Henquet C, Krabbendam L, Spauwen J *et al.*
BMJ, 2005; **330**: 11

This study of nearly 2500 young people aged 14–24 years found that use of cannabis moderately increased psychotic symptoms at follow up 4 years later. The effect was not exclusive to but was more pronounced in those with a predisposition for psychosis (such as paranoid ideation), but independent of use of other drugs, tobacco or alcohol.

This supports the accumulation and converging evidence of a pro-psychotic effect of cannabis which followed a dose–response pattern. The study was able to establish the association as causal.

Cannabis use and risk of psychotic or affective mental health outcomes: a systematic review
Moore THM, Zammit S, Lingford-Hughes A *et al.*
Lancet, 2007; **370**: 319–328

This comprehensive Department of Health sponsored review found that published evidence indicated that cannabis is likely to cause psychotic illnesses. They adjusted for dozens of confounding variables and found a clear and persistent dose–response effect. This may be as close as we get to the truth, as randomised trials are impossible.

One estimate suggests that if all cannabis consumption ceased we would prevent 800 cases of schizophrenia per year. Public warnings are warranted. There may also be a link with anxiety and depression but this was less clear.

DECRIMINALISATION

Should drugs be decriminalised? Yes
Chand K
BMJ, 2007; **335**: 966

Chand, a GP, proposes legalisation, regulation and taxation of the entire drugs market. The downgrading of cannabis to a Class C drug – widely seen as a mistake and currently being re-examined – is seen by Chand as a "tiny step in the right direction".

Prohibition has failed, he argues, and drugs fuel violent gangs and gun crime. We need to regulate and tax it. Using the revenue gained to educate children to avoid drugs is the way to go he tells us, completely missing the paradox he is presenting. The drug money would "give children the tools to make healthy choices in the future".

He tells us that legislation could eliminate the allure of drugs but offers no specifics that tell us how decriminalisation has 'paid off' in term of health outcomes in The Netherlands.

With monitoring, we will know just how toxic the drugs we are authorising are. We can then empty the prisons and watch the revenue roll in. People over 18 can then make their own mind up how they spend their spare time.

Should drugs be decriminalised? No
Califano JA
BMJ, 2007; **335**: 967

What we should be concentrating on is more research into prevention and treatment, argues this US expert. Legalisation or decriminalisation would make the drugs cheaper, more available and more acceptable.

The US has 46 million adult smokers, up to 20 million alcoholics, but only 6 million drug addicts. Legalisation opens up a huge marketing opportunity to get the numbers up. Keeping the market to adults only would be an impossible dream if our experience of smoking and alcohol is anything to go by.

Italy, which has tended not to prosecute personal possession of a small

LIFESTYLE

amount of heroin, has ended up with one of the highest rates of heroin addiction in Europe.

Adolescent use of marijuana has massively increased in The Netherlands where coffee shops sold it like ice cream. Amounts have recently been limited and age of admission increased to 18.

Sensible use of the legal system means an arrest can be seen as an opportunity to treat, educate and plan on-going care with regular screening. Restrictive policies in Sweden have made their drug use just one-third of the European average.

The increased potency of modern cannabis and the mounting evidence of psychosis and other mental illness are well documented. Califano notes that "Drugs are not dangerous because they are illegal; they are illegal because they are dangerous".

OPIATE ABUSE

The effectiveness of community maintenance with methadone or buprenorphine for treating opiate dependence
Simoens S, Matheson C, Bond C, *et al.*
Br J Gen Pract, 2005; **55**: 139–146

This systematic review of maintenance therapy in primary care found that methadone and the lesser used buprenorphine were both effective and that higher doses were associated with better treatment outcomes.

This is important as a recent survey showed that almost half the GPs surveyed were prescribing substitute medication – three times as many as 16 years previously. However, most doses were too low to constitute optimal methadone maintenance risking adverse patient behaviours and poor outcomes (*Br J Gen Pract,* 2005; **55**: 444–451). Primary care could truly be an effective setting to expand high quality substitute prescribing in treatment of opiate dependence.

Incidence of hepatitis C virus and HIV among new injecting drug users in London: prospective cohort study
Judd A, Hickman M, Jones S *et al.*
BMJ, 2005; **330**: 24–25

This recent reassessment of prevalence rates of HIV and hepatitis C infection in injecting drug users shows that our harm reduction strategies have not been as successful as first thought. Testing users mostly from London who had started their habit within the previous 6 years showed baseline prevalence to be 44% for hepatitis C and 4.2% for HIV.

Over the year of study, the incidence of new cases of hepatitis C virus among new injecting drug users was 42 per 100 person years and of HIV was 3.4 cases per 100 person years. The suggestion is that transmission may have recently increased perhaps due to greater injection of crack and riskier behaviour in the new recruits.

LIFESTYLE

PRESCRIBING HEROIN

Should heroin be prescribed to heroin misusers? Yes
Rehm J, Fischer B
BMJ, 2008; **336**: 70

Arguing in favour of using heroin to treat heroin addiction, the authors quote Swiss studies which show feasibility and effectiveness for a hardcore group of users refractory to previous treatment. Treatment retention improved and benefits were seen in mental health, physical complications and a decrease in criminal activity. It was cost-effective compared with methadone maintenance and the trials have been extended to allow continuation of the practice under appropriate safeguards.

So what's the problem? Well, there has been an expansion of the public debate on the ethics, safety and clinical value of prescribing heroin and the whole idea of maintenance treatment in general.

The authors argue that maintenance overall (with buprenorphine or methadone) is more successful than abstinence. Concerns over safety are not backed up by the Swiss studies where mortality is lower than other maintenance programmes and heroin dependence is decreasing.

They argue that using this as one tool of a comprehensive programme is a useful approach for a subgroup of refractory addicts with severely compromised health and previous failed attempts with methadone.

Should heroin be prescribed to heroin misusers? No
McKeganey N
BMJ, 2008; **336**: 71

This author points to heroin prescription as an approach borne of frustration at our inability to tackle an escalating drug problem. Can we really call this exertion of social control a treatment?

Although the Swiss showed some success they also admit it may have reduced some patients' inclination to stop using heroin. A London study did not find the same health benefits as the Swiss and it is difficult to say if the value comes from aspects of the therapeutic programme other than the heroin itself.

The author here points out that the cost of heroin maintenance is 3–4 times that of methadone treatment and that UK doctors in private clinics have been accused of careless prescribing and investigated by the GMC.

Does such as approach cede authority to the patient? What do you say to the patient who requests cocaine? When requests escalate, where do you find yourself?

The approach only makes sense if the aim is not to treat dependency but tackle the complications. It may protect health and reduce criminality, but the right services can do so much more. Most addicts want services to help them become drug-free. Abstinence programmes can attain very good results especially with residential rehabilitation. Health services need to be sure they are supporting them in this aim rather than maintaining their dependency.

CLINICAL ISSUES

LIFESTYLE

VITAMINS

The Challenge

Neural tube defects and oral clefts are among the most common congenital malformations, but folic acid supplementation in the periconceptional period reduces the risk of these defects massively. In addition, folate intake, at least as part of the diet, appears to have a protective effect on stroke. For these reasons, there is an ongoing interest regarding mandatory folate fortification of foods.

Folate and B vitamins bring down blood homocysteine levels. We know that homocysteine in the blood is clearly associated with cardiovascular disease. So for more than a decade, researchers have been trying to show that supplementation with folate, B6 and B12 vitamins can reduce cardiovascular disease. However, higher concentrations of these vitamins in the blood have not been shown to reverse the disease processes, so the role of supplementation is far from clear.

Oxidative stress is implicated in most human diseases, leading to high hopes for antioxidants as a bit of a cure-all. Health food outlets have been promoting the supposed benefits direct to the consumer and at least 25% of older people in the UK now take nutritional supplements.

But there is a lot of controversy about the role of vitamin supplements for prevention of vascular disease and cancer. They are not as harmless as many would like to believe.

What we know already:

- Meta-analysis of 17 000 people from 12 RCTs found that folic acid supplementation had no value in reducing the risk of cardiovascular events or reducing all-cause mortality in those with a history of vascular disease.
- The largest randomised trials we have conclude that antioxidant supplementation with vitamin E, vitamin C and beta-carotene cannot be recommended for CHD prevention. Wasting more time on them may reduce compliance with proven medications such as aspirin, ACE inhibitors and statins.
- A meta-analysis of 14 randomised trials ($n = 170\,525$) looked at the effects of supplementation with vitamins A, C and E on oesophageal, gastric, colorectal, pancreatic, and liver cancer incidences – none were shown to be protective.
- Beta carotene (even in over-the-counter formulations) leads to a small but significant increase in all-cause mortality and cardiovascular death.
- A combination of beta-carotene with vitamin A is associated with a 30% increased risk of death. Combination of beta-carotene with vitamin E led to a 10% increase.
- Reports suggest that use of multivitamin supplements in early life could leads to a higher risk of asthma and food allergies.

LIFESTYLE

Recent Papers

FOLIC ACID

Lowering homocysteine with folic acid and B vitamins did not prevent vascular events in vascular disease or after myocardial infarction. *Evidence-Based Medicine,* 2006; **11**: 104–105
The following papers are reviewed
Homocysteine lowering with folic acid and B vitamins in vascular disease
Lonn E, Yusuf S, Arnold MJ *et al.*
N Engl J Med, 2006; **354**: 1567–1577
and
Homocysteine lowering and cardiovascular events after acute myocardial infarction
Bønaa KH, Njølstad I, Ueland PM *et al.*
N Engl J Med, 2006; **354**: 1578–1588

Does folate really help to reduce cardiovascular disease by lowering homocysteine?

Good observational evidence and some small trials said yes. These two large randomised trials provide a clear 'no'. Confidence intervals were tight enough to rule out an important effect.

The first study – HOPE-2 – randomised 5522 patients over 55 with cardiovascular disease in 145 centres in 13 countries. A combined pill with folic acid, vitamin B6 and B12 did increase the blood concentrations of these vitamins and lowered plasma homocysteine by around 22%. But it failed to have a positive effect on a combined end point of CVD death, MI, or stroke.

However, in analyses of each outcome separately, a beneficial effect of the intervention on stroke was observed. The commentator thinks this is unlikely to be a causal association, since such an effect was not observed in other trials. Like the authors of HOPE-2, he thinks this finding is an overestimate of the effect or due to chance.

Similarly, the NORVIT (Norwegian Vitamin) trial of 3749 patients with recent MI were randomised to various combinations of the same vitamins or to placebo. Again they lowered homocysteine to a similar degree but after 3 years there was no evidence of improvement in end-points. The combination tablets that contained all three ingredients even showed a trend towards an increase in fatal or non-fatal MI in stroke and sudden cardiac death.

It seems the one untested element of the 'polypill' can now be dropped.

The commentator espouses how similar the pattern is to the fallen arguments for vitamin E and HRT. It seems that in CVD prevention there is 'simply no substitute for large randomised controlled trials that measure clinical, not surrogate, end-points'. We end up 'chasing rainbows' when we should be focussing on ensuring that all patients are receiving the therapies that we know work.

Efficacy of folic acid supplementation in stroke prevention: a meta-analysis
Wang X, Qin X, Demirtas H, *et al.*
Lancet, 2007; **369**: 1876–1882

Hang on a minute though! Are we about to throw the baby out with the bath water?

LIFESTYLE

This meta-analysis of eight relevant randomised trials, specifically to discover any potential for folic acid to prevent stroke, found the following:
- folic acid supplementation significantly reduced the risk of stroke by 18%
- the effect was better where treatment was longer, where homocysteine decreased by more than 20% , where there was no fortification in the food supply, and no previous history of stroke

These findings indicate that folic acid supplementation can effectively reduce the risk of stroke in primary prevention, particularly where the food supply has not already been fortified.

Effect of homocysteine lowering on mortality and vascular disease in advanced chronic kidney disease and end-stage renal disease
Jamison RL, Hartigan P, Kaufman JS, *et al.*
JAMA, 2007; **298**: 1163–1170

According to this study of over 2000 high-risk people with high homocysteine and advanced chronic kidney disease, supplementation with folate, B6 and B12 vitamins does not reduce cardiovascular disease.

Most similar work is from the US where there is fortification anyway so the search for the Emperor's clothes will probably continue.

Folic acid supplements and risk of facial clefts: national population based case-control study
Wilcox AJ, Lie RT, Solvoll K, *et al.*
BMJ, 2007; **334**: 464

This well-designed case-control study looked at possible effects of folic acid on facial clefts in Norway, which has one of the highest rates of facial clefts in Europe. After adjusting for confounding factors, they found that:
- folic acid supplementation of at least 400 µg/day during early pregnancy seemed to reduce the risk of isolated cleft lip with or without cleft palate by about one-third
- diets rich in folate-containing foods reduced the risk somewhat
- the lowest risk of cleft lip was among women with folate-rich diets who also took folic acid supplements
- folic acid provided no protection against cleft palate alone

FOLATE FORTIFICATION

Folic acid and birth malformations
Bille C, Murray JC, Olsen SF
BMJ, 2007; **334**: 433–434

This editorial notes the undoubted value of folate and the uncertainty about the optimal dose. Three possibilities for supplementation exist.
- Eat some folate. Even then it is difficult to reach the doses that supplementation provides and such recommendations alone have failed to make much of an impact.
- Take supplements in the periconceptional period. However, low compliance

LIFESTYLE

and high rates of unplanned pregnancy have sabotaged this approach with fewer than 50% of women following the recommendations.

- Fortify staple foods such as corn flour, wheat and rice. A particular dose cannot be guaranteed when fortifying food for obvious reasons.

Worries over theoretical complications have delayed implementation and some feel a population measure that is aiming to reach only women of childbearing age is too sweeping.

More concrete evidence of wider health benefits might seal the deal for fortification in Europe. But that may never happen and, in the meantime, we are missing the chance to decrease the burden of the 4500 neural tube defects each year in the EU alone.

International retrospective cohort study of neural tube defects in relation to folic acid recommendations: are the recommendations working?
Botto LD, Lisi A, Robert-Gnansia E, *et al.*
BMJ, 2005; **330**: 571.

Folic acid supplements consumed before conception can reduce spina bifida and other neural tube defects by over 80%. This retrospective study in 13 countries that issued advice to take folic acid in this way found no detectable improvement in incidence of neural tube defects up to 6 years after the recommendation.

Preventable new cases of neural tube defects are still appearing. The time may be right to join the US and Canada who ensure their citizens get at least some folate by fortifying their flour with it.

Should folic acid fortification be mandatory? Yes
Wald NJ, Oakley GP
BMJ, 2007; **334**: 1252

Delay in fortifying flour with folic acid is unjustified. Here, Wald and Oakley systematically dismantle all the arguments against the practice. They argue that there is now a public duty to act, as withholding a known benefit causes harm.

- It is necessary, safe and effective and could save 250 000 children worldwide from spina bifida and anencephaly each year.
- It has been done in 40 countries so far including the US with no validated adverse effects on health.
- It is important to reach the less affluent. Chile, for example, has reduced its neural tube defects by 43%.
- Most pregnancies remain unprotected as supplements must be taken before pregnancy occurs.
- Evidence indicates other benefits such as a modest protection against cardiovascular disease.
- Meta-analysis has shown a reduction in strokes after supplementation.
- There is no convincing evidence of carcinogenesis, if anything folic acid intake is associated with protection against colorectal cancer.
- Worries that it masks B12 deficiency are a misnomer. We have better tests nowadays than just observing macrocytosis.

CLINICAL ISSUES

LIFESTYLE

- Worries about the synthetic folic acid that we use to fortify foods are invalid. It has higher bioavailability and is stable when cooked.

Should folic acid fortification be mandatory? No
Hubner RA, Houlston RD, Muir KR
BMJ, 2007; **334:** 1253

The counter position expresses concern that folate supplements may have cancer-promoting effects and that the use of synthetic folate may further complicate the effects on DNA synthesis.

The authors mention a number of weak associations that do not reach significance and wonder about the possibility of promoting tumour growth in pre-existing adenomas of the colon. Certainly this would be a major worry if substantiated, but even they admit that the low levels in food fortification may not be enough to cause this, assuming that an effect even exists.

They recommend further investigation to confirm these worries prior to mandatory fortification.

Other than that there really is very little substance to this supposed counter-argument.

ANTIOXIDANTS

Meta-analysis: high-dosage vitamin E supplementation may increase all-cause mortality
Miller ER, Pastor-Barriuso R, Dalal D, *et al.*
Ann Intern Med, 2005; **142:** 37–46

A meta-analysis of 1 135 000 subjects in 19 trials indicated increased mortality with increasing doses of vitamin E, further refuting suggestions of a benefit for heart disease or cancer.

About 11% of adult Americans consume at least 400 IU of vitamin E daily, more if they are older and take other antioxidants. Doses above this can kill and those who choose to take vitamin E for the reasons above should be aware of the risk to their health or better still, just stop (*Ann Intern Med,* 2005; **143:** 116–20). It probably leads to heart failure in the long run and it may be time to finish with this discredited supplement. (*JAMA,* 2005; **293:** 1338–1347).

Mortality in randomised trials of antioxidant supplements for primary and secondary prevention: systematic review and meta-analysis
Bjelakovic G, Nikolova D, Gluud L, *et al.*
JAMA, 2007; **297:** 842–857

Up to one-fifth of adults in the US and Europe use antioxidant supplements thanks to early observational studies which were heavily trumped up by manufacturers.

We now know they are wasting their money and probably harming their health.

This meta-analysis adds to the data by reviewing 68 trials in nearly a quarter of a million people. They confirmed that supplements containing beta carotene,

LIFESTYLE

vitamin A, and vitamin E increased mortality overall by about 5% compared to placebo.

Vitamin C and selenium had no significant effect on mortality and need further study.

MULTIVITAMINS

Effect of multivitamin and multimineral supplements on morbidity from infections in older people (MAVIS trial): pragmatic, randomised, double blind, placebo controlled trial
Avenell A, Campbell MK, Cook JA, *et al.*
BMJ, 2005; **331**: 324–329

> This placebo-controlled trial of the effect of multivitamin and multimineral supplementations was done in Scotland over a period of a year.
>
> There was no effect on self-reported infections, prescriptions, admission rates, quality of life or contacts with primary care. The study was of good quality and largely confirms previous research but biases can creep in. The doses used were low and the populations were relatively fit.

Role of multivitamins and mineral supplements in preventing infections in elderly people: systematic review and meta-analysis of randomised controlled trials
El-Kadiki A, Sutton AJ
BMJ, 2005; **330**: 871

> Older people are susceptible to infection and vitamin supplements have been used on an *ad hoc* basis. This review looked at the available evidence for and against and found little evidence to suggest that multivitamin and mineral supplements actually prevent infections in elderly people.
>
> Overall, a lot of the evidence was weak, flawed and conflicting. It does not support a policy of routine supplementation in all elderly people as things stand.

LIFESTYLE

EXERCISE

The Challenge

Physical inactivity increases the risk of many chronic diseases – notably coronary heart disease, type 2 diabetes, and cancer of the colon.

Interventions promoting physical activity can give massive health benefits in reducing cardiovascular risk factors, diabetes, obesity, osteoporosis, and symptoms of depression. But it is hard to bring the message home.

Most adults in the UK do not reach the 30 minutes of moderately intense physical activity on most days that is sufficient to provide most of the anti-inflammatory and anti-atherosclerotic health benefits.

General practice is ideally placed to identify sedentary adults and deliver brief interventions, and physical activity is "today's best buy in public health". But changing longstanding and complex patterns of physical inertia is a huge challenge for healthcare and government.

What we know already:

- Young adults assessed by treadmill test as having low fitness were twice as likely to develop diabetes, high blood pressure, and the metabolic syndrome than participants with high fitness levels, even after accounting for body mass index.
- Research has shown that for both sexes, moderate physical activity delays cardiovascular disease and extends life in the over fifties by 1.3 years. High physical activity extends life by 3.7 years.
- In a study of Welsh men, light and moderate intensity exercise, such as walking, golf and dancing, had inconsistent and non-significant effects on mortality but habitual vigorous intensity extended life.
- The Nurses Health Study showed that those who walked faster for longer had half the cardiovascular risk, diabetic risk and all cause mortality than those doing the least.
- Walking can probably improve metabolic control and other health parameters, and politicians and doctors need to work towards getting that advice out there.
- Coronary benefits are gained relative to the individual's perceived level of their own exertion. This reduces the urge to prescribe a certain intensity of exercise that has not taken individual capacity into account.
- Getting people on to healthy modes of transport is difficult. Motivated subgroups could be influenced on around 5% of all trips.
- Meta-analysis by the ExTraMATCH Collaborative found that exercise training improved survival in patients with chronic heart failure to a similar degree (risk reduction 32%) as the best pharmacological agents. It also increased the median time to hospital admissions.

Guidelines

At least five a week: Evidence on the impact of physical activity and its relationship to health (April 2004). This report from the Chief Medical Officer recommends that adults do at least

30 minutes a day of moderately intense activity on five or more days a week. It also advises that children and young people do at least 60 minutes every day. Walking, golf, mowing the lawn, decorating and cycling are considered examples of moderate physical activity.

Recent Papers

IN CHILDREN

Effectiveness of interventions to promote physical activity in children and adolescents: systematic review of controlled trials
Van Sluijs EMF, McMinn AM, Griffin SJ
BMJ, 2007; **335**: 703
and
Encouraging children and adolescents to be more active
Giles-Corti B, Salmon J
BMJ, 2007; **335**: 677–678

> Three out of 10 boys and 4 out of 10 girls are estimated not to take the recommended hour a day of moderate to vigorous intensity physical activity.
>
> This systematic review and the accompanying editorial tell us that most strategies to promote activity in children do not seem to work very well. The most effective have many components and take place in many settings, with school-based interventions likely to be more effective when involving families.
>
> Most of the interventions provide information alone and that is seldom effective. None have examined the influences of gender, culture or socioeconomic status.
>
> How to create environments that support the safety of active transport such as walking to school and cycling is under-researched.
>
> Clearly complex interventions which influence populations are needed. Some argue that this limits the conclusions we can draw from randomised controlled trials in limited areas.

IN THE ELDERLY

Exercise is associated with reduced risk for incident dementia among persons 65 years of age and older
Larson EB, Wang L, Bowen JD *et al.*
Ann Intern Med, 2006; **144**: 73–81

> This study followed 1740 subjects over the age of 65 years who were clear of cognitive impairment at baseline. Those who exercised regularly over a mean follow-up period of 6 years reduced their risk of developing dementia by 38%. The elderly have particularly low exercise levels and the most benefit in this large robust study went to those who were the least fit. Walking 15 minutes three times a week was enough to delay dementia.

CLINICAL ISSUES

LIFESTYLE

Exercise program for nursing home residents with Alzheimer's disease
Rolland Y, Pillard F, Klapouszczak A, *et al.*
J Am Geriatr Soc, 2007; **55:** 158–165

This exercise programme in five US nursing homes slowed up the decline in activities of daily living in patients with Alzheimer's disease. The trial was randomised, controlled and its effects persisted after 12 months. Training in strength, balance and flexibility of just 1 hour twice a week was enough to show the benefit.

WALKING

Regular brisk walking improves cardiovascular risk factors in healthy sedentary adults.
Evidence-Based Medicine, 2007; **12**: 171
The following paper is reviewed
The effect of walking on fitness, fatness and resting blood pressure: a meta-analysis of randomised, controlled trials
Murphy MH, Nevill AM, Murtagh EM, *et al.*
Prev Med, 2007; **44:** 377–385

A review of 23 randomised controlled trials to assess programmes to increase walking found that regular brisk walking led to improvement in cardiovascular fitness, body weight and diastolic BP. No effect on systolic BP was noted.

Although actual improvements were small (e.g. 1.5 mmHg diastolic drop), the benefits may still have been overestimated as drop out rates were high due to the motivation required. But compliance rates are often even lower in everyday practice. So either the interventions motivated them or they were already highly motivated groups.

Even so, these apparently small benefits could be considerable when extended across a population, particularly in those with pre-existing compromise.

Brisk walking is now an evidence-based intervention we can recommend.

Interventions to promote walking: systematic review
Ogilvie D, Foster CE, Rothnie H, *et al.*
BMJ, 2007; **334:** 1204

This systematic review of walking trials included 19 randomised and 29 non-randomised trials to examine how best to promote walking.

Successful interventions can increase walking by up to 30–60 minutes per week on average. When targeted at the most sedentary or the most motivated, interventions are effective. However, there is very little good evidence on the sustainability, generalisability, or clinical benefits of such approaches.

Effects of aerobic training, resistance training, or both on glycaemic control in type 2 diabetes
Sigal RJ, Kenny GP, Boulé NG, *et al.*
Ann Intern Med, 2007; **147:** 357–369

Regular exercise can assist glycaemic control in type 2 diabetics.

The DARE (Diabetes Aerobic and Resistance Exercise) clinical trial participants were 251 adults aged 39–70 years with type 2 diabetes who exercised three times a week for 6 months. They were quite heavy and averaged a BMI of 35. This study looked at combining aerobic and resistance training and found the approach better than either type of exercise alone.

- Aerobic exercise reduced their HbA1c concentrations by 0.5 of a percentage point compared with inactive controls.
- Resistance training with weights had a similar effect at 0.4 percentage points.
- Participants who did both forms of exercise achieved an extra reduction of about another 0.5 of a point.
- The exercise had no effect on their serum lipids or blood pressure.

As each percentage point reduction means 15–20% fewer cardiovascular events, the benefit could be large. However, because of the study design the combined effect could be due to longer exercise duration in the combined exercise group.

Nevertheless the importance of exercise in diabetes is clearly demonstrated.

LIFESTYLE

SMOKING

The Challenge

Smoking is the leading preventable cause of death in the UK. It is a chronic condition requiring long-term management plans, but we are still unsure about which of the 4000 ingredients in cigarette smoke lead to the harm.

Deaths from second-hand smoke following exposure at work are estimated at more than 600 each year in the UK. The British regional heart study showed that passive smoking (in non-smokers) leads to an excess risk of CHD of 50–60%. They used measurements of serum cotinine (a nicotine metabolite that reflects the past 24 hours of exposure) but only half the amounts found were explained by domestic exposure alone. Exposure at home accounts for 2700 deaths in those aged 20–64 and 8000 in those aged ≥65. The remaining risk is presumed to come from pubs, restaurants and the workplace.

Children with less mature immune, nervous, and respiratory systems are particularly vulnerable to the health effects of passive smoking. The main sources of exposure to second-hand smoke in children are usually the home or the car, which are areas out of legislative control. But they could also be exposed anywhere smoking is allowed.

Effects of second-hand smoke on platelet and vascular endothelial function are almost immediate. This explains the rapid reductions in hospital admissions for acute myocardial infarction observed in areas after implementation of smoke-free legislation. We also know that the risks of second-hand smoke exposure are greater for ex-smokers than for never smokers, perhaps due to susceptibility of already existing mutations.

Enforcement of smoke-free work environments and public places eliminates exposure to second-hand smoke and is a public health priority throughout the world. On July 1st 2007, England followed Scotland and Ireland and introduced a new law to make virtually all enclosed public places and workplaces smoke-free.

What we know already:

- There is no safe threshold for smoking. Follow-up of over 42 000 Norwegian men and women found that smoking 1–4 cigarettes per day was associated with triple the risk of dying from ischaemic heart disease and lung cancer.
- About 27% of the UK population smokes – about 25% of 15 year olds smoke regularly.
- Nicotine is extremely addictive but two-thirds of smokers want to quit.
- One-third of smokers try to quit each year and most need several attempts (typically up to seven). Half quit eventually. Each 10 years of age increases the chances of success by one-third.
- Challenging any suggestions that smoking rates would not be improved, smoke-free legislation has been shown to be associated with an increase in smoke-free homes, a tendency to smoke less, and more successful cessation attempts among adults.
- A sharp increase (estimated at 28%) in quitting since the 2007 ban has dropped the cost of the NHS Stop Smoking Services to £164 per quitter.
- Varenicline is a partial nicotinic agonist and is the first new smoking cessation agent in nearly a decade that does not contain nicotine. It is currently the most successful smoking

cessation aid followed by bupropion, then NRT. Nortiptyline and clonidine have also been shown to be effective.

- Brief advice to stop smoking is successful in 1 in 40 cases making it one of the most cost-effective interventions in medicine.
- Combining drugs with counselling using a CBT approach yields the best results but the style and depth of counselling in studies varies greatly. The more intense the intervention, the higher the quit rates.
- Positive predictive indicators for success in quitting smoking are a low nicotine dependence score and those with previous attempts to stop who are 80% more likely to quit.
- Hardcore smokers with increased nicotine dependence, no desire or intention to quit in the future, and who smoke daily, represent 16% of all UK smokers. The tendency increases with age affecting one-third of smokers ≥65 years. They were more likely to be recalcitrant in their attitudes and deny the risks. Benefits of giving up at this age are actually enhanced. Doing so at age 65 years can extend life by 2 years. Specific interventions may be needed.
- Smoking is associated with lower body mass but relatively increases abdominal girth (a better measure of health risk), implying that smoking is actually associated with an adverse fat distribution profile.

Recent Papers

GENERAL

Mortality in relation to smoking: 50 years' observations on male British doctors
Doll R, Peto R, Boreham J *et al.*
BMJ, 2004; **328**:1519–1528

The fifty year results of this most famous of all papers were published in 2004. Sir Richard Doll's analysis of smoking habits in nearly 35 000 male British doctors since 1951 has concluded that:

- long-term cigarette smokers die on average 10 years earlier than non-smokers
- the full mortal effects of smoking can take 50 years to mature
- about half of all persistent smokers are killed by their habit (this figure has even reached two-thirds for this particular cohort)
- stopping smoking at age 60, 50, 40, or 30 years gains, respectively, about 3, 6, 9, or 10 years of life expectancy
- stopping at age 50 halves associated risks. Stopping at 30 avoids almost all of the elevated risk
- medical progress has reduced mortality rates in the last fifty years but persistent smokers do not qualify for these improvements
- on current patterns of uptake and in the absence of widespread cessation, there will be about one billion deaths from smoking this century

LIFESTYLE

LEGISLATION

Changes in child exposure to environmental tobacco smoke (CHETS) study after implementation of smoke-free legislation in Scotland: national cross sectional survey
Akhtar PC, Currie DB, Currie CE, Haw SJ
BMJ, 2007; **335:** 545

Scotland brought in smoke-free legislation in enclosed public spaces in March 2006.

Salivary cotinine measurement in non-smoking children (mean age 11.4 years) approximately halved among pupils living in households in which neither parent-figure smoked (51% fall) or in which only the father-figure smoked (44%).

There was no evidence of any increases in second-hand smoke exposure as a result of displacement of smoking patterns from public places into the home and the effect of the legislation was entirely positive for children.

Changes in exposure of adult non-smokers to secondhand smoke after implementation of smoke-free legislation in Scotland: national cross sectional survey
Haw SJ, Gruer L
BMJ, 2007; **335:** 549

According to this study of Scottish adults under 75 years, since the legislation:
- mean cotinine concentrations in adult non-smokers fell by 39%
- cotinine concentrations halved in those living in non-smoking households
- the lesser 16% fall in cotinine concentrations in non-smokers from smoking households was not statistically significant
- the reduced exposure in public places did not seem to displace to the home despite no detected reduction in exposure in homes or cars

SMOKING CESSATION

'Catastrophic' pathways to smoking cessation: findings from national survey
West R, Sohal T
BMJ, 2006; **332:** 458–460

Behavioural approaches are the prevailing model for smoking cessation courses. They use a trans-theoretical model to identify a sequence of stages:
- precontemplation – where an anti-smoking seed may be planted for the future
- contemplation – an opportunity to build on the patient's dissatisfaction with his habit
- preparation – where the smoker is making plans to break the habit
- action – the time of the attempt when as much support as possible is required
- maintenance – to keep the ex-smoker motivated and try to avoid ......
- relapse – which is all too common and starts the cycle off again

However, many feel this is too arbitrary. This study of nearly 2000 smokers found that almost half had made no organised plan to quit. This spontaneous group

LIFESTYLE

kicked the habit abruptly and were more likely to succeed for 6 months than those who planned ahead regardless of age, sex or socioeconomic group.

The authors offer us a catastrophe theory whereby a tiny trigger leads to a sweeping change when the proper tensions are right. They describe the 3Ts – tension (personal dissatisfaction creating motivation), trigger (to activate the change when the smoker is 'on the cusp') and treatments (nicotine patches and counselling immediately available to support the attempts).

Should doctors advocate snus and other nicotine replacements? No
Macara AW
BMJ, 2008; **336:** 359

Snus is the Swedish word for snuff, somewhat superceded by cigarettes and defined as "A finely ground moist tobacco, either loose or in tiny sachets – a bit like tiny teabags – that are placed under the upper lip and typically held in the mouth for about 30 minutes before being discarded".

Although Sweden gained an exemption from the 1992 EU ban, there have been calls for snus and other alternative nicotine sources to be expanded to offer more options to cigarettes.

Evidence is incomplete as snus are often used by people who also smoke tobacco. They cause cancers of the oral cavity and there is also an association with pancreatic cancer. It is widely accepted that smokeless tobacco also has a significant effect on myocardial infarction. Although less addictive than smoked tobacco, nicotine is delivered in higher quantities than usual nicotine therapy.

As a harm reduction measure it can be considered but it may lead to harm potentiation. Some 60% of those using snus to quit smoking become chronic users. There is no evidence that snus affects smoking prevalence and they may increase tobacco use in the population.

Should doctors advocate snus and other nicotine replacements? Yes
Britton J
BMJ, 2008; **336:** 358

Nicotine is relatively harmless. It is the hundreds of toxins in tobacco smoke that make smoking so deadly. Although snus cause pancreatic cancer and cardiovascular disease they do not cause lung cancer or COPD, making them less hazardous overall. In addition, substitution with snus has led to lower levels of smoking in Sweden.

Regulations currently prohibit the supply of tobacco products that are not to be chewed or smoked, so snus are illegal in the UK unless you get someone in Sweden to post them to you. Although not the ideal option, for those unlikely to quit it is probably the next best approach. A switch to less hazardous sources of nicotine could save millions of lives. As a last resort, they must make sense.

The Royal College of Physicians has released *Harm Reduction in Nicotine Addiction: Helping People Who Can't Quit.* The RCP supports expanded availability and promotion of stronger products to satisfy the nicotine addiction without killing so many people, ideally but not necessarily as a step to quitting. These products would deliver as much nicotine as quickly as cigarettes and be more attractive and cheaper.

LIFESTYLE

OBESITY

The Challenge

The prevalence of obesity has been increasing in developed countries and it has been predicted that it will soon overtake smoking as the leading health problem in the UK. It currently affects over 1.1 billion individuals worldwide and more than half of British adults are overweight. Nearly one-third of 11-year-olds are overweight and 17% are obese. Obesity in pre-school children has increased by over 70% in the last generation.

The consensus is that the cause is environmental – easy access for the modern human to food and little need for exercise. Interventions to date have focused on dietary behaviour and exercise, but as a whole have had little or no impact on the growing epidemic.

Obesity shortens lifespan and the role of primary care in managing obesity is linked to the aims of the national service framework for coronary heart disease. The Department of Health requires primary care to deliver obesity management services, but attempts so far have proved to be labour intensive and with modest results at best. There are serious questions of feasibility and new models may be needed.

The UK House of Commons Health Committee report on obesity (May 2004) recommended measures such as simpler labelling of food, categorising healthfulness, and stopping school sponsorship by fast food chains. The WHO calls for immediate bans of advertising junk food to children and restriction of sugar content.

Body mass index is becoming discredited as a parameter. Abdominal obesity is more closely related to physical activity and probably reflects both visceral and subcutaneous fat and so total fatness. It is therefore a better predictor of coronary risk than BMI which gives no indication of fat distribution.

The 'metabolic syndrome' is proposed as the common antecedent of cardiovascular disease and type 2 diabetes. The syndrome is characterised by the co-existence of obesity (especially central), dyslipidaemia (especially high triglycerides and low levels of HDL), hyperglycaemia and hypertension. Specific thresholds are currently elusive. Diagnosing such a syndrome might have screening potential but this seems a long way off.

Insulin resistance has been put forward as the unifying pathophysiology as has obesity, but the argument still seems incomplete.

Is the metabolic syndrome a real entity which predicts a cardiovascular endpoint greater than the sum of its parts? Evidence is unclear. Inactivity fuels obesity fuels diabetes fuels cardiovascular disease. Prevention of obesity could break the vicious circle. More research on the metabolic syndrome is needed before targets can be identified and effective interventions tailored.

Currently part of our response is to treat with anti-obesity drugs. Global sales in 2005 were estimated at $1.2bn and are increasing all the time.

What we know already:

- A large primary care study estimates that obesity more than doubles prescribing in most drug categories.
- Ultimately as weight loss is so hard to achieve and even harder to sustain, public and personal approaches should head rapidly towards prevention.
- No randomised controlled trials have evaluated the efficacy of screening for obesity.
- Small changes in energy intake and output can have a major impact on the risk of obesity. Two hours spent watching TV can raise the risk of obesity by 23% and of diabetes by 14%. Two hours of sitting at work is associated with increases of 5% and 7% respectively. But 2 hours of standing or walking around at home reduced obesity by 9% and diabetes by 12%.
- Only a few treatments have been shown to work. They include drug treatment, complex multicomponent weight loss programmes and surgery in extreme cases.
- Counselling and behavioural interventions promoting exercise and dietary change achieve small weight reductions of 2–3 kg.
- Apart from surgical intervention, weight loss tends to be modest. Surgical techniques reported weight loss up to 40 kg, with the main adverse effects being re-operation and wound infection.
- In one study, GPs primarily believed obesity to be the responsibility of the patient, rather than a problem requiring a medical solution. They felt that obese patients wanted to hand them responsibility creating possible friction.

Guidelines

Obesity: the prevention, identification, assessment and management of overweight and obesity in adults and children. *NICE*, Dec 2006.

The first NICE clinical guideline to outline strategies to prevent and tackle obesity in adults and children was released in December 2006.
- Coordinated efforts are needed to maximise the effectiveness of interventions. Primary care trusts will be required to implement recommendations with audit criteria.
- BMI should be used to classify the degree of obesity bearing in mind it is less reliable in Asians, the elderly and highly muscular people.
- Waist circumference should be used to assess health risks but is unreliable when BMI exceeds 35 kg/m^2.
- Weight management programmes should include behavioural change strategies to increase activity and reduce energy intake with ongoing support and realistic targets. Guidance is also given on the role of drugs and bariatric surgery.

The National Audit Office (www.nao.org.uk) has issued a report 'Tackling Obesity in England'. This is a detailed account of the costs of the problem, management strategies in the NHS and population initiatives to address all aspects of obesity.

LIFESTYLE

Recent Papers

THE SCALE OF THE PROBLEM

Is the obesity epidemic exaggerated? Yes
Basham P, Luik J
BMJ, 2008; **336:** 244

These authors feel that those who warn of impending doom are premature. They tell us in this head to head argument that there is too much uncertainty in the evidence. They worry about the reliability of data that go back decades and note that as populations grow healthier and more prosperous, they live longer and gain weight.

They find some statistics which show little change in the number of overweight children in recent consecutive years casting doubt on the claims for an epidemic. BMI as an index has already been discredited as an index of diagnostic value. Despite increasing levels of obesity, life expectancy continues to increase and the diseases that it is blamed for have largely multifactorial causes. They even express scepticism that obesity causes insulin resistance and diabetes.

They claim that some in the public health community believe in knowingly exaggerating the message on the assumption that it is so important to get the message out. They find the implications of this to be too high a price for evidence based medicine to pay.

Is the obesity epidemic exaggerated? No
Jeffery RW, Sherwood NE
BMJ, 2008; **336:** 245

On the other hand, an abundance of observational data show the rising prevalence of obesity with rates increasing from 6% to 23% in England between 1982 and 1999, reflecting similar rises in many other countries.

The adverse effects of obesity include many serious health conditions, including hypertension, hypercholesterolaemia, diabetes, coronary heart disease, and some forms of cancer. The dose–response relationship with BMI even appears among adults in the upper half of the 'healthy' weight range. As weight loss has proved to be difficult to achieve, a potential crisis is in the offing. The burden of diabetes has almost doubled between 1994 and 2005.

With such evidence, we can either hope the science is wrong or develop public health measures to avert the deteriorating situation.

However, a reduction in cardiovascular disease has admittedly occurred alongside rising bodyweights. Why? Better treatments of risk factors?

Lifetime medical costs of obesity: prevention no cure for increasing health expenditure
van Baal PHM, Polder JJ, Ardine de Wit G
PLoS Med, **5:** e29

This paper questions the idea that treating obesity is going to save money in the long run.

They modelled healthcare costs for three cohorts of 20-year-old men and women – committed smokers, people with a body mass index over 30, and healthy controls. They estimated costs over a lifetime.

- Smokers cost least because smoking kills people relatively cheaply and quickly.
- The healthy group cost most as they carry on living and developing the numerous diseases of old age that make them expensive to treat.
- Obese people fell in the middle as savings from the complications of obesity would be spent on the complications of living longer.

So programmes to treat obesity are not going to save us money in the long run.

But governments should still remember that living longer along with preventing suffering are the worthy goals of public health measures.

PARAMETERS

Association of bodyweight with total mortality and with cardiovascular events in coronary artery disease: a systematic review of cohort studies
Romero-Corral A, Montori V, Somers V *et al.*
Lancet, 2006; **368**: 666–678

A systematic review of 40 studies with 250 152 patients and 4 years of follow up, looked at the association between obesity, and total mortality and cardiovascular events in cardiac patients (following angioplasty, bypass or MI).

- Morbidly obese people (BMI ≥35) had the highest risk for cardiovascular mortality but did not have increased total mortality.
- Obese patients (BMI 30–35) did best of all and had no increased risk for cardiovascular or total mortality.
- Overweight people (BMI 25–30) had the lowest risk for total mortality and cardiovascular mortality compared with those for people with a normal BMI.
- Patients with a low BMI <20 had an increased risk for total and cardiovascular mortality.

This all appears bizarre and paradoxical. It is unlikely weight protects against cardiac disease. The authors tell us that using BMI as an indicator of cardiovascular risk should stop. It may not distinguish between fat and lean mass.

A previous *Lancet* study of over 27 000 people covered a wide ethnic variation in 52 countries. They found that waist and hip circumferences (adjusted for BMI) and waist-to-hip ratio were closely and independently associated with risk of MI even after adjustment for other risk factors. Waist-to-hip ratio had the strongest association worldwide so in most ethnic groups it might be more clinically valuable to redefine obesity in this way. BMI had the worst correlation and the authors suggested it should perhaps become obsolete as a measure of risk for heart attack (*Lancet,* 2005; **366**: 1640–1649).

LIFESTYLE

OBESITY AND CANCER

Cancer incidence and mortality in relation to body mass index in the Million Women Study: cohort study
Reeves GK, Pirie K, Beral V, *et al*.
BMJ, 2007; **335**: 1134

This paper looked at incidences of cancer in 1.2 million women aged between 50 and 64 years in the Million Women Study.

Increased BMI is already known to increase the risk of adenocarcinoma of the oesophagus, endometrial cancer, kidney cancer, and post-menopausal breast cancer in women, but this study went further. It illustrated that obesity or being overweight in post-menopausal women:
- accounts for 5% of all cancers (about 6000 annually)
- accounts for half of all cases of endometrial cancer and adenocarcinoma of the oesophagus
- may increase the risk of multiple myeloma, leukaemia, pancreatic cancer, non-Hodgkin's lymphoma, and ovarian cancer

These incidences were generally reflected in the mortality data.

CHILDHOOD OBESITY

Parents' awareness of overweight in themselves and their children: cross sectional study within a cohort (EarlyBird 21)
Jeffery AN, Voss LD, Metcalf BS *et al.*
BMJ, 2005; **330**: 23–24

This study of the parents of 277 children found that:
- only one-quarter recognised when their child was overweight
- even when the children were obese, one-third of mothers and over one-half of fathers saw their child's weight as about right
- nearly half the overweight parents judged their own weight to be about right
- the apparent lack of parental concern probably stems from a lack of awareness
- this gap must be addressed as parents are crucial partners in the fight against childhood obesity
- the adults' obesity and perception of their children's weight was independent of socioeconomic grouping

Early life risk factors for obesity in childhood: cohort study
Reilly JJ, Armstrong J, Dorosty AR, *et al.*
BMJ, 2005; **330**: 1357

This study of 9000 children in Avon, UK, was set up to identify risk factors in the early life environment for childhood obesity at age seven. It found associations with birth weight and weight gain in the first year, adiposity rebound by age 43 months, parental obesity, more than 4 hours a week watching the television at age 3 years and short (<10.5 hours) periods of sleep at age 3.

There was a relationship with maternal smoking *in utero* but no protective effect of breast-feeding.

METABOLIC SYNDROME

Metabolic syndrome
Khunti K, Davies M
BMJ, 2005; **331**: 1153–1154

Insulin resistance seems still to be the main underlying factor that leads to the metabolic syndrome, type 2 diabetes and cardiovascular disease. But different definitions now exist for metabolic syndrome with one body proposing a simpler definition – raised BP, low HDL-cholesterol, high serum triglycerides, high FPG and abdominal obesity – with no direct mention of insulin resistance.

In a recent joint statement, the American Diabetes Association and European Association for the Study of Diabetes questioned the diagnosis of metabolic syndrome and argued that too much emphasis has been given to this so-called 'syndrome' when there is so much uncertainty about its definition, pathogenesis, and known risk factors without regard for whether they can be clustered into a definition of 'metabolic syndrome' (*Diabetes Care,* 2005; **28**: 2289–2304).

This editorial finds the label a practical and useful one though. Definitions that omit the likes of a glucose tolerance test allow us to consider metabolic syndrome without too much increased workload.

MEDICATIONS

Long term pharmacotherapy for obesity and overweight: updated meta-analysis
Rucker D, Padwal R, Li SK, *et al.*
BMJ, 2007; **335:** 1194–1199

This meta-analysis of 30 randomised trials of three anti-obesity drugs found that:
- all 3 drugs modestly reduce weight (less than 5 kg) – rimonabant by nearly 5 kg, sibutramine by 4 kg and orlistat by 3 kg
- there were differing effects on cardiovascular risk factors
- side effect profiles included increased mood disorders for rimonabant, raised BP and pulse in those taking sibutramine, and increased GI disturbances in the orlistat group
- there were no data on the effects of anti-obesity drugs on morbidity or mortality end points, although studies are ongoing

Orlistat over the counter
Williams G
BMJ, 2007; **335**: 1163–1164

Orlistat inhibits gut lipases and reduces absorption of dietary fat. Systematic review shows that up to one-third of people taking a standard dose three times a day lose 10% of their weight. The main side effect is steatorrhea and faecal incontinence – dubbed "the oops factor".

LIFESTYLE

It has been available over the counter without prescription in the US since 2006 and its makers would like to do the same in Europe. After all, it is safe and people should be able to choose how to spend their own money.

However, this editorial argues that such a measure will not benefit health. Even in optimised trials, with whatever additional support and follow up were offered, the effect of 2–5 kg per year weight loss is modest, declines with time and reverses on stopping the drug.

In the real world people rarely persevere and will have unrealistic expectations, failing to make the necessary change to their lifestyle risks. It will perpetuate the myth that the answer is not in diet and exercise but in a magic bullet.

Advertising the "body of your dreams" in pill form will attract and disappoint a cosmetic rather than a medical market. Faecal incontinence does not fit in nicely with a short term fix. Neither will there be proper follow up surveillance so the manufacturers will continue to make lots of money without needing to prove real-world efficacy.

SURGERY

Effects of bariatric surgery on mortality in Swedish obese subjects
Sjöström L, Narbro K, Sjöström CD, *et al.*
N Engl J Med, 2007; **357:** 741–752

The prospective, controlled Swedish Obese Subjects study involved over 4000 severely obese subjects. The half that received the bariatric surgery had maximum weight losses after 1 to 2 years of 32% for gastric bypass, 25% for vertical-banded gastroplasty and 20% for banding.

Overall mortality decreased. The hazard ratio for death adjusted for sex, age, and risk factors was 0.71. After 10 years, those that had the surgery had 25% less body weight compared with just 2% weight loss for those on conventional treatment programmes.

Long-term mortality after gastric bypass surgery
Adams TD, Gress RE, Smith SC, *et al.*
N Engl J Med, 2007; **357:** 753–761

Some 8000 people who had gastric bypass surgery were matched with severely obese controls in this cohort study. Long-term mortality from any cause decreased by 40% in the surgical group. Death in the surgical group decreased by 56% for coronary artery disease, by 92% for diabetes and by 60% for cancer.

ATRIAL FIBRILLATION

The Challenge

Atrial fibrillation (AF) is the most common cardiac dysrhythmia and a source of considerable morbidity and mortality. The prevalence of atrial fibrillation rises with age from 1.5% in people in their 60s to more than 10% in those over 90. Patients with AF have twice the mortality of those without AF and have a risk of thromboembolic stroke of 5% per year – about five times the normal risk. About one-quarter of all strokes in elderly people are caused by AF and the strokes are often severe with high mortality or a low quality of life.

The AFFIRM Investigators (Atrial Fibrillation Follow-up Investigation of Rhythm Management) and other studies found similar effects on mortality and cardiovascular morbidity for both rate and rhythm control strategies. Rate control should therefore be first choice for many (expect perhaps the young), avoiding the failure rates of rhythm control procedures. The cost of struggling to keep someone in sinus rhythm with all its attendant hospital days, pacemaker procedures, cardioversions, short-stay and A&E visits, makes rate control a clear economic winner.

Long-term anticoagulation reduces stroke in high risk individuals but warfarin is massively underprescribed, with decisions being poorly based on evidence and fuelled by exaggerated fears. Common reasons for not anticoagulating include non-compliance, fear of bleeding risk, dementia, risk of falls, and patient refusal. Prior GI bleeding and old age are not contraindications in themselves.

Costs of related hospital admissions, outpatient consultations, GP consultations, and drug treatment (including the cost of anticoagulant monitoring) are huge, and with increased pick-up rates will expand greatly. Nearly a million people in the UK are on warfarin and this is predicted to rise fivefold in the next decade.

The number of deaths associated with the use of anticoagulant drugs needs to be addressed as a high priority. In 2006 alone there were 120 deaths and 480 incidents of serious harm related to warfarin which were reported to the National Patient Safety Agency.

What we know already:

- Over 100 000 Europeans monitor their own oral anticoagulation but studies sometimes show a lack of interest or confidence in doing this and high dropout rates.
- SMART – Self Management of Anticoagulation: a Randomised Trial of patients in the West Midlands assesses home testing of their INR with a point of care coagulometer. Some 76% chose not to undertake self management showing that it is not desirable to all. Of those that did, three-quarters completed training and preferred it to usual care. The main reason for dropping out was difficulty with getting enough blood from the pinprick but it appears to be a safe and reliable approach in a well-trained minority.
- After more than 50 years, a new oral anticoagulant – the first oral thrombin inhibitor, ximelagatran, has been developed; in a fixed dose, it may be as effective as adjusted dose warfarin without the need for close monitoring and the fears of drug interactions.
- More severe strokes and the risk of death are the rewards for INRs that dip below 2.0.

CLINICAL ISSUES

- The risk of intracranial haemorrhage increases by a factor of 2.5 at age 85 years but does not seem to be eased by lower target ranges.
- Warfarin has not been shown to benefit heart failure patients in sinus rhythm.
- In a small study of adults with stable INRs, a majority of those randomised to paracetamol 2–4 g daily moved above the therapeutic INR range within 3 weeks.

Recent Papers

SCREENING

Accuracy of diagnosing atrial fibrillation on electrocardiogram by primary care practitioners and interpretative diagnostic software: analysis of data from screening for atrial fibrillation in the elderly (SAFE) trial
Mant J, Fitzmaurice DA, Hobbs FDR, *et al.*
BMJ, 2007; **335**: 380

This study in 29 practices looked at 2595 patients over 65 years of age as part of the SAFE study – Screening for Atrial Fibrillation in the Elderly.

12-lead ECGs were read by software, nurses or GPs whose abilities varied widely. The machine was most accurate but all three methods shared a not terribly good sensitivity of around 80%, meaning that 20% of AF cases would be missed.

At least diagnosis of AF by GPs was more specific than nurses, but it was still more likely to be wrong than right (positive predictive value 41%). A one-lead ECG was found to be just as reliable as a 12 lead.

Sadly, the bottom line is that doctors in the community cannot be trusted to recognise AF on an ECG and training did not seem to help. Better trained people are required to do this.

Diagnosing atrial fibrillation in general practice
van Weert H
BMJ, 2007; **335**: 355–356

An accompanying editorial defends GPs by claiming that they would scrutinise the ECG better if they had the clinical information to know what they were looking for. So real-life sensitivity might improve.

Palpation of a pulse has a sensitivity of 94% for AF, but further tests are indicated due to a lower specificity of 72%. A new case of AF could be found for 70 pulses taken and five ECGs if they were read by somebody suitably competent. For paroxysmal cases, a patient-activated loop recorder would be necessary.

Screening versus routine practice in detection of atrial fibrillation in patients aged 65 or over: cluster randomised controlled trial.
Fitzmaurice DA, Hobbs FDR, Jowett S, *et al.*
BMJ, 2007; **335:** 383–386

This study also from the SAFE group looked at nearly 15 000 patients over 65 years of age in 50 primary care centres. They were randomly allocated direct to ECG to look for AF, or opportunistic screening (going on to perform ECG only if the pulse was irregular) over a period of 12 months.

Opportunistic screening proved to be just as effective as more systematic screening in patients aged 65 or over. It is safe, acceptable and becomes the preferred method for case detection as long as pulse taking is done conscientiously by health professionals.

SYMPTOM CONTROL

Rate control in permanent atrial fibrillation
Nikolaidou T, Channer KS
BMJ, 2007; **335:** 1057–1058

New NICE guidelines from June 2006 recommend beta blockers or calcium antagonists in preference to digoxin for AF except for mainly sedentary patients. This editorial takes issue with the down-regulation of digoxin, noting that the aim is to improve symptoms and exercise tolerance.

- The AFFIRM investigators reported no significant difference in heart rate in rest or exercise between beta blockers or digoxin alone although some other studies did.
- The positive inotropic effect of digoxin leads to worsening symptoms when it is withdrawn from patients with heart failure.
- There is clear evidence that beta blockers can worsen exercise capacity particularly if uncovering heart failure.
- Verapamil and diltiazem are negatively inotropic drugs with dose-related side effects.

The authors recommend the combination of digoxin and a beta blocker, starting with digoxin first.

Some patients with paroxysmal atrial fibrillation should carry flecainide or propafenone to self treat
Camm AJ, Savelieva I
BMJ, 2007; **334:** 637

Often episodes of AF resolve spontaneously within 48 hours but there may be distressing symptoms such as palpitations or chest pains. This *BMJ* 'Change Page' suggests that patients with infrequent symptomatic episodes of paroxysmal AF might carry flecainide or propafenone with them for such times, using the 'pill in the pocket' approach. For patients without underlying heart disease this is likely to lead to a safe, simple chemical cardioversion and avoid admission to hospital.

CLINICAL ISSUES

CARDIOVASCULAR

At the moment, however, the drugs are not licensed for self-treating single attacks and a cardiologist should make the decision.

WARFARIN

Self monitoring increases the efficacy and safety of anticoagulant therapy. *Evidence-Based Medicine,* 2006; **11**: 103
The following paper is reviewed
Self-monitoring of oral anticoagulation: a systematic review and meta-analysis
Heneghan C, Alonso-Coello P, Garcia-Alamino JM, *et al.*
Lancet, 2006; **367**: 404–411

This meta-analysis of 14 randomised trials involving 3000 adults shows how successful the approach can be.

If patients are able to monitor their own INR, they spend more time in the therapeutic range and benefit from fewer thromboembolic events, fewer major bleeding episodes and a longer life. If they are capable enough to adjust their dose, they are likely to be better at it than their physician and benefit even more.

Not everyone can however. Some would not or could not. You need good manual dexterity, adequate vision and strong motivation as well as extensive education, a suitable device and lots of expensive test strips.

Impact of adverse events on prescribing warfarin in patients with atrial fibrillation: matched pair analysis
Choudhry NK, Anderson GM, Laupacis A, *et al.*
BMJ, 2006; **332**: 141–145

A doctor who has prescribed warfarin to a patient who goes on to have a major haemorrhage is less likely to prescribe appropriate anticoagulants for atrial fibrillation in the future. Patients treated in the 90 days following such an experience had reduced odds of receiving warfarin compared with prescribing before the event occurred. The odds reduced further in the following 90 days. The result was equivalent to a 12% absolute reduction in the likelihood that they would receive warfarin.

However, if patients suffered a thromboembolic stroke when they were not on warfarin, this did not instigate a change in the doctor's prescribing patterns for future patients.

Dramatic events are easily remembered and regretted. When those are acts of commission rather than acts of omission, physicians receive a harsh reminder of their 'do no harm' ethic. Future strategies should address physicians' perceptions of risk.

Warfarin reduced major stroke more than aspirin in elderly patients with atrial fibrillation in primary care. *Evidence-Based Medicine,* 2007; **12:** 172.

The following paper is reviewed

Warfarin versus aspirin for stroke prevention in an elderly community population with atrial fibrillation (the Birmingham Atrial Fibrillation Treatment of the Aged Study, BAFTA): a randomised controlled trial

Mant J, Hobbs FDR, Fletcher K, *et al.*

Lancet, 2007; **370:** 493–503

> This study of nearly 1000 elderly patients over 75 years (mean age 81 years) found that over a mean of 2.7 years, warfarin was more effective than aspirin at preventing major stroke in those with no contraindications. Target INR was 2.5. A low rate of bleeding was reassuring and the evidence confirms that in the elderly we are underutilising warfarin. All cause mortality was unaffected.

CARDIOVASCULAR

ASPIRIN

The Challenge

The complexity of the aspirin debate continues with many patients choosing to take daily preventative aspirin despite lack of clarity in the evidence. In low risk patients there is no proven mortality benefit. Any reduction in the risk of coronary disease events tends to be offset by the increased risk of major gastrointestinal bleeding. British Hypertension Society guidelines recommend low dose aspirin in high risk controlled hypertensives over 50 years old with a 10 year risk of cardiovascular disease of 20%.

Increased cardiovascular and all cause mortality in those on aspirin and ibuprofen has been demonstrated. Aspirin and NSAIDs bind to the same place on the COX-1 enzyme, but NSAIDs take priority. Ibuprofen may therefore reduce or negate the antiplatelet cardioprotective effects of aspirin in people who take it before the aspirin or who take it regularly. This is a problem as they are two of the world's most commonly used drugs. There is currently insufficient evidence for or against concomitant use of ibuprofen in patients needing prophylactic aspirin. But of the two, only aspirin should be used to specifically prevent MI. Further studies are awaited for a definitive answer, but there are difficulties in doing this well. They include the fact that prescription records do not record drugs bought over the counter, use of ibuprofen may be sporadic, compliance with taking aspirin is suboptimal, and ibuprofen may turn out to have good antiplatelet properties in itself.

What we know already:

- Low doses of aspirin seem to be as effective as high doses for primary and secondary prevention of vascular events.
- The Warfarin/Aspirin Study in Heart Failure (WASH) showed no evidence that aspirin is effective or safe in patients with heart failure alone. This group had higher risk of adverse events due mainly to increased hospitalisation. Antithrombotics contribute to polypharmacy in these patients.
- Regular use of aspirin reduces the risk of a colorectal neoplasm, but the mechanism by which aspirin affects carcinogenesis in the colon is not well understood.
- Research from the Women's Health Study looked at the use of low dose aspirin (100 mg on alternate days) in 6377 women over 65 years of age to see if it protected against cognitive decline. It didn't.

Recent Papers

PRIMARY PREVENTION

Aspirin dose for the prevention of cardiovascular disease – a systematic review
Campbell CL, Smyth S, Montalescot G, Steinhubl SR
JAMA, 2007; **297**: 2018–2024

> With a wide range of aspirin dosage – up to 1300 mg per day – this systematic review of eight randomised trials and three observational studies in around 10 000 people found that:
> - low doses (75–81 mg) of aspirin are better than high doses in the setting of cardiovascular disease prevention
> - buffered or enteric coated aspirin showed no advantages
> - widespread usage of a 325 mg daily dose would increase major bleeds by 900 000 annually over that caused by a low dose

---

Aspirin for the primary prevention of cardiovascular events in women and men: a sex-specific meta-analysis of randomized controlled trials
Berger JS, Roncaglioni MC, Avanzini F, *et al.*
JAMA, 2006; **295**: 306–313

> To determine if the benefits and risks of aspirin treatment in the primary prevention of cardiovascular disease vary by sex, this meta-analysis of randomized controlled trials included almost 95 000 people.
> In the women, aspirin:
> - reduced cardiovascular events by 12%
> - reduced ischaemic stroke by 24%
> - had no significant effect on MI
>
> In the men, aspirin:
> - reduced cardiovascular events by 14% and MI by 32%
> - had no significant effect on ischaemic stroke
>
> In both men and women in this low risk group (who did not have pre-existing cardiovascular disease):
> - there was no apparent effect on cardiovascular mortality or all-cause mortality
> - aspirin treatment increased the risk of major bleeding equally (by around 70%)
>
> So, if aspirin reduces myocardial infarction in men and not women, and reduces ischaemic stroke in women and not men, we need to refer to sex-specific sets of data to help us discuss the risk and merits of taking aspirin as primary prevention.

Aspirin for everyone older than 50? "FOR"
Elwood P, Morgan G , Brown G, *et al.*
BMJ, 2005; **330**: 1440–1441

> Whether or not to take aspirin for primary prevention of cardiovascular disease is still a thorny question. A pair of "FOR" and "AGAINST" articles appears in this *BMJ*.

CLINICAL ISSUES

CARDIOVASCULAR

The FOR article supports its use but covers the information void by suggesting the public should be given the evidence we have and should make their own decision on whether or not to take it. They consider that the crucial question is "at what age does benefit outweigh risk?" But is it clear that even this question is valid?

They also consider side effects of aspirin to be 'unusual and seldom serious' and that for '[asymptomatic] people to consult a doctor before starting aspirin prophylaxis is unreasonable and places the doctor in an impossible position'. Everybody should evaluate the risks and benefits for themselves.

This reads as an extraordinary argument. They use the fact that many high-risk people are still undetected and therefore not on aspirin as a reason to consider a single low dose pill for larger populations.

Aspirin for everyone older than 50? "AGAINST"
Baigent C
BMJ, 2005; **330**: 1442–1443

High-risk patients with occlusive arterial disease can expect a benefit of about a quarter of their baseline risk for a vascular event. But in those without disease it is not so clear.

This "AGAINST" argument is much more scientifically rooted.

The balance of benefits for aspirin in people over 70 has not been clearly defined. Neither do the benefits clearly exceed risk of a major GI bleed in people younger than 60 without vascular disease. Age thresholds therefore seem illogical at present.

Meta-analysis of five of the six primary prevention trials performed show that aspirin reduces myocardial infarction by about one-third but, crucially, has little or no effect on stroke or death from vascular causes.

In 2005, data from the Women's Heath Study suggested low-dose aspirin protects against stroke in healthy women but has no effect on myocardial infarction.

SECONDARY PREVENTION

Aspirin plus dipyridamole versus aspirin alone after cerebral ischaemia of arterial origin
The ESPRIT Study Group
Lancet, 2006; **367**: 1665–1673

Patients who have a stroke do better on aspirin and dipyridamole than on aspirin alone according to ESPRIT – the European/Australasian Stroke Prevention in Reversible Ischemia Trial.

In this vulnerable group, combined treatment reduced the combined mortality from vascular death, further stroke, heart attack and serious bleeding by 3 percentage points from 16% to 13%, with an NNT of 104 per year. Age, gender, race, and type of vessel involved did not seem to matter, but in the first week following the primary event, aspirin alone seemed preferable.

Adding the result to an existing meta-analysis gave a risk ratio for the combination of 0.82.

Results are about as clear as we can hope for and show that combination treatment (75 mg of aspirin and 200 mg b.d. of dipyridamole) is an effective option for ischaemic stroke or TIA. It caused no more serious bleeding than aspirin alone.

Dipyridamole with aspirin is better than aspirin alone in preventing vascular events after ischaemic stroke or TIA
Sudlow C
BMJ, 2007; **334**: 901

This *BMJ* 'Change Page' re-examines the previous data in the light of the ESPRIT study above and concludes that dipyridamole should be added to low dose aspirin after ischaemic stroke or TIA. Further risk of vascular events could be reduced by one-fifth compared with aspirin alone, assuming a baseline risk of vascular events of 5% per year. Trials have not found bleeding to be a problem and although dipyridamole causes headache in up to one-third of people, it usually settles in a week or two.

It is 20 times more expensive than aspirin, however. At a NNT of 104 and pointing to several weaknesses in the new trial, some perceive the small benefit as non-existent or not worthwhile *(BMJ,* 2007; **334:** 1020).

COLORECTAL CANCER

Routine aspirin or nonsteroidal anti-inflammatory drugs for the primary prevention of Colorectal cancer
U.S. Preventive Services Task Force Recommendation Statement
Ann Intern Med, 2007; **146:** 361–364

Temptations to prescribe aspirin or other NSAIDs as primary prevention for colorectal cancer have been quashed after two systematic reviews failed to show a net benefit. Although aspirin at higher doses appears to be effective at reducing the incidence of colonic adenoma and colorectal cancer, it also causes a dose-related increase in gastrointestinal complications and possibly haemorrhagic stroke.

It is unclear whether such an approach will saves lives, whereas the downside of these drugs is well known including renal impairment and cardiovascular disease. Chemoprevention with aspirin should not be used for anyone at average risk, even if they have a family history of cancer (unless associated with familial polyposis coli).

Aspirin and the risk of colorectal cancer in relation to the expression of COX-2
Chan AT, Ogino S, Fuchs CS
N Engl J Med, 2007; **356:** 2131–2142

This observational study implies that the benefits of aspirin are probably confined to cancers that express the cyclo-oxygenase-2 (COX-2) enzyme.

There was a 36% reduction in such a group, but aspirin had no impact where there was no such expression. Significant benefit was not illustrated until after 5 years of use. This long duration implies that the influence may be on the early stages of adenoma or cancer.

As we know, the side effects are too much of a price to pay, but in the long run a cleaner agent could help target the problem.

HYPERTENSION

The Challenge

Hypertension is the most common treatable risk factor for cardiovascular disease in patients over 50 years of age. It affects about one billion people worldwide and in the UK fills 8% of total bed capacity of the NHS. It accounts for 30% of all UK deaths. Cost to the NHS of antihypertensives in 2001 was around £840 million – 15% of total annual cost of all primary care drugs.

The value of detection and treatment are not in doubt but surveys still show massive underdiagnosis, undertreatment (with extensive use of monotherapy), and poor rates of BP control. In the UK, it is controlled in only 10% of the hypertensive population and only one-third of those on medication.

How do we define it? The relationship with vascular mortality persists to pressure as low as 115/75 mmHg and exists for any incremental increase in systolic or diastolic pressure throughout ages from 40 to 89 years in adults with no history of vascular disease.

Even the term prehypertension (120/80 to 139/89 mmHg) has now entered our vocabulary and is recognised as an independent risk factor for major cardiovascular events and an early warning light according to analysis of the Framingham data.

Targets get ever stricter and have a less compelling evidence base. They can be felt to be somewhat arbitrary and feel unachievable to doctors and patients.

How do we detect it? Research has suggested that pulse pressure and systolic BP are better predictors of eventual development of congestive heart failure than diastolic blood pressure, independent of age. Measures of night-time BP and morning surges have also been proposed as possible preferable parameters to record.

Measurement is problematic. Blood pressure measured at home and ambulatory readings provide additional and different data to episodic clinic visits. 'White coat' hypertension is real and important and not a research artefact and should be factored in. 'Masked' hypertension is the reverse of 'white coat' hypertension. Here, BP is lower in clinical measurements than during ambulatory monitoring.

And how do we treat it? Treatment can be sabotaged by factors such as lack of adherence to drugs, errors of measurement, antagonising drugs, and secondary hypertension.

Effective implementation of lifestyle measures (weight and salt reduction, dietary change and exercise) requires time, effort, patience and reinforcement. Programmes can work but are best supported by well-trained health professionals such as practice nurses, and should be supported by clear written information. Needless to say, such interventions are intensive and expensive.

A glut of research has pitted one antihypertensive against another, but in recent times the mists have begun to clear and guidelines are helping us to choose the right approach for our patients. Recently the discreditation of atenolol with regard to preventing MI in primary hypertensives has been a major development.

Still, one conclusion seems to scream louder than the others. Getting blood pressure down is overwhelmingly more important than the drug cocktail used.

CARDIOVASCULAR

What we know already:

- Lowering blood pressure by 10/5 mmHg reduces stroke by about a third and that of ischaemic heart disease events by about 25% at age 65 across all BP levels in Western populations.
- False positives and false negatives are realities for all screening tests but low positive predictive values for BP measurement means that routine measurement of BP in those under 35 without other risk factors is more likely to misdiagnose than to diagnose hypertension correctly.
- Home blood pressure monitoring can improve hypertensive control by increasing compliance devoid of the white coat effect. It may improve control and could reduce health costs by reducing visits and involving patients more closely in the management of their blood pressure. However, inaccuracy of electronic devices is a problem and self-monitoring may increase anxiety or lead to patients adjusting their own doses illogically; training is needed.
- Conventional BP measurement fails to identify some individuals at high or low risk, but these cases may be 'unmasked' by the use of ambulatory BP.
- Low-dose thiazides can be as effective, or more effective, than any other antihypertensive agent. Studies have shown diuretics to be unsurpassed in decreasing cardiovascular outcomes, meaning they maintain a very strong claim as first-line therapy.
- Atenolol is cheap and has different pharmacokinetic properties to other beta blockers. Good data have shown it to be inferior to non-atenolol beta blockers but evidence is not yet concrete enough to lead to a mandate to use a substitute in all patients.
- Beta blockers have tended to be no better than placebo in the elderly and should be avoided unless another condition indicates their use. Those under 60 years have different pathophysiology and some beta blockers may be as good as other antihypertensives in this group.
- Systematic review involving around 20 000 black patients in 30 trials has shown that beta blockers and ACE inhibitors are no more effective than placebo in reducing blood pressure.

Key Trials

*HOT – The Hypertension Optimal Treatment Trial (**Lancet**, 1998; **351:** 1755–1762)*
This large trial of nearly 19 000 people provides our best evidence for blood pressure targets. Although it was underpowered, it reports an optimal blood pressure for reduction of major cardiovascular events as 139/83 mmHg. However a target of 150/90 was not disadvantageous and the British Hypertension Society still uses this as an 'audit standard' target blood pressure.

*ALLHAT – The Antihypertensive and Lipid-Lowering Treatment to Prevent Heart Attack Trial (**JAMA**, 2002; **288:** 2981–2997)*
When it comes to deciding health policy, there is no substitute for a high quality randomised trial and ALLHAT was excellent. It was the largest anti-hypertensive trial to date and included 33 357 people including large numbers of women, black people, Hispanics and diabetics. Its conclusions are valid irrespective of sex, ethnicity or diabetes. It compared the calcium channel blocker amlodipine, the ACE inhibitor lisinopril, the thiazide diuretic chlorthalidone and the alpha blocker doxazosin. The alpha blocker arm was stopped early due to excessive mortality particularly due to heart failure.

ALLHAT looked at fatal coronary heart disease and non-fatal MI in patients over 55 with hypertension and at least one other risk factor.

It is well recognised that ACE inhibitors are less effective in lowering blood pressure in the elderly or black people as the renin-angiotensin system is more suppressed.

The thiazide was the best performer, reducing blood pressure more effectively and preventing cardiovascular end-points better than amlodipine or lisinopril with no evidence of impaired glycaemic control even in diabetics. It beat the ACE inhibitor group in terms of prevention of stroke and cardiovascular disease. Thiazides stake their claim to be the first line medication but there is an increasing lobby to start patients on combination therapy.

Further analysis of the ALLHAT data shows that diuretics may be more effective at reducing the incidence of heart failure than ACE inhibitors or calcium blockers, particularly during the first year of treatment. CCBs are known to cause fluid retention so that's not too surprising. The association with lisinopril was weaker and not statistically significant and may be due to delayed effects, confounding therapies, less effective BP reduction or chance (*Evidence-Based Medicine*, 2007; **12**: 17).

ALLHAT included patients as young as 55 and fewer than 50% were white, compared with 95% of patients in ANBP2 – the Second Australian National Blood Pressure Study – which looked at over 6000 elderly Australians between 65 and 84 years of age. It seemed to contradict the ALLHAT finding that ACE inhibitors were more effective than diuretics for reducing a composite outcome of all cardiovascular events and all-cause mortality. We know that ACE inhibitors are less effective in the black population so this could explain the difference. Some doubt the clinical significance of these statistically significant results in comparison to our poor record on treatment in general.

LIFE – Losartan Intervention for Endpoint Reduction (*Lancet*, 2002; **359**: 995–1003)

This study looked at patients with hypertension and LVH and showed superiority of losartan in cardiovascular morbidity and particularly stroke prevention compared to atenolol despite similar drops in blood pressure. Recent work has indicated this is due to a lack of performance from atenolol due to its specific properties (*Lancet*, 2004; **364**: 1684–1689). It is now accepted that we should no longer have to use beta blockers for hypertension as liberally as we should after MI.

SCOPE – The Study on Cognition and Prognosis in the Elderly (*J Am Coll Cardiol*, 2004; **44**: 1175)

This study supported LIFE's results. As part of antihypertensive therapy, it used candesartan or placebo in 1500 patients over 70 years old who had isolated systolic hypertension. There was 42% relative risk reduction in stroke with a candesartan-based regime compared with a mostly thiazide approach. Blood pressure reduction was the same but the ARB appeared to show specific vascular protective effects of AT1-receptor blockade in this age group.

STOP-2 – Swedish Trial in Old Patients with Hypertension-2 (*Lancet*, 1999; **354**: 1751–1756)

This trial randomised elderly hypertensives aged over 70 years to older drugs (thiazide or beta blocker) or to the newer drugs (ACE inhibitor or calcium channel blocker). It found no differences between older antihypertensives and newer more expensive drugs in terms of blood pressure control, heart failure or other major events.

CARDIOVASCULAR

ASCOT – *Anglo-Scandinavian Cardiac Outcomes Trial: Blood Pressure-Lowering Arm* (*Lancet*, 2005; **366**: 895–906)

Preliminary results from the large ASCOT open label trial were presented in 2005. Some 19 000 higher risk patients with hypertension were randomised either to atenolol 50–100 mg, with bendroflumethazide 1.25–2.5 mg if needed, or to amlodipine 5–10 mg, with perindopril 4–8 mg per day if needed. The groups did not differ for the primary outcome which was non-fatal MI and fatal coronary heart disease. But ASCOT was still stopped early because the amlodipine-based arm had significantly lower rates of all cause mortality and all coronary events. Amlodipine plus perindopril also seemed to prevent onset of diabetes and may be a promising combination.

It was better than atenolol plus bendroflumethiazide for reducing strokes, cardiovascular mortality and all cause mortality (*Lancet*, 2005; **366**: 895–906).

However, commentators claim that the atenolol may be only marginally inferior to amlodipine and the main lesson of ASCOT–BPLA is to aim for tight blood pressure control and close monitoring of other risk factors. For example, a further 1% relative risk reduction in coronary events and stroke (from 9% to 8%) is significant but "not inspiring" with a NNT of 220 to prevent one cardiovascular event over a year and to prevent one death the NNT is 650. Non-atenolol beta blockers may be just as good as other antihypertensives in preventing stroke, MI and total mortality (*BMJ*, 2007; **334**: 946–949).

Thiazides are still well-supported as first line therapy but this research supports existing data that beta blockers should not be used first line for hypertension without other compelling indications (*Evidence-Based Medicine*, 2006; **11**: 42).

Further analysis discovered that addition of atorvastatin to amlodipine can reduce fatal and non-fatal cardiac events by more than 50% and stroke by over 25%. The effect is potent, appears within only 3 months and does not appear when atorvastatin is added to atenolol. A theory is that these two drugs work synergistically to help stabilise atherosclerotic plaques (*Eur Heart J*, 2006; **27**: 2982–2988).

Guidelines

In 2006 the guidelines from the British Hypertension Society and NICE were updated with regards to advice on medications.

British Hypertension Society guidelines for hypertension management 2004 (BHS-IV): summary (*BMJ*, 2004; **328**: 634–640)

These guidelines from the British Hypertension Society (www.bhsoc.org):
- recommend routine screening at least every 5 years for all adults and annually if high–normal blood pressure
- emphasise formal assessment of total risk of cardiovascular disease
- advise use of multifactorial interventions, including statins and aspirin, to reduce risk
- recommend a treatment algorithm based on the AB/CD rule

Risk assessment

A new chart has been produced to calculate risk of cardiovascular disease. The aim is now to assess 10 year risk of all cardiovascular disease events rather than risk of CHD alone.

It has been simplified since 1999 by including only three age strata and now there is no separate chart for type-2 diabetics because their risk of cardiovascular disease is taken to be equivalent to people who have had an MI. Therefore they follow the secondary prevention approach.

Drug treatment

Targets are 140/85 mmHg for most patients but for diabetics and those with established cardiovascular disease a lower target of 130/80 mmHg is recommended.

Medication is recommended in patients with:

- sustained grade 2 hypertension (>160/100 mmHg)
- grade I hypertension (systolic blood pressure 140–159 or diastolic blood pressure 90–99 mmHg, or both), if there is any complication of hypertension, target organ damage or diabetes, or if there is an estimated 10 year risk of cardiovascular disease of 20%

The AB/CD algorithm

Clinical trials have shown that treatment algorithms deliver better blood pressure control than current clinical practice. We also know most people need more than one drug for blood pressure control. This algorithm classifies hypertensives into 'high renin' or 'low renin'.

A – ACE inhibitors or ARBs

B – beta blockers

C – calcium channel blockers

D – diuretics

A and B inhibit the renin–angiotensin system whereas C and D do not affect that system making them more effective first line agents for older white people or black people. New guidance downgrading beta blockers came in during 2006 in agreement with NICE (*see below*).

Particular caution is advised when using beta blockers and diuretics in patients at especially high risk of developing diabetes, e.g. strong family history of diabetes, obesity, impaired glucose tolerance, features of the metabolic syndrome, or of South Asian and African–Caribbean descent.

A paper by the BHS President in the *BMJ* (2006; **332**: 833–836) discusses ethnic variations and tells how hypertension could be usefully divided, like diabetes, into Type 1 and Type 2. Hypertension in black people is more prevalent than in whites and the different pathogenesis denotes the need for different approaches.

Hypertension: management in hypertension in adults in primary care

NICE – Updated June 2006 (www.nice.org.uk)

This set of guidelines from NICE also emphasises the need for formal risk assessment to include all cardiovascular treatments. They recommend monitoring of blood pressure over 140/90 mmHg, formal assessment of risk to identify those with a 10 year cardiovascular risk of >20%, and lifestyle advice. However, they follow the ALLHAT trial in that drug therapy can often begin with a low-dose thiazide.

In response to current research, NICE has removed beta blockers from their birthright of first line treatment for hypertension. Good evidence has indicated they are less effective than alternatives in the elderly at preventing stroke and in reducing the risk of diabetes (especially if also taking a thiazide).

For those aged 55 or for black patients a calcium channel blocker or thiazide should be used. For those under 55, ACE inhibitors are first line.

Recent Papers

USE OF GUIDELINES

Reassessing normal blood pressure
Nash IS
BMJ, 2007; **335:** 408–409

This paper reminds us of the need to treat blood pressure in a context of overall cardiovascular risk rather than getting obsessed with thresholds which are abstract from the full clinical picture – a picture which may fail to recognise the important areas of age and smoking, for example. Treatment of blood pressure is much more valuable in those with a higher baseline risk. Applying a new threshold and enforcing it with guidelines and audit may draw us away from the bigger picture.

We know this but we do not factor it in as much as we should to lower total atherothrombotic risk with a combination of interventions.

Applicability to primary care of national clinical guidelines on blood pressure lowering for people with stroke: cross sectional study
Mant J, McManus RJ, Hare R
BMJ, 2006; **332:** 635–637

British Hypertension Society guidelines for lowering BP after stroke or TIA to 140/85 are based on the PROGRESS trial. But the research was on hospital patients.

This Birmingham study found the following in a primary care population with confirmed stroke and TIA:

- they averaged 12 years older than those in the trials – important because over the age of 80, reduction in risk of stroke through lowering BP may be offset by an increase in mortality
- they were twice as likely to be women
- the median time elapsed since stroke was 2.5 years rather than 8 months – important as risk of further cerebrovascular event declines with time

These factors undermine the applicability of the research to primary care in a very important area.

MEDICATION

Should beta blockers remain first choice in the treatment of primary hypertension? A meta-analysis
Lindholm LH, Carlberg B, Samuelsson O
Lancet, 2005; **366:** 1545–1553

Beta blockers are not as effective as other antihypertensive drugs in the absence of overt heart disease, according to this Swedish meta-analysis (also reviewed in *Evidence-Based Medicine,* 2006; **11:** 85).

They have been a popular first choice for treating hypertension over the years

CARDIOVASCULAR

but this has recently come under renewed scrutiny and they may not have the same excellent benefits that they have in secondary prevention.

They identified seven RCTs involving 27 000 subjects with primary hypertension that compared beta blockers with placebo or no treatment, and 13 trials with 106 000 participants that compared beta blockers with other antihypertensives.

The risk of stroke was reduced by 19% when compared with placebo, less than half that previously assumed. When compared with other antihypertensive medications, beta blockers were associated with a 16% higher risk of stroke. It is suggested that reduction in brachial BP may not reflect reductions in central systolic BP as well as other antihypertensives.

The authors conclude that beta blockers should not be used as first line drugs when there are thiazides, calcium channel blockers, and ACE inhibitors, which seem to have advantages. Nor should they be used as a reference in trials. Beta blockers should be reserved for where there are comorbidites such as post-MI, heart failure, arrhythmia, and stress. Sudden discontinuation should be avoided – reduce the dose while substituting the alternative.

Available evidence does not support the use of ß blockers as first line treatment for hypertension. *Evidence-Based Medicine,* 2007; **12**: 112
The following article is presented
Beta-blockers for hypertension
Wiysonge C, Bradley H, Mayosi B, *et al.*
Cochrane Database Syst Rev 2007

This review included 13 RCTs and over 90 000 patients and concluded that we should not be using beta blockers first-line for hypertension.

As a group, beta blockers do not reduce mortality or coronary heart disease more than placebo or other drugs and they can increase adverse effects. They can reduce overall cardiovascular disease and stroke more than placebo but when compared directly to CCBs they seemed to increase the risk of mortality and stroke.

Atenolol was the principal agent used in the research assessed and we cannot extend these conclusions automatically to other beta blockers with better reputations.

It was noted that there were still reductions in BP readings which may have a useful effect. We do know that those with clinically evident coronary disease or heart failure benefit from beta blockers and they were excluded from these trials.

Thiazide diuretic prescription and electrolyte abnormalities in primary care
Clayton JA, Rodgers S, Blakey J *et al.*
Br J Clin Pharmacol, 2006; **61**: 87–95

In this large study in UK general practice, only one-third of those on thiazides had a record of their electrolytes being tested and 20% of those tested were hypokalaemic and/or hyponatraemic.

The incidence of morbidity from hyponatraemia relates to the absolute level and speed of change. Thiazide-induced hyponatraemia typically occurs within 2–12 days of drug initiation. Chronic hyponatraemia is generally asymptomatic until the sodium concentration falls below 125 mmol/l. Approximately 1% of the patients in this study dropped their sodium concentration below that level and it is likely that they will have been symptomatic and perhaps required hospitalisation.

Just over 1% of the patients tested had severe hypokalaemia (potassium <3.0 mmol/l). In the majority the thiazide was discontinued and in those who continued the thiazide, the potassium concentration was normal when repeated. The evidence linking thiazide-induced hypokalaemia and cardiac complications is conflicting.

Still, this is a reminder to increase testing and monitoring and use low doses wherever possible.

Gout, not induced by diuretics? A case-control study from primary care
Janssens HJEM, van de Lisdonk EH, Janssen M *et al.*
Ann Rheum Dis, 2006; **65**: 1080–1083

Fears of provoking gout have led some to be shy of using diuretics but this case-control study reassures us. Patients with their first case of gout were matched by age and gender with controls. The relative risk of gout in those who had ever had a diuretic was 1.56 but this was accounted for by higher associations of gout with those suffering from hypertension and heart failure. (There was no association with MI.)

The authors tell us there is no need to avoid diuretics or substitute them in those with or at risk of gout. We should be focussing on hypertension and cardiovascular morbidity when we see a patient with gout.

Comparative effectiveness of angiotensin-converting enzyme inhibitors and angiotensin II receptor blockers for treating essential hypertension
Matchar DB, McCrory DC, Olando LA *et al.*
Ann Intern Med, 2008; **148**: 16–29

This systematic review of evidence from over 50 studies showed strong evidence that ACE inhibitors and ARBs are equally effective in controlling essential hypertension in the long term. No differences were noted in terms of mortality, cardiovascular end points, quality of life or indeed any other parameter looked at, including lipid levels and progression to diabetes.

The review does confirm that ACE inhibitors were less well tolerated as they are more likely to cause cough (9.9% vs. 3.2% in a pooled analysis of 26 randomised trials).

However, further large, long trials are needed as most studies lasted less than 6 months and they were unable to identify any subgroups which would respond better to one drug than another.

COMBINATION THERAPY

Value of low dose combination treatment with blood pressure lowering drugs: analysis of 354 randomised trials

Law MR, Wald NJ, Morris JK *et al.*
BMJ, 2003; **326**: 1427

This fascinating meta-analysis takes the argument in an entirely new direction. The authors examined 354 randomised trials in 40 000 treated patients on thiazides, beta blockers, ACE inhibitors, ARBs, and calcium channel blockers. They found:

- all five categories of drug produced similar reductions in blood pressure and the effects were additive
- the average reduction was 9.1 mmHg systolic and 5.5 mmHg diastolic at standard dose and only 20% lower at half standard dose
- the drugs reduced blood pressure more so from higher levels

Regarding side-effects:

- symptoms attributable to thiazides, beta blockers, and calcium channel blockers were strongly dose related, but were not dose-related for ACE inhibitors (mainly cough)
- angiotensin II receptor antagonists caused no apparent side-effects
- using two drugs in combination, side-effects were less than additive
- adverse metabolic effects (such as changes in cholesterol or potassium) were negligible at half standard dose

The authors conclude that combination low-dose drug treatment increases efficacy and reduces adverse effects. Three drugs at half standard dose are estimated to lower blood pressure by 20/11 mmHg on average and thereby reduce the risk of stroke by 63% and IHD events by 46% at age 60–69. Low-dose combination therapy should be considered first line. Three such drugs are preferable to one or two drugs at standard dose. Drug selections should still be tailored for the patient.

Angiotensin-converting enzyme inhibitors and calcium channel blockers for coronary heart disease and stroke prevention

Verdecchia P, Reboldi G, Angeli F, *et al.*
Hypertension, 2005; **46**: 386–392

This review of 28 trials compared ACE inhibitors and calcium channel blockers (CCBs) in terms of serious cardiovascular end-points and stroke. This included a total of 179 000 patients suffering 9500 cardiac cases and 6000 cases of stroke.

Protective effects are mainly due to improvements in BP and any of the four classes of drug can deliver this well. However, two classes appear to have additional benefits beyond these effects:

- ACE inhibitors appeared superior to CCBs for prevention of MI and cardiac death
- CCBs appeared superior to ACE inhibitors for prevention of stroke

The authors propose the combination of ACE inhibitor and calcium blocker as a promising rationale for a broad spectrum of cardiovascular prevention.

CARDIOVASCULAR

SELF-MONITORING

Self-measurement of blood pressure at home reduces the need for antihypertensive drugs: a randomized, controlled trial
Verberk WJ, Kroon AA, Lenders JW, *et al.*
Hypertension, 2007; **50:** 1019–1025

This study randomized 430 hypertensive patients to doctor's office measurement, ambulatory monitoring (start and end of trial), and self-measurement with follow up at one year.

It found that monitoring blood pressure at home led to reduced use of medication and saved money with no adverse effects on outcomes such as left ventricular mass index and proteinuria. Systolic and diastolic blood pressure levels were similar although there was a slight increase in ambulatory readings in the self-measurement group.

However, this is more research to confirm that self-monitoring is a highly practicable and useful tool.

Targets and self monitoring in hypertension: randomised controlled trial and cost effectiveness analysis
McManus RJ, Mant J, Roalfe A, *et al.*
BMJ, 2005; **331**: 493

A Birmingham study compared usual care to visits by patients to the practice to use the facilities to monitor their own BP, the location of the measurements providing a nice safety net in case of persistently high readings. They showed that self-monitoring is feasible in a community setting, is popular with patients and has negligible costs. It can bring the benefits of home monitoring to individuals without the means to purchase their own equipment. After a year there were no differences between the groups except that patients who self monitored lost more weight. The authors recommend GPs should offer this option to their hypertensive patients.

An accompanying editorial agrees that the professional measurement data we use can be applied to self monitoring. This study showed cost-effectiveness while reaching targets more effectively than usual care through absence of the white coat effect and possibly better adherence. Whether it can be sustained over time is yet to be shown. Self selection by enthusiastic participants may mean it is not suitable for all (*BMJ,* 2005; **331**: 466–467).

LIPIDS

The Challenge

NICE recommends statin therapy for individuals with established cardiovascular disease or for primary prevention in people estimated to have a 10-year CVD risk of 20% or higher. It has been estimated that about 14% of adults in England (over 5 million people) meet these eligibility criteria. Statins represent the largest prescribing cost to the NHS at around £600 million a year – 8% of the total drug budget.

Why? Well, their use is known to reduce further coronary events and improve survival in patients with coronary heart disease. Meta-analysis makes it clear that lowering LDL cholesterol is predicted to decrease all stroke in the general population by 10% for a 1 mmol/l reduction (due to benefits in thromboembolic rather than haemorrhagic stroke).

They work best where absolute reductions in cholesterol are greatest so those with high pre-treatment levels receive most benefit. There is a strong argument for starting high-risk people on high doses rather than a start slow and go slow approach.

And their safety profile is very good. Meta-analysis tells us that 1% fewer treated patients than placebo patients reported problems. The only serious effects are rare – rhabdomyolysis and liver failure from hepatitis.

So what is the problem? Less than half of those taking statins achieve recommended target levels of cholesterol. About half the patients that might benefit actually receive statins, a third take sub-optimal doses and there is significant underprescribing in the elderly.

The main barriers to prescribing within general practice are organisational: confusing guidelines, errors and omissions by GPs, problems communicating with secondary care and reluctance by patients to take medication.

One of the biggest current debates in developed-world medicine is the extent to which we should identify risk groups or go for whole-population solutions. Uncertainty regarding choice and dose of statin remains.

What we know already:

- Low density lipoprotein (LDL) cholesterol and high density lipoprotein (HDL) cholesterol are both important and independent determinants of cardiovascular risk.
- Aggressive lowering of lipids with atorvastatin 80 mg improves cardiovascular outcomes after hospitalisation for acute coronary syndrome (PROVE IT-TIMI trial). Significantly lower markers of inflammation may account for the very early benefits, within 30 days, whereas the reduction in longer-term events are probably due to improvements in LDL cholesterol.
- Meta-analysis shows that statins reduce stroke but may not reduce fatal stroke. Each 10% reduction in LDL cholesterol corresponds to a risk reduction of all stroke of 16% (with no effect on haemorrhagic stroke). Sharing a common pathology with coronary artery disease, statin use after ischaemic stroke is almost certainly cost effective and is a good idea even if it is just to prevent MI.
- A "therapeutic crossover" of effects has been noted whereby statins appear to have antihypertensive effects particularly where blood pressure is higher.

- Some muscle symptoms are common with statins and are often well tolerated. Significant myopathy is rare and the usefulness of routine measurement of transaminase and CK levels in all patients taking statins is questionable. However, the 80 mg dose of simvastatin carries a risk of myopathy of approximately 1 in 250.
- Fears of cancer are unsubstantiated but cholesterol is important in brain function and some have suggested statins may promote cognitive decline. Low levels of total and LDL cholesterol in the elderly seem to be associated with higher mortality but this may reflect frailty, malnutrition or subclinical disease.
- Observational studies suggest that statins may promote bone formation and reduce fracture risk in the elderly.
- Triglyceride levels are closely linked to obesity and best treated by losing weight and taking more exercise. Fasting triglyceride levels look increasingly likely to have an independent role in predicting coronary heart disease.

Key Trials

There are some classic trials regarding lipids that it is important to know.

Primary prevention

WOSCOPS – The West of Scotland Coronary Prevention Study (1995)
WOSCOPS was a randomised controlled trial involving 6595 men aged 45–64 years with high total cholesterol levels (above 6.5 mmol/l) and no previous history of MI or CHD. They received either pravastatin or placebo and were followed up for 5 years.
    Treating 1000 patients for 5 years would prevent 7 deaths from CHD and 20 non-fatal MIs. Pravastatin was shown to reduce:
- total cholesterol by 20%
- death from CHD by 31%
- death from any cause by 22%
- revascularisation procedures by 37%

The Air Force/Texas Coronary Atherosclerosis Prevention Study (1998)
This trial involved men and women without a history of cardiovascular disease. It randomised 5608 men and 997 women, with average cholesterol levels of 5.7 mmol/l, to either placebo or lovastatin, and followed up for over 5 years.
    Lovastatin reduced the risk of:
- New cardiovascular disease by 54% in women and 34% in men
- Revascularisation procedures by 33%

The group treated with a statin benefited most when individual cardiovascular risk was higher but cholesterol level alone was found to be a poor indicator of that risk.

Secondary Prevention

The 4S Trial – The Scandinavian Simvastatin Survival Study (1994)
This large randomised double-blinded trial of 4444 men (81%) and women (19%) was a milestone in the secondary prevention of cardiovascular disease. Patients between 35 and 70

years who already had angina or a previous MI and had a cholesterol between 5.5 and 8.0 mmol/l were given either simvastatin or a placebo. Doses were adjusted over a median of 5.4 years follow up.

There were no significant differences in non-cardiovascular death, including death from cancer, trauma or suicide, and the drug was well tolerated.

In the simvastatin group, total cholesterol, LDL cholesterol, and triglycerides reduced by 25%, 35% and 10%, respectively; HDL cholesterol increased by 8%.

Simvastatin was shown to reduce the risk of:
- total mortality by 30%
- coronary death by 42%
- major coronary events by 34%
- revascularisation procedures by 37%

Ten-year follow up confirmed that the survival advantage persists. Importantly there was no validation of concerns regarding cancer. No difference was noted in its incidence or mortality between the simvastatin group and the placebo group (*Lancet*, 2004; **364**: 771–777).

CARE – Cholesterol and Recurrent Events (1996)

This was a 5-year mission to explore the effect of pravastatin (or placebo) on over 4000 men and women under 75 years. They were all post-MI patients who had a total cholesterol under 6.2 mmol/l (average 5.4 mmol/l).

Pravastatin was found to reduce the risk of:
- Cardiac events (both fatal and non-fatal) by 24%
- Stroke by 28%
- Revascularisation procedures by 26%

LIPID – The Long-term Intervention with Pravastatin in Ischaemic Disease (1998)

This was similar to CARE but with over 9000 subjects. They were under 75 years with cholesterol under 7 mmol/l. The trial was a double-blinded, randomised controlled trial and compared the effects of 40 mg of pravastatin with those of placebo with a mean follow-up period of 6.1 years.

Pravastatin was found to reduce the risk of:
- cardiac events (both fatal and non-fatal) by 24%
- MI by 29%
- overall mortality by 22%
- stroke by 19%
- revascularisation procedures by 20%

For every 1000 patients assigned to pravastatin, death from any cause would be avoided in 30 patients, death due to coronary disease avoided in 19, and death due to stroke avoided in 8.

The Heart Protection Study (*Lancet*, 2002)

This was an important trial (also mentioned in the diabetes chapter) that looked at over 20 000 patients aged 40–80 years. Men accounted for 75% and subjects either had vascular disease (whether coronary, cerebral or peripheral) or a risk factor such as diabetes. All were therefore at high risk and had a broad range of baseline total cholesterols averaging 5.9 mmol/l. The benefits of simvastatin in this group were conclusive on all counts. In addition, there was no difference in nonvascular mortality or cancer incidence.

Doubt has even been cast on the need to test lipids before starting statins in these groups as 40 mg of simvastatin has been shown to be so beneficial and targets so questionable. However, testing could increase concordance with therapy as well as identify particularly high triglycerides or low HDLs for special attention.

Extrapolation of the data showed that the benefit could extend 5 years either side of the 40–80 range and that 40 mg of simvastatin is cost-saving in most age ranges and vascular risk groups studied. Costs were favourable in every risk and age category of the study but the population of this study had a relatively high baseline level of disease. Routine use of statins in otherwise low risk patients still needs further exploration (*BMJ*, 2006; **333**: 1145).

Further analysis found benefits in stroke reduction were significant by the second year and an overall 30% reduction in ischaemic stroke was measured in high-risk individuals. The groups did not differ for haemorrhagic stroke. The evidence supports starting statins in all patients who can tolerate them after non-haemorrhagic stroke or TIA, regardless of age, gender, BP or anything else. As yet, death from stroke is still unimproved (*Lancet*, 2004; **363**: 757–767).

Recent Papers

GENERAL USE OF STATINS

Primary prevention of cardiovascular diseases with statin therapy
Thavendiranathan P, Bagai A, Brookhart MA, Choudhry NK
Arch Intern Med, 2006; **166**: 2307–2313

This meta-analysis sought to clarify the role of statins in primary prevention in patients without cardiovascular disease. Seven trials comprising 42 848 patients were included with a mean follow up of 4.3 years.
- Major coronary events and revascularisations decreased significantly by around 30%.
- Major cerebrovascular events significantly decreased by 14%.
- The 22% risk reduction in coronary heart disease mortality was non-significant.
- There was no significant reduction in overall mortality.

So stroke and heart attacks are prevented but they do not seem to extend life when used in primary prevention.

Rosuvastatin in older patients with systolic heart failure
Kjekshus J, Apetrei E, Barrios V, *et al.*
NEJM, 2007; **357**: 2248–2261

Over 5000 heart failure patients aged over 60 were randomised to 10 mg of rosuvastatin or placebo in the CORONA trial – COntrolled ROsuvastatin MultiNAtional Study in Heart Failure. LDL cholesterol decreased and there was a small reduction in hospital admissions for cardiovascular causes, mostly heart failure, in the rosuvastatin group.

But the drug surprisingly failed to improve coronary outcome or death from cardiovascular causes. Perhaps disease was too advanced in this group or could it be that not all statins are the same?

Which statin, what dose?
Drug and Therapeutics Bulletin, 2007; **45**: 33–37

This excellent review summarises many key points about statins.
- Each 1 mmol/l reduction in LDL cholesterol concentration by statin therapy is associated with a fall of around 20% in major vascular events (MI, coronary death, coronary revascularisation, or stroke) and of around 12% in mortality rate.
- The absolute benefit is smaller in individuals at lower baseline risk, with 'diminishing returns' for statin therapy as baseline risk falls.
- In addition to the NICE target group, the revised Joint British Societies (JBS)2 guidelines advocate statin therapy if the total-cholesterol to HDL-cholesterol ratio is 6 or more, irrespective of other risk factors, as well as for diabetics who are over 40 years or have other risk factors. However, due to incomplete evidence about primary prevention, this advice may include low risk groups who benefit little.
- Is high dose therapy desirable? The additional benefit in primary prevention is likely to be small, and would be expected to be associated with a higher likelihood of unwanted effects leading to discontinuation rates. In addition, very strict targets may not be achievable, more intensive monitoring is required, long-term safety has not been established, and cost-effectiveness diminishes.
- They recommend that many patients could be switched to generic simvastatin to reduce costs.

Switching statins
Moon JC
BMJ, 2006; **332**: 1344–1345

Around 85% of all statins prescribed are simvastatin or atorvastatin. In May 2003 simvastatin's patent expired and the cost reduced eightfold for the 40 mg dose and 20-fold for the 20 mg dose. Simvastatin 40 mg can cost less than £1 per month per patient when purchased in bulk.

Simvastatin 40 mg and atorvastatin 10 mg and 20 mg have been shown to be equally effective. Meta-analysis using simvastatin 40 mg and atorvastatin 10 mg showed no significant differences in mortality, death from coronary heart disease, or stroke.

The only important difference is cost.

It is time, the authors argue, for the UK to implement therapeutic substitution of simvastatin 40 mg nationally by switching patients currently taking atorvastatin 10 mg and 20 mg, and prescribing generic simvastatin. If simvastatin is not tolerated or considered inappropriate, the alternative is pravastatin 40 mg, another cheap generic statin. This could save the NHS £1 billion over the next 5 years. Atorvastatin remains on patent until 2011.

CARDIOVASCULAR

Discontinuation of statin therapy and clinical outcome after ischemic stroke
Colivicchi F, Bassi A, Santini M, Caltagirone C
Stroke, 2007; **38**: 2652–2657

An Italian study of 631 stroke survivors who were followed up for 12 months showed that 39% stopped taking their statin within the year. It cost some of them their lives as, having excluded possible confounding factors, stopping statins was an independent predictor of all-cause mortality.

Do statins reduce blood pressure? A meta-analysis of randomized, controlled trials
Strazzullo P, Kerry SM, Barbato A, *et al.*
Hypertension, 2007; **49**: 792–798

Meta-analysis of 20 trials and 828 patients in which concomitant antihypertensive treatment was unchanged during the trial looked at the 'therapeutic crossover' effect previously observed with statins.

Having controlled for age and cholesterol, the mean reduction in systolic pressure was around 2 mmHg which is clinically significant and meaningful. The effect was greater where the baseline systolic blood pressure was higher than 130 mmHg.

PREVENTING STROKE

High-dose atorvastatin after stroke or transient ischemic attack
SPARCL Investigators – Stroke Prevention by Aggressive Reduction in Cholesterol Levels
N Engl J Med, 2006; **355**: 549–559

We know statins reduce the number of strokes in those at increased risk for cardiovascular disease. But are they as effective after a recent stroke or TIA where heart disease is absent?

SPARCL randomly assigned 4731 patients with LDL cholesterol under 5 mmol/l and no known heart disease, but who had had a recent stroke or TIA, to high dose (80 mg) atorvastatin per day or placebo.

Follow up at 5 years showed modest but clear benefit. High doses of the statin:
- reduced the chances of another stroke over 5 years
- slightly increased haemorrhagic stroke
- reduced the risk of major cardiovascular events
- had a similar mortality in the two groups

MANAGEMENT STRATEGIES

High dose statins reduce risk of non-fatal cardiovascular events more than standard dose statins. *Evidence-Based Medicine,* 2007; **12:** 42
The following paper is presented
Meta-analysis of cardiovascular outcomes trials comparing intensive versus moderate statin therapy
Cannon CP, Steinberg BA, Murphy SA, *et al.*
J Am Coll Cardiol, 2006; **48:** 438–445

> Four trials with a total of 27 548 patients with stable coronary heart disease or acute coronary syndromes met the selection criteria for this meta-analysis: PROVE IT-TIMI-22 (n = 4162), A-to-Z (n = 4497), TNT – Treating to New Targets (n = 10 001), and IDEAL (n = 8888).
>
> High dose therapy with simvasatin 40–80 mg or atorvastatin 80 mg was shown to further reduce cardiac mortality and MI by a significant but modest amount over 2–5 years.
>
> It is a safe approach to take. Cardiovascular mortality was not increased and side effects were low. All cardiovascular end-pints in patients with coronary heart disease were improved. Optimum targets still remain to be elucidated, however.
>
> Still the main worry is the relevance in day-to-day practice. Our rates of prescribing of statins at any dose are too low and patients' adherence is poor. Until we are more successful at improving these areas, results such as these seem like the icing on a cake we have not yet made.

Strategies for prescribing statins
Donner-Banzhoff N, Sönnichsen A
BMJ, 2008; **336:** 288–289

> This editorial supports the 'fire and forget' approach to lipid-lowering, such as was used in the 4S trial, over the rigorous implementation needed for a 'treat to target' strategy. The diminishing returns from spending more effort using higher more toxic doses to achieve ever smaller increments towards the dubious target may not be the best approach. There is so much work to be done in working on other modifiable risk factors.
>
> UK and SIGN guidelines advocate the importance of measuring cholesterol and adjusting to targets, but this intensive effort may not work so well as tight targets are rarely met in reality. Complex strategies also encourage errors and imperfections. Titrating a dose according to defined targets of LDL was not the strategy laid down by the large statin trials. Even the 80 mg high-dose atorvastatin trials did not adjust their dose. 'Targeteers' may feel like using a drug such as ezetimibe to help them hit the bulls-eye, but where is the evidence of clinical outcome for that approach?
>
> Two types of trials to evaluate treatments are defined. Explanatory trials use highly compliant study centres with narrow inclusion criteria to measure specific outcomes. However, pragmatic trials such as the early statin trials are performed in the real world and are also needed to illustrate an effective treatment policy.
>
> Prescribing a statin at a standard dose – 'fire and forget' – without further testing or dose adjustment is a lot simpler and we should focus on doing this well first.

Should women be offered cholesterol lowering drugs to prevent cardiovascular disease? Yes
Grundy SM
BMJ, 2007; **334**: 982

This head to head feature looks at the debatable area of whether all the benefits of statins extend to women. With most of the evidence from the primary prevention trials belonging to men, we do not really know if the same benefits will prevail in women.

Grundy makes no claim to treat low-risk women, but advises that estimating risk before starting drugs will identify good candidates. He refers to the concepts of primary and secondary prevention as an "artificial distinction" that should be replaced by a strategy of absolute risk estimation regardless of whether previous events have occurred. As we have no large scale trial of giving statins to women at moderately high risk, say 10–20% 10-year risk, simply excluding women until there is such a trial seems to be pushing the point. There is even less evidence for treatment with diet alone.

Raised cholesterol is known to be a major risk factor for women and atherosclerotic plaques look the same in women as in men. A high risk of heart disease should be targeted rather than waiting for it to establish.

Should women be offered cholesterol lowering drugs to prevent cardiovascular disease? No
Kendrick M
BMJ, 2007; **334**: 983

Cardiovascular disease affects men at an earlier age and men and women respond differently to statins, argues Kendrick. No secondary prevention trials have shown statins to reduce mortality in women. Primary prevention trials have not even managed a reduction in cardiovascular end points in women never mind affecting mortality.

With unproven benefits, Kendrick believes women should not be prescribed statins at all when we can get evidence-based value for money elsewhere.

He argues side effects are greatly under-reported with three more women dying in the statin arm of the 4S study than in the placebo arm. He also finds a US Food and Drug Administration report that simvastatin was reported as a direct cause of 416 deaths between 1997 and 2004.

With statins increasingly prescribed to young women, the potential for teratogenicity and severe neurological abnormalities is also of concern.

Proven harm and lack of proven benefit dictates that the evidence-based approach is not to prescribe.

CORONARY HEART DISEASE

The Challenge

Coronary heart disease (CHD) is already the major cause of illness and death in Western countries. Some 80–85% of affected men and women have at least one of the big four conventional risk factors – smoking, diabetes, hyperlipidemia, and hypertension.

We know that heart disease in British women over 60 is more common than previously thought and is being underdiagnosed and undertreated. There is room for improvement in patients over 70 years who are less likely to be taking a statin, beta blockers post-MI, or have well controlled blood pressure. In addition, CHD is associated with depression, social isolation or lack of social support, as well as catastrophic life events.

Doctors have tended to struggle to make logical decisions about preventative treatment. The challenge is great but the news is not all bad. We know that we can reduce the risk of cardiovascular disease with lifestyle measures such as smoking cessation, regular exercise and maintenance of normal weight. We can adopt dietary measures including reducing intake of total and saturated fats, increasing consumption of fish, reducing salt, limiting alcohol consumption, and eating at least five portions of fresh fruit and vegetables per day.

Meta-analysis shows that exercise-based cardiac rehabilitation reduces all cause and cardiac mortality. Multidisciplinary disease management programmes for patients with CHD improve processes of care, reduce admissions to hospital, and enhance quality of life or functional status.

Cardiac liaison nurses offering people the choice of home or hospital-based rehabilitation and nurse-led clinics bridge the gap between primary and secondary care. They help optimise secondary prevention to reach long-term government targets.

And we are finally having an impact. CHD mortality has halved since 1981 in the UK, resulting in 68 000 fewer deaths in 2000. More than half the reduction is attributable to reductions in major risk factors, principally smoking but also blood pressure and cholesterol. This is despite (and offset by) negative trends in levels of obesity, physical activity and diabetes. Around 40% of this reduction is attributable to improved treatments in individuals (such as thrombolysis, improved treatments in heart failure and in secondary prevention measures). Since the implementation of the National Service Framework for prevention of CHD in 2000, prescription of drugs to men and women with established heart disease has improved markedly.

Still, after MI, much more work is needed to improve exercise-based rehabilitation, uptake of antiplatelets, statins, ACE inhibitors and beta blockers, monitoring of risk factors, and structured long-term care assisted by validated registers of high risk patients. Comprehensive strategies that promote primary prevention, particularly for smoking and dietary change, and that maximise population coverage of effective treatments are crucial, especially for secondary prevention and heart failure.

We also aim to target high risk people. There are many guidelines and tools to help us, but refinement of these tools for use within specific populations is much needed. The National Service Framework criteria, Sheffield tables, treatment by age threshold or fixed parameter values, offer different risk assessments from the highly adopted Framingham equation. Currently, national guidelines for prevention of CHD recommend the use of absolute risk profiles to guide treatment. They set explicit standards for secondary prevention and cardiac rehabilitation.

What we know already:

- Screening the entire population is not considered cost-effective so we target sub-groups.
- In one study population, the NSF guidelines selected 43% for cholesterol measurement and identified 81% of those at 15% or greater risk. The Sheffield tables selected 73% and identified 99.9% of those at high risk. The cost of this high sensitivity was a false positive rate of 68%. Estimating risk using fixed cholesterol values selected just 18% and identified 76% of those at 15% or greater risk.
- However, an age threshold of 50 years selected 46% and identified 93% of the high-risk group. It has been suggested therefore that measuring the cholesterol concentration of everyone over 50 is a simple and efficient population screening tool. Its simplicity and transparency should increase uptake to screening and outweigh the costs of extra cholesterol testing.
- Various inflammatory risk markers are being researched for the future to help in risk stratification of ischaemic heart disease as well as provide new targets for intervention. CRP, fibrinogen, plasma viscosity, and white cell count have all found limited practical relevance so far.
- Prescribing of statins has improved most with new initiatives, doubling in usage since 2000. But even by 2003, only about 80% of men and women with a history of MI were taking antiplatelets, only two-thirds were receiving statins, and less than half were taking beta blockers and ACE inhibitors.
- In one US study, discontinuation of therapy at 6 months occurred in 8% of those taking aspirin, 12% of those taking beta blockers, 13% of those taking statins, and 20% of those taking ACE inhibitors.
- Nurse-led clinics for the secondary prevention of CHD seem to be cost effective in primary care. At a cost per patient of £136, a QALY has been shown to cost just over £1000.
- Patients with stable coronary artery disease who are already on intensive standard therapy show no additional benefit from using an ACE inhibitor in CHD that is not complicated by heart failure (PEACE Trial – Prevention of Events with ACE Inhibition).

Guidelines

The British Hypertension Society has published guidelines on use of aspirin and statins in patients at risk of cardiovascular complications.

- Aspirin: use 75 mg daily if patient is aged 50 years with blood pressure controlled to <150/90 mmHg and target organ damage, diabetes mellitus, or 10 year risk of cardiovascular disease of 20% (measured by using the new Joint British Societies' cardiovascular disease risk chart).
- Statin: use sufficient doses to reach targets if patient is aged up to at least 80 years, with a 10 year risk of cardiovascular disease of 20% (measured by using the new Joint British Societies' cardiovascular disease risk chart) and with total cholesterol concentration at least 3.5 mmol/l.

Recent Papers

INCIDENCE

Modelling the decline in coronary heart disease deaths in England and Wales, 1981–2000: comparing contributions from primary and secondary prevention
Unal B, Critchley JA, Capewell S
BMJ, 2005; **331**: 614

> The authors used a validated model to estimate how much of the recent cardiovascular improvements were attributable to control of risk factors in apparently healthy people (primary prevention) and in patients with CHD (secondary prevention).
>
> Changing the risk factors of the healthy was responsible for four times the mortality benefit than these changes in those with established CHD, that is 81% versus 19% of lives saved.
>
> The risk factors they were referring to were smoking, cholesterol, and blood pressure.
>
> Comprehensive population-wide strategies for tobacco control and healthier diets are what really matters.

Trends in rates of different forms of diagnosed coronary heart disease, 1978–2000: prospective, population based study of British men
Lampe FC, Morris RW, Walker M, *et al.*
BMJ, 2005; **330**: 1046

> A big drop in the rate of major coronary events in the last two decades has been largely offset by the increase in diagnosing angina according to a study of nearly 8000 middle-aged men.
>
> The rate of major coronary events fell by an average of 3.6% a year, whereas the rate of first diagnosed angina increased by an average of 2.6% a year. These effects almost balance each other out when looking for an impact on the overall incidence of CHD. But the apparent increase in angina may well may be due to increased diagnosis of previously hidden disease and more aggressive management. The figure may settle in the future so we can see that tackling risk factors prevents angina as well. Until then, this study confirms prevention of more serious events such as MI.
>
> It also highlights the need for continued emphasis on the primary prevention of coronary heart disease and a good angina service.

CLINICAL ISSUES

CARDIOVASCULAR

DETECTION

Derivation and validation of QRISK, a new cardiovascular disease risk score for the United Kingdom: prospective open cohort study
Hippisley-Cox J, Coupland C, Vinogradova Y, *et al*.
BMJ, 2007; **335:** 136

New cardiovascular disease risk scores are needed. The Framingham cohort study is well established as a point of reference in the UK, but refers to an American population which was almost entirely white and was undertaken at a time of very high levels of cardiovascular disease. It is known to tend to over-estimate risk in affluent areas and underestimate risk in deprived areas.

This proposed model, called QRISK, was based on data drawn from the EMIS clinical computer system, which is extensively used in general practice, and was able to include data on social deprivation, body mass index and family history, as well as use of antihypertensives to create a more accurate risk prediction for a UK population.

Data covered about 7% of the UK population which the authors claim was likely to be suitably representative. The study was validated and found to discriminate better than the Framingham algorithm particularly for women from deprived areas. Overall, QRISK would reclassify about 1 in 10 patients from high to low risk or vice versa.

The authors feel that the QRISK is an important next step in reducing health inequalities in cardiovascular disease, particularly in identifying high risk patients on the basis of age sex and social deprivation.

Families of patients with premature coronary heart disease: an obvious but neglected target for primary prevention
Chow CK, Pell ACH, Walker A, *et al*.
BMJ, 2007; **335:** 481–485

First degree relatives of patients with premature MI have twice the risk of the condition due to sharing lifestyle risk factors and genetic predisposition. So maybe we should make more of an effort to seek them out.

Despite recommendations in several guidelines, surveys suggest that we do not get round to doing this formally in daily practice. Relatives at risk could easily be identified at the time the patient presents to hospital argue the authors. They can then be flagged up for counselling and screening. Motivation tends to be high, but an emphasis on genetic risk may reduce motivation to improve lifestyle factors.

Some have shed doubt on the choosing of patients on the basis of one risk factor alone. Identifying patients from multiple risk factors before their relatives present may be a better way to go (*BMJ*, 2007; **335:** 577).

ASSOCIATIONS

Job strain and risk of acute recurrent coronary heart disease events
Aboa-Éboulé C, Brisson C, Maunsell E, *et al.*
JAMA, 2007; **298**: 1652–1660

Stress or strain at work has two components – high workload or low autonomy. This Canadian study of nearly 1000 men and women under 60 who returned to work after their first MI found that chronic job strain doubled the risk of recurrent heart disease.

They adjusted for 26 potentially confounding factors but found that stress and strain seemed to independently increase the likelihood of a cardiac death or progression of cardiac disease. Only around 10% of the group were women so the picture was not clear there.

MEDICATION

Effect of combinations of drugs on all cause mortality in patients with ischaemic heart disease: nested case-control analysis
Hippisley-Cox J, Coupland C
BMJ, 2005; **330**: 1059–1063

Combinations of statins, aspirins, and beta blockers are associated with the greatest reduction in all cause mortality – about 83% – in patients with a first diagnosis of ischaemic heart disease. This was the first large study to assess the effects of drugs combined in this way and identified 13 000 cases of ischaemic heart disease in a new UK database, QRESEARCH. Controls were matched for ischaemic heart disease, age, sex, and year of diagnosis and were alive at the time their matched case died.

The addition of an ACE inhibitor provided no additional benefit.

A strategy to reduce cardiovascular disease by more than 80%
Wald NJ, Law MR
BMJ, 2003; **326**: 1419–1423

Papers from this important issue of the *BMJ* bang the drum for the Polypill. Wald and Law propose this neologism as a panacea for heart disease.

They have synthesised over 750 trials with 400 000 participants and the argument goes like this.

- The strategy was to reduce simultaneously the four cardiovascular risk factors (low density lipoprotein cholesterol, blood pressure, serum homocysteine, and platelet function) regardless of pretreatment levels.
- The challenge is to develop a single daily pill combining effective drugs to achieve a large effect in preventing cardiovascular disease with minimal adverse effects.
- Changing all four risk factors together potentially reduces IHD events by 88% and stroke by 80%.

- The recommended combination is a statin (e.g. atorvastatin 10 mg or sim-vastatin 40 mg), three blood pressure lowering drugs (e.g. a thiazide, a beta-blocker, and an ACE inhibitor) each at half standard dose, folic acid (0.8 mg), and aspirin (75 mg).
- The components of the Polypill would cause adverse symptoms in 8–15% of people (depending on the precise formulation). Aspirin has the most side-effects but the advantages for thrombotic stroke outweigh those of increased haemorrhagic stroke.
- Withdrawal due to side-effects would occur in 1–2 per 100 and fatal side-effects in less than 1 in 10 000 users.
- There may be some contraindications to the Polypill, e.g. beta-blockers in asthma, aspirin if not tolerated.

With these caveats, they propose giving this combination pill to anyone at high risk but also to **all** over 55s. One-third of people taking this pill from age 55 would benefit, gaining on average about 11 years of life free from an IHD event or stroke.

They propose that this would have a greater impact on the prevention of disease in the Western world than any other single intervention.

- Cost would be low with generic ingredients that are all off-patent.
- There is no need to measure risk.
- There is no need for investigations.
- They propose a new model where we recognise that in Western society risk is high in all of us.
- Targeting single risk factors has so far produced only modest reductions in disease so there is much to gain and little to lose.

All the ingredients are proven effective in randomised controlled trials except folic acid whose evidence is observational but still compelling. The maximum observed effect of folic acid lowers serum homocysteine by about 25% and reduces IHD events by about 16% and stroke by 24%.

A combination of three low-dose drugs from different groups has greater efficacy and fewer adverse effects than using one or two drugs in standard dose.

The blood pressure reduction with three drugs in combination at half standard dose is about 11 mmHg diastolic, reducing coronary events by 46% and stroke by 63%.

Other than the statin, omitting a single component has a relatively minor effect. Aspirin prevents 32% of IHD events when used alone but only prevents an additional 5% when added to other ingredients of the Polypill.

The most important BMJ for 50 years?
Smith R
BMJ, 2003; **326**

Richard Smith's playful editorial piece describes the Polypill as 'genius'.

The use of multiple low-dose antihypertensives to lessen side-effects and maximise benefit is praised.

The inexpensive ingredients make it good news for the developing world but not for pharmaceutical companies. Perhaps a large generic company in India could supply us? (It has been claimed that manufacturers in India plan to forge ahead without further study in order to bring a Polypill to market quickly.)

Yes, there are issues of medicalisation but then the plan does circumvent the need for screening so nicely. And then of course what are we going to do with all the cardiologists and cardiac surgeons?

A cure for cardiovascular disease?
Rodgers A
BMJ, 2003; **326**: 1407–1408

This editorial agrees that large reductions in risk are likely with the Polypill.

The argument that three blood pressure lowering agents at half the standard dose are the best way to achieve large reductions in blood pressure is found convincing.

The author agrees that the drugs involved, contrary to modern perceptions, have remarkably few side-effects and pharmacological reasons for stopping treatment are rare. He calls for more information on the adverse effects of the combination but recognises that all the drugs involved have been extensively studied.

A wide debate on the new paradigm is called for. Treating risk rather than risk factor threshold is the new concept here and treating vast asymptomatic populations using age alone as a variable is controversial to say the least. It will involve a challenge to cardiovascular disease being a 'natural' cause of death.

Further trials will also be needed to look at issues such as tolerability and adherence as well as technical issues of production.

The preventive polypill – much promise, insufficient evidence
Reddy KS
NEJM, 2007; **356:** 212

This article reminds us that the polypill would be a cost effective antidote to cardiovascular disease, particularly in low and middle income countries where drugs have not been widely used and adherence is poor.

India's active generic drug industry would keep costs low. Already the World Heart Federation has declared support for a polypill with aspirin, an ACE inhibitor and a statin. Two Indian manufacturers have a product which also contains a beta blocker.

Indians have had rapid increases in CHD, hypertension and diabetes due to unhealthy living and inactivity – a problem still worsening in deprived areas. Focussing on ill people has been a negligent approach he argues. Population measures are needed.

Trials will help to show whether the polypill lives up to its press or not.

CLINICAL ISSUES

CARDIOVASCULAR

HEART FAILURE

The Challenge

Heart failure accounts for 5% of admissions to medical wards, with enormous healthcare costs from high readmission rates. It is preceded by hypertension in over 90% of cases and the treatment of hypertension can prevent more than 40% of heart failure events.

Unfortunately diagnosis by clinical assessment of symptoms and signs is difficult. It tends to be incorrect in more than half of cases. Unrecognised hypervolaemia is common as blood volume does not correlate well with physical signs. Indeed JVP may be the most useful, so many of us could be in trouble there. In addition, it presents with symptoms shared with many other conditions, such as COPD. Heart failure is largely poorly managed in general practice. Even in hospital, there are major deficiencies in prescribing ACE inhibitors and beta blockers and even recording of an ECG.

Some suggest that a National Service Framework for chronic heart failure is urgently needed as only a systematic overhaul and a multidisciplinary approach can stop heart failure being the 'Cinderella of cardiology'.

UK general practitioners are not alone in still struggling with uncertainty when trying to make a symptomatic rather than pathophysiological diagnosis. They tend to worry about using ACE inhibitors in the elderly and there is confusion surrounding the resurgence of spironolactone and beta blockers previously regarded as dangerous. Lack of time and availability of diagnostic tests compound the situation and local organisational factors such as access to echocardiography and, most importantly, interpretation of its results compound the situation. New, conjoint models of care to straddle primary and secondary care are needed.

There is far to go but the Healthcare Commission has shown that progress has been made with waiting times for echocardiography falling in the last 2 years. More than 70% of patients now have this test within 13 weeks. Additionally, some 82.5% of patients now receive an ACE inhibitor compared to less than 50% in 2003/4. More than 80% of communities have some form of specialist heart failure service, but less than one-quarter of those admitted to hospitals were referred to them (www.healthcarecommission.org.uk).

What we know already:

- Beta blockers improve prognosis in all grades of symptomatic heart failure and may be as important as ACE inhibitors in treatment. Bisoprolol, metoprolol and carvedilol all reduce mortality but not all beta blockers are the same. There is no evidence to support the use of atenolol in heart failure or after MI.
- B-type natriuretic peptide is a red flag in heart failure indicating volume overload and a stretched ventricle. Levels above 500 pg/ml are accepted as diagnostic but it is a strong prognostic indicator regardless of the stage of heart failure. Each 100 pg/ml increase in BNP was associated with a 35% increase in the relative risk of death. Even in asymptomatic patients, BNP > 20 pg/ml was associated with twice the risk of death.
- Assays of BNP and N-terminal pro-BNP variant in primary care reduced referrals to a cardiology clinic by 25% in nearly 300 patients in South Durham who had symptoms and signs suggestive of heart failure.

- Evaluation of BNP in the emergency department leads to quicker treatment, fewer hospitalisations, a shorter length of stay and lower costs, actually improving outcomes.
- Even when ejection fraction is preserved, in so-called diastolic heart failure, there is also substantial mortality.
- Portable echocardiography can detect cardiac abnormalities and assess ventricular function with a sensitivity higher than that of clinical examination and reaching 70–90% compared with conventional echocardiography. New approaches such as this may perhaps best be used in a team with ongoing specialist feedback to recognise limitations.
- Concerns about side effects of beta blockers linger, but an overview of randomised trials in patients up to 67 years of age showed small but significant absolute risks of hypotension (11 per 1000), dizziness (57 per 1000), and bradycardia (38 per 1000). There was no significant fatigue associated with therapy and fewer patients were withdrawn from beta blocker therapy than from placebo. This should alleviate concerns about prescribing this life-saving therapy to patients with heart failure.
- Are these results generalisable to an older group? A meta-analysis with 12 000 subjects looking at all cause mortality data from five completed trials revealed that elderly and non-elderly heart failure patients both derive considerable and similar mortality reduction from the use of beta blockers.
- Digoxin is useful in heart failure. It helps to keep patients out of hospital but the level should be kept low. In men the optimal range seems to be 0.5–0.8 ng/ml, with mortality being lower in this group.
- For post-MI patients with some degree of heart failure, additive effects mean that the combination of statins and beta blockers can reduce mortality by close to 50%.
- Poor prescribing of ACE inhibitors and beta blockers on hospital discharge sacrifices a lot of mortality. Overhesitation in prescribing to the elderly (who have most to gain) may be to blame.

Key Trials

MERIT-HF: Effect of metoprolol in chronic heart failure: Metoprolol Randomised Intervention Trial in Congestive Heart Failure (MERIT-HF). Lancet, 1999; **353**: 2001–2007
Nearly 4000 patients with class II–IV heart failure, stable on optimum standard therapy (any combination of diuretics and ACE inhibitor) were assigned increasing doses of slow release metoprolol. The study was halted at mean follow up of 1 year as all-cause mortality was significantly lower in metoprolol group (34% risk reduction). There were significantly fewer cardiovascular deaths and the drug was well tolerated.

It improved survival in stable patients, preventing 1 death per 27 patients treated per year.

CHARM: Effects of candesartan on mortality and morbidity in patients with chronic heart failure: the CHARM-Overall programme. Lancet, 2003; **362**: 759–771
This was a prospective study of 7599 patients with chronic heart failure (NYHA class II–IV) given placebo or candesartan – an angiotensin II receptor blocker (ARB).
- Cardiovascular death significantly reduced in the candesartan group (18% vs. 20%).
- Hospital admission due to heart failure was significantly reduced (20% vs. 24%).
- Non-cardiovascular death was not significantly different but overall mortality was reduced.

- Benefit was greatest where there was reduced left ventricular ejection fraction and occurred even if the patients were already on an ACE inhibitor.

ValHEFT (The Valsartan Heart Failure Trial) has shown similar benefits for losartan but a retrospective analysis implied that adding an ARB on to an ACE inhibitor and a beta blocker was associated with an increased mortality. CHARM is a prospective study and contradicts this saying it is safe in mild to moderate left ventricular failure.

RALES: The effect of spironolactone on morbidity and mortality in patients with severe heart failure. N Engl J Med, 1999; **341**: 709–717.
In patients with severe heart failure, an aldosterone blocker might be the preferred agent to add to an ACE inhibitor and a beta blocker rather than an ARB based on the results of the Randomized Aldactone Evaluation Study (RALES). However, only a relatively small proportion of patients were receiving both an ACE inhibitor and a beta blocker. Direct comparative studies of an ARB and an aldosterone blocker in patients with left ventricular failure on this regime are needed.

Guidelines

NICE – *Management of Chronic Heart Failure in Adults in Primary and Secondary Care* (http://www.nice.org.uk)

NICE guidance now recommends:
- Full evaluation of all patients suspected of having heart failure using 12-lead ECG or testing B-type natriuretic peptide (BNP), to exclude a diagnosis of heart failure
- ACE inhibitors should be given in the presence of left ventricular dysfunction
- Diuretics are used for symptoms
- Beta blockers licensed for use in cases of heart failure are used in a carefully monitored 'start low, go slow' manner after treatment with diuretics and ACE inhibitors, regardless of whether or not symptoms persist
- All patients with chronic heart failure should be monitored at least every six months with clinical assessment of function, fluid status, cardiac rhythm, medication review, and measurement of urea, electrolytes, and creatinine

Recent Papers

DETECTION

Public awareness of heart failure in Europe: first results from SHAPE
Remme WJ, McMurray JJ, Rauch B, *et al.*
Eur Heart J, 2005; **26**: 2413–2421

The Study of Heart failure Awareness and Perception in Europe (SHAPE), found poor awareness among the general public of what heart failure actually is.

- Only 3% could correctly identify heart failure from a description of typical symptoms and signs.
- Most thought that these patients should reduce all physical activity.
- Most thought it was less serious than it is.
- One-third also wrongly thought heart failure was a normal consequence of getting older.
- Nearly one-third thought modern drugs could not prevent the condition.

It could be time to rebrand heart failure and sell it to the public.

Management of chronic heart failure in the community: role of a hospital based open access heart failure service
Shah S, Davies MK, Cartwright D *et al*.
Heart, 2004; **90**: 755–759

This Birmingham study evaluated an open access heart failure service based at a teaching hospital. They assessed nearly 1000 GP referrals of patients with suspected heart failure.

- Only 31% were found to have left ventricular systolic dysfunction (LVSD denotes an ejection fraction < 50% on echocardiography).
- Risk factors for this were male sex, age over 60 years, diabetes, ischaemic heart disease or atrial fibrillation.
- Abnormal ECG and cardiothoracic ratio > 0.5 were good predictors of LVSD.
- A normal ECG had a negative predictive value of 80%
- A cardiothoracic ratio of < 0.5 on CXR had a negative predictive value of 82%.
- A combined negative predictive value of 88% make ECG and CXR good predictors with which to identify lower risk patients.
- The authors suggest that this type of model is a cost-effective service to community referrals.

Medical history, physical examination, and routine tests are useful for diagnosing heart failure in dyspnoea. *Evidence-Based Medicine,* 2006; **11**: 58
The following paper is reviewed
Does this dyspnoeic patient in the emergency department have congestive heart failure?
Wang CS, FitzGerald JM, Schulzer M *et al*.
JAMA, 2005; **294**: 1944–1956

A review of 18 high quality studies on patients with acute dyspnoea showed the following. The findings useful for ruling in heart failure were (in decreasing order) pulmonary venous congestion and interstitial oedema on CXR, a third heart sound, a history of heart failure, and jugular venous distension.

For ruling out heart failure the best findings were a serum BNP <100 pg/ml, absence of cardiomegaly and pulmonary venous congestion on CXR, crepitations, exertional dyspnoea, and a negative history of heart failure.

Prevalence and prognostic implications of electrocardiographic left ventricular hypertrophy in heart failure: evidence from the CHARM programme

Hawkins NM, Wang D, McMurray JJ *et al.*
Heart, 2007; **93**: 59–64

ECG is a simple, cheap tool which has been shown to be a significant independent predictor of worsening clinical outcome in heart failure even when systolic function is preserved.

Further analysis of the CHARM study showed that LVH was present on ECG in 15% of those patients with heart failure, with and without reduced left ventricular fraction. It proved to be associated with a 78% increase in cardiovascular death and major cardiovascular events overall.

A relationship with hypertension had previously been recognised but was inconclusive in heart failure.

Accuracy of electrocardiography in diagnosis of left ventricular hypertrophy in arterial hypertension: systematic review

Pewsner D, Jüni P, Egger M, *et al.*
BMJ, 2007; **335**: 711

This systematic review concludes that ECG alone is not a good enough tool to rule out left ventricular hypertrophy in hypertensive patients. While it is desirable to identify such patients, because LVH increases cardiovascular risk 5–10-fold, ECG is a poor screening tool because sensitivity is so low.

Echocardiography is a more comprehensive tool when the ECG voltages suggest LVH as recommended by the 2004 guidelines of the British Hypertension Society.

Diagnosing left ventricular hypertrophy in arterial hypertension

Nielsen OW, Sajadieh A
BMJ, 2007; **335**: 681–682

The accompanying editorial reminds us that ECG changes do remain a specific sign of organ damage and a marker of increased risk, as well as pointing to other things such as atrial fibrillation or ischaemic heart disease. Expert evaluation has been shown to be better than by GP alone, however, and increases sensitivity and specificity.

Even echocardiography has its faults. Sometimes image quality is poor in some patients and inter-observer variation is typically 15%. However, it should be done when the history or ECG indicates.

Screening for left ventricular systolic dysfunction using GP-reported ECGs

Goudie BM, Jarvis R, Donnan PT, *et al.*
Br J Gen Pract, 2007; **57**: 191–195

This survey gave 123 Scottish GPs the opportunity to review 180 ECGs for abnormality – 41 had changes of left ventricular hypertrophy. Although most GPs had the skill to identify an abnormal ECG, the differences exposed would result in such discrepancies in local referral rates for specialist care, that they would have a great impact in appropriate and fair use of any secondary diagnostic resources. This information would need to be factored into the development of such services.

MEDICATION

Detrimental effects of beta-blockers in COPD: a concern for nonselective beta-blockers
van der Woude HJ, Zaagsma J, Postma DS, *et al.*
Chest, 2005; **127**: 818–824

This study may look as though it is in the wrong chapter but unless we think of our heart failure patients who also suffer with COPD, we may offer them a treatment that does them a great disservice. The authors compared different beta blockers – propranolol, metoprolol and celiprolol and showed different types of beta blockers have different pulmonary effects:

- propranolol reduced FEV_1, increased airway hyperresponsiveness, and reduced the effect of formoterol
- metoprolol increased airway hyperresponsiveness but did not affect FEV_1
- celiprolol seemed safe at the doses used with no pulmonary effects

Reminders in echocardiography reports increased use of β blockers in reduced left ventricular ejection fraction. *Evidence-Based Medicine,* 2007; **12**: 185.
The following paper is reviewed
Clinical reminders attached to echocardiography reports of patients with reduced left ventricular ejection fraction increase use of β-blockers. A randomized trial
Heidenreich PA, Gholami P, Sahay A, *et al.*
Circulation, 2007; **115**: 2829–2834

Where the ejection fraction is reduced on echo, a simple process like a written reminder in the report helps to resolve physician lapses about acting on the results with appropriate medication like beta blockers. Including specific guidelines for recommended drugs such as metoprolol and carvedilol was a useful move.

The process is simple, cheap and can contribute immensely to morbidity and mortality rates. When used with monitored titration, beta blockers are tolerated with very few complications and fears of making a bad situation worse tend to be unfounded.

Angiotensin receptor blockers and myocardial infarction
Verma S, Strauss M
BMJ, 2004; **329**: 1248–1249

This is a useful editorial summarising the current controversy over the role of angiotensin receptor blockers looking at their effects in the following trials.

- VALUE – this trial showed a 19% increase in fatal and non-fatal MI compared to amlodipine in high-risk hypertensives.
- CHARM-Alternative – showed a 36% increase in MI with candesartan despite lowering blood pressure.

CARDIOVASCULAR

- CHARM-Preserved – reduced admissions for chronic heart failure but did not prevent death.
- SCOPE – candesartan showed a non-significant increase in fatal and non-fatal MI in the elderly despite lowering blood pressure.
- LIFE – showed no reduction in MI.
- RENAAL – in diabetics with nephropathy, losartan offer renal protection but no reduction in cardiovascular mortality.

So ARBs reduce blood pressure but may increase MI. ACE inhibitors on the other hand have consistently produced at least a 20% reduction in MI in high risk patients. Large trials are awaited (ONTARGET/TRANSCEND) but in the meantime the authors warn, should we get fully informed consent before using these drugs and forget about thinking of them as ACE inhibitors without the cough?

However, a systematic review in 2005 of all available data on ARBs shows a neutral impact on MI. While more data are awaited, we need not worry about the risk of MI if we think our patients need an ARB in preference to an ACE inhibitor. *BMJ,* 2005; **331**: 873.

Angiotension receptor blockers do not differ from ACE inhibitors in chronic heart failure or acute MI. *Evidence-Based Medicine,* 2005; **10**: 76.
The following paper is reviewed
Meta-analysis: angiotensin-receptor blockers in chronic heart failure and high-risk acute myocardial infarction
Lee VC, Rhew DC, Dylan M, *et al.*
Ann Intern Med, 2004; **141**: 693–704

A review of 24 RCTs found that in patients with chronic heart failure, ARBs do not differ from ACE inhibitors for all cause mortality or hospital admission.

The commentary reminds us that there is no evidence that ARBs are any better, and ARBs cost much more than generic ACE inhibitors. They tell us 'ARBs *are* great drugs; their misfortune is that ACE inhibitors are too' and suggest that the pharmaceutical industry so keen to show superiority for their latest offerings are 'probably close to giving up'.

FOLLOW UP CARE

Telemonitoring or structured telephone support programmes for patients with chronic heart failure: systematic review and meta-analysis
Clark RA, Inglis SC, McAlister FA, *et al.*
BMJ, 2007; **334**: 942

This review of 14 RCTs and over 4000 patients incorporated recent evidence of a higher quality than was previously available to evaluate the impact of remote monitoring of heart failure patients. This included interventions such as telephone contact and transfer of physiological data to the healthcare provider.

The conclusion was that such programmes produced a 21% reduction in admissions to hospital for heart failure (but not for total admissions) and a 20% reduction in all cause mortality as well as improving quality of life. The methods were likely to be cost effective. Few trials had follow up longer than 6 months but that is the period of highest risk anyway. This method of organising follow up care may therefore be useful, particularly in remote communities.

Telephone interventions for disease management in heart failure
Grancelli HO, Ferrante DC
BMJ, 2007; **334:** 910–911

This accompanying editorial tells us that similar studies have shown different results, such as a failure to improve mortality. However, trials differ on many points such as the inclusion of sicker patients as well as choice of the recipe for these complex interventions. There are many components of different disease management strategies which may look at diet, education, medication and surveillance. Any intervention that includes a few of these is likely to be effective as an adjunct to the clinician–patient relationship.

STROKE

The Challenge

At over 5 million kills per year, stroke is the second leading cause of death in the world and the largest single cause of major disability in the UK. Each year 100 000 people in England and Wales have a stroke. The UK has poor survival rates for stroke. Thirty per cent die in the first month and one-third are still significantly disabled at 1 year – a huge burden to individuals and society as a whole. Five per cent require long term residential care. The cost to the NHS is around £2.8 billion per year.

The risk of stroke soon after a TIA or minor stroke is much higher than commonly quoted. Around 15% of ischaemic strokes are preceded by a TIA and, unless these seemingly minor episodes are taken as red alerts, a stroke may occur before the patient is fully assessed.

Concepts of hypertension and hypercholesterolaemia may have become irrelevant or even harmful in this group as almost all stroke/TIA patients will benefit from treatment for cholesterol and blood pressure regardless of actual levels. Given the benefits of these medications, clinicians must avoid over-worrying about polypharmacy and concentrate on improving their diagnostic accuracy. Only half the patients referred as TIAs have actually had one. Other neurological diagnoses are made in 30%.

The National Service Framework for Older People Standard 5 outlines the recommended approach to stroke. Stroke units are the gold standard of care and organised inpatient care has enduring benefits. Mortality improves as does recovery from stroke. However, access is limited and the ageing demographic means the burden of stroke is set to rise.

In England many patients are compromised by failure to access these services and claims of overt and covert rationing have led to shouts of inherent ageism. National guidelines now recognise stroke as a medical emergency requiring urgent hospital admission to allow the best possible outcome. We need educational measures to tell doctors the best practice, streamlining of local services, and the redesigning of stroke services in a similar way to heart disease programmes, to reduce the horrendous disability of stroke.

What we know already:

- Haemorrhagic stroke accounts for 20% of strokes but are more likely to be fatal.
- The Face Arm Speech Test which assesses facial droop, arm strength, and normal conversation, can accurately diagnose stroke with good agreement between paramedics and physicians. FAST may facilitate rapid triage of stroke to urgent specialist care.
- Therapeutic benefits have been shown for aspirin, antihypertensives, statins and treatment for atrial fibrillation. The results of the US Field Administration of Stroke Therapy-Magnesium (FAST-MAG) pilot trial showed the viability of giving magnesium sulphate as a neuroprotective agent in the prehospital setting in the first hour or two after stroke. Further work on the value needs to be undertaken.
- OXVASC showed that incidence of stroke in Oxfordshire fell by 40% over the last 20 years due to the increased use of antiplatelets, statins, and antihypertensives, and reductions in risk factors; 28% more strokes were expected in OXVASC due to an increase in the elderly

population but the observed number actually fell. Incidence declined by more than 50% for primary intracerebral haemorrhage.

- Survival rates 10 years following a stroke are higher for those who went to a stroke unit rather than a general ward – possibly due to early reduction in disability. Complex multi-disciplinary programmes maximise potential in re-enabling patients.
- Caregivers are a neglected group but a simple practical training programme in basic nursing and facilitation of personal care has been shown to lower the burden of the caregiver. It even reduced anxiety and depression in the patients themselves. Quality of life improved and effect persisted at one year. Hospital costs were lower and there was a trend to use less respite care.

Key trials

The Heart Protection Study and other major trials have confirmed that stroke risk halves for every 10 mmHg fall in diastolic pressure even at conventional normotensive values. The effect is regardless of baseline BP and there seems to be no demonstrable floor to this benefit.

The HOPE study (2000)
This involved 9297 subjects from 19 countries. They were all high-risk but had controlled BP.
- Ramipril reduced fatal stroke by 61% and non-fatal stroke by 24%, independent of BP. The reduction in BP was quite small (3.8/2.8 mmHg) but the reduction in stroke risk was greater than expected at 32%
- The effect of 10 mg ramipril is stronger than 2.5 mg, so titrating the dose upwards will be important to realise maximum benefit
- It is unknown how much of this benefit will translate to other ACE inhibitors
- Patients already taking aspirin have less benefit and this interaction needs further study
The authors of HOPE recommend that patients at high risk of stroke should be treated with ramipril for primary and secondary prevention irrespective of their initial BP levels.

PROGRESS (2001)
In the perindopril protection against recurrent stroke study, a combination of perindopril and the diuretic indapamide reduced the risk of stroke over 4 years by 28%, with BP reduction of 9/4 mmHg. This benefited intracerebral haemorrhage perhaps more than ischaemic events.

Recent Papers

Improving the outcome of stroke
Markus H
BMJ, 2007; **335**: 359–360

This editorial claims that the UK has some of the worst outcomes for stroke mortality in Europe and poor processes of care might be to blame.

CARDIOVASCULAR

Stroke has tended to fall between the two stools of neurology and general medicine. Claims that underinvestment has caused the problems seem unfounded as costs are similar to other European countries, but our outcomes are inferior. This may be because good early care reduces hospital stay – the major reason for the costs.

Thrombolysis given within 3 hours of ischaemic stroke (after a quick CT scan) reduces disability and improves outcome. Currently only 1% of patients receive it. Better organisation could save £20 million per year, avoid 550 deaths and allow 1700 full recoveries.

We need to challenge the traditional perception of stroke so that it is viewed as a medical emergency and dump the bias that "treatment won't make any difference anyway" and avoid using phrases like "just a TIA".

In the best units, still only a minority will be eligible for carotid endarterectomy and thrombolysis but techniques will hopefully improve to better target those who will benefit. Intensive medication is very important too and a CT is still needed to exclude haemorrhage before the antiplatelets can be started.

MEDICATION

Effect of urgent treatment of transient ischemic attack on early recurrent stroke (EXPRES) study: a prospective population based sequential comparison
Rothwell PM, Giles MF, Chandratheva A, *et al*.
Lancet, 2007; **370**: 1432–1442

As many as one in ten people who have a TIA will go on to have a disabling stroke, often in the first week.

Research from nine primary care practices in Oxfordshire started patients very early on aspirin, statins, antihypertensives, and anticoagulants. The incidence of stroke fell by 80%. Initial figures had 10% of those attending going on to have a stroke within 90 days. But over the course of the intervention, the proportion fell to 2%.

If this model was replicated in all UK sufferers of a TIA, 10 000 strokes a year could be prevented.

Thrombolysis with alteplase for acute ischaemic stroke in the Safe Implementation of Thrombolysis in Stroke-Monitoring Study (SITS-MOST): an observational study
Wahlgren N, Ahmed N, Dávalos A, *et al*.
Lancet, 2007; **369**: 275–282

Alteplase seems to be safe in clinical practice which should reassure doctors who fear the drug's potential for haemorrhage.

An observational study in 6483 patients across Europe found that mortality at 3 months was 11% – less than the 17% from the original clinical trials. The risk of intracranial haemorrhage was also lower in practice than the original clinical trials.

CARDIOVASCULAR

RISK ASSESSMENT

A simple score (ABCD) to identify individuals at high early risk of stroke after transient ischaemic attack
Rothwell PM, Giles MF, Flossmann E *et al.*
Lancet, 2005; **366**: 29–36

> This team from Oxford have validated a simple scoring system to predict the risk of stroke in the 7 days following a TIA. The system is called ABCD and has a maximum of 6 points according to:
> - Age (≥60 years = 1),
> - Blood pressure (systolic > 140 mmHg or diastolic ≥90, or both = 1),
> - Clinical signs (unilateral weakness = 2, speech disturbance but no weakness = 1, other = 0),
> - Duration of symptoms (≥60 minutes = 2, 10–59 = 1, < 10 = 0).
>
> The seven day risk of stroke was 0.4% for those who scored less than 5, 12% for patients who scored 5, and 31% for patients who scored 6. A score of 6 should be treated as a medical emergency, they suggest.
>
> Commentary in *Evidence-Based Medicine* (2006; **11**: 27) reminds us that other factors sometimes considered predictive of risk, such as crescendo pattern, carotid stenosis and multiplicity, were not considered, and without further validation the score is not quite ready for clinical use. And whom should we admit? There is no intervention proven to decrease stroke risk in the short term, so perhaps only those who are being considered for thrombolysis. How often is that happening in your local hospital? That aside, once the cause is established, early initiation of secondary prevention should logically decrease ongoing risk.

The ABCD, California, and unified ABCD² risk scores predicted stroke within 2, 7, and 90 days after TIA. *Evidence-Based Medicine,* 2007; **12**: 88.
The following paper is presented
Validation and refinement of scores to predict very early stroke risk after transient ischaemic attack
Johnston SC, Rothwell PM, Nguyen-Huynh MN, *et al.*
Lancet, 2007; **369**: 283–292

> A 7 point score that unified the predictive abilities of the ABCD and California scores was assessed here. The ABCD² score is the most externally validated tool currently available for predicting the risk of stroke at 2, 7 and 90 days after a TIA. It can be used to triage patients into low and high risk to assist in prioritising interventions, and perhaps even inpatient observation to avoid future stroke and maximize benefit from thrombolysis should a stroke occur.
>
> Overall, 3.9%, 5.5%, and 9.2% of patients had stroke within 2, 7, and 90 days of TIA. The ABCD² score classified 34% of patients as low risk, 45% moderate, and 21% at high risk of stroke.

CARDIOVASCULAR

Underinvestigation and undertreatment of carotid disease in elderly patients with transient ischaemic attack and stroke: comparative population based study
Fairhead JF, Rothwell PM
BMJ, 2006; **333**: 525–527

An expansion of the OXVASC population looked at secondary care services in Oxfordshire.

They found that patients over 80 years who suffer a TIA or minor ischaemic stroke have a steep increase in incidence of symptomatic carotid stenosis (> 50% stenosed). However, that age group is substantially underinvestigated with carotid imaging and undertreated with carotid endarterectomy.

Accusations of ageism have appeared and in investigating whether or not this is ageism, the authors found there is good evidence of benefit for endarterectomy in the elderly with little increased risk from the surgery. The decision not to refer or go through with imaging the carotids might be being made in primary or secondary care. The study could not tell us. But it could say this was not likely to be due to contraindication or the patient's own choice.

DIABETES

The Challenge

Diabetes is a chronic progressive disease that affects 2 million people in the UK with perhaps another million cases undetected. It is the fourth leading cause of death in the UK and is responsible for 5% of all NHS expenditure. By 2025, it has been estimated that 300 million people will be diabetic – a global pandemic. Even if obesity levels remain constant which seems unlikely, the most important factor is the increasingly elderly demographic.

Diabetes fulfils many of the criteria for screening yet important uncertainties remain, making the validity of this approach questionable. The burden of such a task is enormous and we do not even have agreement on what test to use. Do we use fasting plasma glucose (FPG) levels, determination of HbA1c, urine tests, or an oral glucose tolerance test (OGTT)? The best screening tool may depend on the local population, as well as cost. The OGTT is still the gold standard investigation, offering better sensitivity and specificity for development of the macrovascular and microvascular complications of diabetes.

Some GPs already actively engage in case-finding but, given the current pressures on primary care, others think this is more the remit of government agencies and others in the area of health promotion and education. If we ever get a widespread programme, primary care is likely to have a role in this large task and healthcare practitioners will need to be motivated and sufficiently well resourced. Unfortunately, many health workers feel as though diabetes is difficult to treat and requires more time and resources than they have available. Patients with type 2 diabetes have been shown not to view their condition as seriously as the healthcare professionals who are trying to help them manage it. As a result, poor control of risk factors is widespread particularly in the young.

In addition, there is concern over overmedicalisation of another 'precursor condition' such as impaired glucose tolerance.

Maybe we could prevent diabetes then? There are two strategies on the table – lifestyle interventions and drugs.

We know that intensive support and training can prevent diabetes in those with impaired glucose tolerance as well as improve the control of those already diagnosed. But less than intensive support tends to fail and effects are difficult to replicate in the real world.

Which brings us to drugs. Most anti-diabetic drugs reduce glycosylated haemoglobin by around 1%. The older drugs, it seems, are the best. Metformin is hard to beat as a first choice in type 2 diabetes with effects that seem to go beyond an effect on blood glucose. It is cheap, has few side effects, less tendency to hypoglycaemia and can be used in heart failure with none of the drama of the glitazones. Orlistat has been shown to reduce the incidence of diabetes but doubts have plagued the glitazones.

What we know already:

- A population strategy for screening for type 2 diabetes does not appear to fulfil WHO criteria – universal screening is impractical and too expensive. High-risk groups should be sought more intensively and screened opportunistically.

CARDIOVASCULAR

- People at high risk of diabetes and cardiovascular complications should be closely followed even if fasting glucose is normal. Targeting should include considerations such as ethnic origin, obesity, and family history.
- Meta-analysis has shown that the relative risk for CHD associated with diabetes is 50% higher in women than it is in men. This may be due to treatment bias that favours men or to a more adverse risk profile in women who do tend to have higher BP and worse lipids, particularly if diabetic.
- Various diabetic risk scores looking at combinations of risk factors in specific populations have been developed. A US study found a cost-effective strategy for diabetes screening was to target hypertensives over the age of 55.
- One US study found that only 7% of the diabetic participants were within recommended targets for HbA1c, cholesterol and blood pressure.
- Beta blockers can be used for diabetics in cardiac failure without worrying about worsening glycaemic control.
- Meta-analysis found that metformin is not associated with an increased risk of lactic acidosis or with an increase in lactate levels.
- Dyslipidaemia is a consistent finding in those with type 2 diabetes and the risk of MI in diabetics is as high whether or not they have had an MI in the past. Routine prescription of statins particularly in older patients should now be considered.
- The DIAD Study – Detection of Ischaemia in Asymptomatic Diabetics – detected signs of coronary disease in 22% of type 2 diabetics who were asymptomatic for cardiovascular disease, perhaps supporting a role for more intensive medication.
- Meta-analysis supports the use of statins even in primary prevention of cardiovascular disease in diabetics. Target cholesterol thresholds remain to be clarified.
- Evidence only supports the use of ACE inhibitors in type 1 diabetes with nephropathy and the use of ACE inhibitors or ARBs in type 2 diabetes with nephropathy.
- Nephropathy has been shown to be an independent risk factor for early cardiovascular death in diabetic patients. Microalbuminuria is associated with a twofold to fourfold increase in the risk of deaths. Overt proteinuria and hypertension compound the risk.
- A coffee intake of seven cups per day seems to halve the chance of developing diabetes compared to drinking one or two cups per day, mechanism unknown.
- NICE only recommends self-testing of blood glucose as part of integrated self care and does not advocate routine testing. Glycaemic control has not been shown to improve and it can amplify a sense of failure and self-blame.

Key trials

The United Kingdom Prospective Diabetes Study (UKPDS)

This was a landmark study of over 5000 diabetics. It was published in 1998 and showed the value of tight blood pressure control in type 2 diabetics. Heart failure was reduced by 56% and strokes by 44%. Although reduction in myocardial infarction alone was not significant, when combined with other vascular end points (i.e. sudden death, stroke, and peripheral vascular disease) reduction was 34%.

Tight control also had considerable benefits on the development of retinopathy and proteinuria.

Other lessons were that:

- Drug treatment is markedly better than diet in terms of any diabetic related end-point
- Metformin should be the drug of choice especially in the obese as it is the only oral hypo-glycaemic agent proved to reduce cardiovascular risk in this group
- The group treated with metformin had no hypoglycaemia and less weight gain
- Intensive glycaemic control resulted in reduced microvascular complications and fewer diabetic end-points than less intense control but no difference in mortality
- Further analysis showed that the level of glycaemic control is more important than the nature of the therapy and that even small reductions in HbA1c will prevent diabetic deaths

DCCT (Diabetes Control and Complications Trial)
Another landmark study showed that intensive efforts in glycaemic control benefited type 1 diabetics by reducing microvascular complications. But it also increased the number of hypoglycaemic episodes and the need for monitoring.

HOPE (Heart Outcomes Prevention Evaluation) and microHOPE study
This 5 year study included 9297 patients who were aged 55 years or older with a history of vascular disease or diabetes, plus one other cardiovascular risk factor. It included 3577 mainly type 2 diabetics and participants were given the ACE inhibitor ramipril or placebo.

Systolic blood pressure decreased by 2–3 mmHg in the ramipril group and reduced combined myocardial infarction, strokes, and deaths from cardiovascular diseases by 25%. The relative risk reduction for myocardial infarction was 22%, stroke 33%, and cardiovascular death 37%. It was reported in 2005 that the benefits observed in HOPE were maintained during 2.6 years of post-trial follow-up for cardiovascular death, stroke, and hospitalisation for heart failure.

The Microalbuminuria, Cardiovascular, and Renal Outcomes in HOPE (MICRO-HOPE) substudy showed that ramipril treatment was also associated with a reduced risk of developing nephropathy. It was concluded that ACE inhibitors should be first-line treatment for blood pressure control in diabetics and may have a role in normotensive patients.

As well as protecting against complications of diabetes, ramipril also significantly lowered the number with a new diagnosis of diabetes by 34%.

Two meta-analyses (*Diabetes Care,* 2005; **28**: 2261–2266 and *J Am Coll Cardiol,* 2005; **46**: 821–826) confirmed that either ACE inhibitors or ARBs at a pre-diabetic stage reduce the incidence of type 2 diabetes by approximately 25%. These medications may find an increasing role in areas such as metabolic syndrome, impaired fasting glucose and those with a family history of diabetes.

Heart Protection Study
This was a randomised placebo-controlled trial designed to determine whether the lipid-lowering agent simvastatin reduced mortality and vascular events in 20 536 high risk patients aged 40–80 years with and without coronary disease. Patients had a broad range of baseline cholesterol levels. It showed that in high-risk patients including diabetics without previous coronary heart disease, simvastatin reduced all-cause mortality, coronary deaths, strokes and major vascular events. The authors suggest a role for routine use of statins in high-risk diabetics regardless of cholesterol level.

CARDIOVASCULAR

DREAM (the Diabetes REduction Assessment with ramipril and rosiglitazone Medication)

Looking prospectively into the possibility that ACE inhibitor treatment with ramipril may prevent new diabetes, DREAM has so far failed to confirm that it reduced the risk of diabetes in non-diabetic patients at high risk of the disease.

However, rosiglitazone at 8 mg per day substantially reduced the incidence of type 2 diabetes and increased the likelihood of regression to normoglycaemia Follow up research has shown that it too led to 'relapse' on withdrawal, implying it is a treatment rather than a preventative (*Lancet,* 2006; **368**: 1096–1105).

Guidelines

The National Service Framework (NSF) on Diabetes laid out 12 standards of care for all aspects of the management of diabetes in December 2001 and produced a delivery strategy in January 2003. These are available on the Department of Health's website.

NICE has a series of guidelines for type 1 and type 2 diabetes. It recommended in August 2003 that treatment with thiazolidinediones (glitazones) for type 2 diabetes should be reserved for those who cannot tolerate the combination of metformin and a sulphonylurea. They should replace the less well tolerated drug. Insulin treatment should not be delayed when treatment with metformin and a sulphonylurea has failed.

Recent Papers

SCREENING

Psychological impact of screening for type 2 diabetes: controlled trial and comparative study embedded in the ADDITION Cambridge randomised controlled trial
Eborall HC, Griffin SJ, Prevost AT, *et al.*
BMJ, 2007; **335**: 486

Would the benefits of screening for diabetes in primary care be outweighed by the terrible psychological stress of being screened?

Not according to this study of 7380 adult in 15 practices in Cambridge. They used a stepwise approach which seemed to 'break it to people gently'.

The Anglo-Danish-Dutch study of intensive treatment in people with screen-detected diabetes in primary care (the ADDITION trial) used random blood glucose, fasting blood glucose and HbA1c and confirmed positive cases with an OGTT.

There were no important psychological costs between those screened and control participants.

Patients' experiences of screening for type 2 diabetes: prospective qualitative study embedded in the ADDITION Cambridge randomised trial
Eborall H, Davies R, Kinmonth A-L, *et al.*
BMJ, 2007; **335**: 490

The main aim of the ADDITION trial is to examine the cost-effectiveness of screening for diabetes and treating positive cases intensively. This small sub-study found that it was the stepwise nature of the programme that reduced psychological harm. Patients were able to adjust and rationalise each step of the way. This seemed to prepare them and minimise the harm from results giving them lower overall anxiety levels.

Hopefully the importance of the disease was not downplayed along the way.

Screening for diabetes
Stolk RP
BMJ, 2007; **335**: 457–458

Although screening for diabetes has been proposed for years as a way of preventing cardiovascular disease, two questions remain:
- will treating asymptomatic hyperglycaemia prevent cardiovascular disease?
- what psychological harm will be caused by screening or diagnosing diabetes and the lifelong use of drugs?

The first question awaits the further results of the ADDITION trial to see if we should start trying to identify those with even so much as a slightly raised blood glucose. Meanwhile we are still waiting for them to present with thirst, polyuria and weight loss, symptoms which may only kick in at relatively high levels of blood glucose.

The two studies above answer the second question in relation to targeted screening as opposed to mass screening. Targeted screening is otherwise known as case-finding or opportunistic screening amongst higher risk groups.

ADDITION targeted those at an increased risk of cardiovascular disease so some may have already been prepared by, say, advice on obesity or their use of antihypertensives. It is possible that the advantages may not translate to a more widespread population approach.

PREVENTION

Pharmacological and lifestyle interventions to prevent or delay type 2 diabetes in people with impaired glucose tolerance: systematic review and meta-analysis
Gillies CL, Abrams KR, Lambert PC
BMJ, 2007; **334**: 299

The value of preventing the growing epidemic of diabetes requires finding interventions that work. This meta-analysis included over 8000 patients and found that both lifestyle and pharmacological measures reduced the rate or progression of type 2 diabetes in those with impaired glucose tolerance. The interventions looked at were lifestyle-related, oral antidiabetic drugs, orlistat, or the herbal jiangtang bushen recipe. The interventions each roughly halved the risk of diabetes.

CARDIOVASCULAR

Interventions which improve diet and exercise are more likely to be sustained than drugs but they still do not last forever. They need to be reinforced. However, they have by far fewer and less serious side effects than drug therapy.

Most of the drugs used to prevent diabetes do so just so long as the drug is taken. In the Diabetes Prevention Programme, stopping metformin caused progression to type 2 diabetes, as did stopping the (now discontinued) troglitazone. Serious side effects of newer drugs have recently come to light and require further research.

The authors wonder whether what is essentially a lifestyle issue should be treated so early with lifelong medication?

The commentary in *Evidence-Based Medicine* (2007; **12:** 108) reminds us of the DREAM trial where rosiglitazone reduced progression to type 2 diabetes by 60%, but washout data suggest a loss of this advantage soon after discontinuation. Given the additional disadvantages of excess fractures, weight gain, and a sevenfold incidence in heart failure, it seems better to hit the gym.

Waking up from the DREAM of preventing diabetes with drugs
Montori VM, Isley WL, Guyatt GH
BMJ, 2007; **334:** 882–884

The results of the DREAM trial promoted aggressive marketing of rosiglitazone as a way of preventing a worldwide epidemic of diabetes. Medicalisation of pre-disease states and risk factors has huge marketing potential.

The trial was stopped early due to benefit in the treatment arm. The trial's primary outcome was a composite endpoint for death and diabetes, but these authors find that approach flawed. Rosiglitazone, they point out, had no effect on all cause mortality – "an outcome of great importance".

The claim is that all the drug is doing is lowering glucose. Is that really the same as preventing diabetes? The DREAM investigators are conducting a discontinuation study to see if diabetes is present after withdrawal of the drug. If so, all it has been doing is treatment of diabetes not prevention. Early indications say this is likely.

Patients may prefer not to develop diabetes. It causes inconvenience to their lifestyle. It may mess up their insurance policy. It might lead to depression. But will early diagnosis and treatment prevent heart disease? Perhaps not. Glitazones increase heart failure. They reduce bone density which may lead to fracture and premature death in older women. (The US released a safety alert regarding excess fractures with pioglitazone in March 2007.)

The benefits then are speculative and the population targeted by marketing is potentially huge. Use of the drugs to prevent diabetes is "impossible to justify".

First do no harm. It's back to the gym.

Rosiglitazone increases risk of MI but does not differ from other drugs for CV death in type 2 diabetes. *Evidence-Based Medicine,* 2007; **12:** 169–170
The following paper is reviewed
Effect of rosiglitazone on the risk of myocardial infarction and death from cardiovascular causes
Nissen SE, Wolski K
N Engl J Med, 2007; **356:** 2457–2471

> Meta-analysis of 42 RCTs with nearly 28 000 participants concluded that rosiglitazone increased the risk of myocardial infarction and cardiovascular death, sparking a huge controversy and calls for regulation for the drug.
> The commentary points to numerous flaws in the data collection which drew on a lot of low quality studies with incomplete access to important data. We are reminded that the results of meta-analysis may fail to predict the results of subsequent definitive trials.

Rosiglitazone evaluated for cardiovascular outcomes – an interim analysis
Home PD, Pocock SJ, Beck-Nielsen H, *et al.*
N Engl J Med, 2007; **357:** 28–38

> The paper above also caused the release of interim results of the RECORD trial – Rosiglitazone Evaluated for Cardiac Outcomes and Regulation of glycaemia in Diabetes. This study of 4458 type 2 diabetic patients in 23 countries found that rosiglitazone increased the risk of heart failure and also inconclusively indicated a tendency towards a higher incidence of MI. However, there was no difference compared to metformin plus sulphonylurea for other cardiovascular outcomes.
> We know about the risk of heart failure from rosiglitazone which results from fluid retention and is reversible on discontinuation. But more data are needed to confirm the risk of cardiac death and MI. In years to come the ACCOR trial and BARI-2D trials should shed some light.

Rosiglitazone and implications for pharmacovigilance
Kazi D
BMJ, 2007; **334:** 1233–1234

> This editorial expresses concern at a risk of misclassification of some data in the meta-analysis by Nissen and Wolski which could alter results markedly. Adding the study of Home *et al.* to the data shows a significant increase in MI. Prospective trials disagree but it may not be possible to prevent an exodus of subjects from these trials.
> Rosiglitazone's popularity has increased steadily with over one million prescriptions in the year ending March 2006 in England alone, a 22% increase over the previous year.
> The editorial expresses dismay at the regulatory processes which monitor drug safety. Pharmacovigilance is the weak link in the chain of drug development. Post-marketing surveillance results in a patchwork of small sponsored trials many of which go unpublished. This is particularly risky for a drug like rosiglita-

zone that comes from a family of drugs notorious for serious side effects and which itself is known to cause heart failure, anaemia and raised LDL. GlaxoSmithKline was never required to conduct a thorough post-marketing survey.

A sea change in the existing culture is needed with more systematic methods to ensure safety. At the moment we will have to weigh up the risk on a case by case basis bearing in mind the fragility of the evidence, but also the availability of cheaper, better drugs.

Long-term risk of cardiovascular events with Rosiglitazone
Singh S, Loke YK, Furberg CD
JAMA, 2007; **298:** 1189–1195

Further meta-analysis of four trials using rosiglitazone for at least 12 months has confirmed an association with a significantly increased risk of MI (by 42%) and twice the risk of heart failure but no sign of any excess deaths as a result.

Pioglitazone and risk of cardiovascular events in patients with type 2 diabetes mellitus – a meta-analysis of randomized trials
Lincoff AM, Wolski K, Nicholls SJ, Nissen SE
JAMA, 2007; **298:** 1180–1188

Pioglitazone on the other hand was associated with a significantly lower risk of death, MI, or stroke (by around 18%) in this meta-analysis of 19 trials enrolling 16 390 diabetics.

Serious heart failure was increased by pioglitazone as expected, although without an associated increase in mortality.

Diabetes and lipid lowering: where are we?
Reckless JPD
BMJ, 2006; **332**: 1103–1104

NICE endorses use of statins in people with an absolute risk of 20% over 10 years as effective and cost-effective, particularly when using generics. This editorial clarifies the situation now that we are sure that statins cut cardiovascular risk in type 2 diabetes.

- All patients with diabetes should be considered for, and most likely receive, a statin if their LDL cholesterol is ≥ 2 mmol/l
- Less research is available about type 1 diabetes, but statins are indicated for those aged 40 years or over
- The role of fibrates is not as clear. They will remain second line agents and fenofibrate beats gemfibrozil as the agent of choice

Impact of self monitoring of blood glucose in the management of patients with non-insulin treated diabetes: open parallel group randomised trial
Farmer A, Wade A, Goyder E, *et al.*
BMJ, 2007; **335**: 132

The DiGEM study – Diabetes Glycaemic Education and Monitoring – in 48 UK general practices had 453 participants with type 2 diabetes and an average age of 66 years. They looked at the effect of self-monitoring of blood glucose three times a day twice a week with or without additional training to interpret the results.

Although commonly recommended for type 1 diabetes, studies in type 2 diabetes had mixed support of this fairly expensive intervention. Compared to usual care, self monitoring made no difference at 12 months to the level of control as measured by HbA1c or any other risk factor.

These patients had reasonably well-controlled diabetes, but only 15% of those eligible entered the study, limiting the generalisability of the findings. Patients who were already testing were excluded.

Commentary in *Evidence-Based Medicine* (2008; **13**: 7) reminds us that there is scepticism in this approach all round. Benefits in diabetics treated with tablets are minimal at best. We can now empower our patients with the confidence to discontinue testing.

Self monitoring of blood glucose in type 2 diabetes: longitudinal qualitative study of patients' perspectives
Peel E, Douglas M, Lawton J
BMJ, 2007; **335**: 493

This small Scottish survey performed in depth interviews with 18 patients over 4 years and found a lack of interest in glucometer readings.

- Few patients used the results to guide and maintain changes in lifestyle.
- There was difficulty in knowing what to do with abnormal readings.
- Patients perceived a lack of interest from health professionals about their results book. They were more interested in HbA1c.
- They perceived health professionals as inconsistent about the value and practicalities of self-management.
- Self monitoring is associated with feelings of personal failure and self blame particularly in female patients.
- If used at all, education needs to be specific and tailored to patient need.

CLINICAL ISSUES

CARDIOVASCULAR

ASTHMA

The Challenge

Asthma causes one in every 250 deaths worldwide. About 300 million people in the world have asthma and with increasing urbanisation and western lifestyles, a further 100 million cases are expected by 2025. Up to 1.4 million asthmatics in the UK are thought to have suboptimal control. It accounts for 8% of self-reported poor health in 18–64 year olds and 18 million working days are lost annually to asthma-related illness.

However, emerging evidence indicates that after years of increasing prevalence, the health-care burden of asthma seems to be levelling off in the UK and falling in some countries. Reasons are unclear and probably multifactorial, perhaps relating to improved use of inhaled cortico-steroids and changes in the incidence of atopy.

Self-management plans are becoming the cornerstone of high quality care. Review clinics to facilitate them are well established in primary care but only about one-third of eligible people attend asthma clinics for their annual review. Different models of review are always being experimented with. Using a trained asthma nurse to conduct telephone interviews to routinely follow up cases tends to be popular and can even reduce costs. Other specialist interventions such as nurse-led clinics targeted at schools and deprived areas can moderately improve uptake of review and symptom control, but such programmes tend to be expensive.

Nearly half of all asthmatics feel limited in their daily life as a result of their condition, putting asthma above diabetes but below arthritis as a chronic health problem. A greater recognition and focus on the psychological aspects of the illness should be a central part of any long-term therapeutic strategy.

What we know already:

- A 20-year longitudinal study of over 3000 patients with active asthma found they were about 12 times more likely to develop COPD than non-asthmatics, even after controlling for smoking. Perhaps these previously distinct entities may share common pathology.
- The START trial – Inhaled Steroid as Regular Therapy in Early Asthma – has demonstrated that early budesonide is both effective and cost-effective in early asthma for all ages.
- Doubling the dose of inhaled corticosteroids does not prevent asthma attacks, reduce symptom scores or reduce the need for oral steroids. Recommendations to double up on inhaled steroids are absent from the latest guidelines.
- Although inhaled steroids reduce the burden of asthma symptoms they do not have a disease modifying effect that persists after discontinuation.
- Smokers display steroid insensitivity. Prednisolone improves asthma control in never-smokers, but not in smokers. Smokers have six times as many exacerbations and barely respond to our most proven weapon.
- Leukotriene receptor antagonists have been found in systematic review to be less effective as a single agent than low doses of inhaled steroid.
- Prevalence of aspirin sensitivity in asthma has been shown to be higher than usually perceived at 21% in adults and 5% in children when determined by oral provocation testing.

- Aspirin-sensitive patients usually suffer cross-reactivity with other NSAIDs: ibuprofen, 98%; naproxen, 100%; and diclofenac, 93%. The incidence of cross-sensitivity to paracetamol among such patients was only 7%.
- The addition of routine peak flow monitoring to symptom-based self management does not improve outcome over symptom-based self-management alone in children.
- Stressful life events in children with chronic asthma lead to both acute and delayed exacerbations. Symptoms increased nearly fivefold within 2 days of a severely negative life event such as illness, death, separation and divorce.
- In a cohort of 199 children followed into adulthood, half did not outgrow asthma. Only 22% achieved complete remission. A further 30% reached clinical remission (no symptoms) but bronchial hyper-responsiveness remained.

Guidelines

British guideline on the management of asthma. British Thoracic Society/Scottish Intercollegiate Guidelines Network. *Thorax*, 2003; **58**: 1–94. May 2008 update at www.sign.ac.uk.

Recent Papers

MEDICATION

Beta agonists

Addition of salmeterol to usual asthma pharmacotherapy may increase respiratory related deaths or life threatening experiences. *Evidence-Based Medicine*, 2006; **11**: 139
The following paper is reviewed
The Salmeterol Multicenter Asthma Research Trial: a comparison of usual pharmacotherapy for asthma or usual pharmacotherapy plus salmeterol
Nelson HS, Weiss ST, Bleecker ER *et al*.
Chest, 2006; **129**: 15–26

The SMART study used more than 26 000 asthma patients in over 6000 sites in the US and sent a few alarm bells ringing when it had to be stopped early. The addition of salmeterol to usual asthma therapy (including steroids) was associated with an increase in asthma-related and respiratory death – an effect which may be more pronounced in African–Americans. Caution is advised when using long acting beta-2 agonists while research continues.

CLINICAL ISSUES

RESPIRATORY

Long acting ß agonists increase severe asthma exacerbations and asthma related deaths in children and adults. *Evidence-Based Medicine*, 2007; **12**: 10
The following paper is reviewed
Effect of long-acting beta-agonists on severe asthma exacerbations and asthma-related deaths
Salpeter SR, Buckley NS, Ormiston TM, *et al.*
Ann Intern Med, 2006; **144**: 904–912

This meta-analysis of 19 RCTs with nearly 34 000 participants looked at the implied dangers of long-acting beta agonists.

- In patients using them, hospital admissions for severe asthma exacerbations increased as did life-threatening asthma attacks.
- There was a small but significant increase in asthma-related death.
- The speculation is that regular use may increase bronchial hyperactivity. Symptoms may worsen without warning and impaired response to the usual beta agonists may cause the trouble.
- Those also taking steroid inhalers were not totally protected as their risk of hospital admission doubled too. The largest study – SMART above – was excluded as it did not look at admission rates.
- This review did not look at the combination of the long-acting beta agonists with steroid in single inhalers which is a more popular approach.
- The commentary concludes that in asthma long-acting beta agonists should not be used alone, only as a component of combined therapy.

Steroids

Use of inhaled corticosteroids during pregnancy and risk of pregnancy induced hypertension: nested case-control study
Martel MJ, Rey E, Beauchesne MF, *et al.*
BMJ, 2005; **330**: 230

Around 5% of women take drugs for asthma in pregnancy. This 10-year study of over 4500 pregnancies in asthmatics reassures us that there is no association between the use of inhaled steroids and pregnancy-induced hypertension or pre-eclampsia.

Markers of poor asthma control and use of oral steroids were each associated with increased risks of these two conditions.

Combination therapy

The correlation between asthma control and health status: the GOAL study
Bateman ED, Bousquet J, Keech ML and the GOAL Investigators
Eur Respir J, 2007; **29**: 56–62

The GOAL Investigators Group – Gaining Optimal Asthma ControL – looked at patients with uncontrolled asthma. It previously showed that step-wise increase of a salmeterol/fluticasone inhaler achieved 'Total Control' of symptoms (defined as being symptom-free for at least 7 out of 8 weeks) in a greater proportion and at lower steroid doses than fluticasone alone. They conclude that the noble aim of 'Total Control' is achievable and was achieved here in 41% compared to 28% with fluticasone alone.

A further study made an assessment using the Asthma Quality of Life Questionnaire and demonstrated improved quality of life with the GOAL method to levels approaching normality. This improvement was even distinguishable between those with Total Control and those with otherwise high levels of control.

Combined budesonide and formoterol for maintenance and relief provided better asthma control than budesonide for maintenance and terbutaline for relief. *Evidence-Based Medicine*, 2006; **11**: 138
The following paper is reviewed
Budesonide/formoterol in a single inhaler for maintenance and relief in mild-to-moderate asthma: a randomized, double-blind trial
Rabe KF, Pizzichini E, Ställberg B *et al.*
Chest, 2006; **129**: 246–256

Budesonide/formoterol in a single inhaler simplifies and improves asthma therapy for both maintenance and symptom relief beyond that of budesonide at a higher dose with terbutaline for relief. This forces patients to take extra doses of steroid when they need their reliever – something that often goes by the wayside in favour of extra rescue medication when symptoms worsen.

The combination more than halved the risk of severe exacerbations, led to 90% fewer asthma-related hospitalisations and 77% fewer treatment days with oral steroids.

It is not clear, however, from this study which ingredient should receive the credit.

Budesonide-formoterol for maintenance and as needed reliever treatment reduced asthma exacerbations. *Evidence-Based Medicine*, 2007; **12**: 9
The following paper is reviewed
Effect of budesonide in combination with formoterol for reliever therapy in asthma exacerbations: a randomised controlled, double-blind study
Rabe KF, Atienza T, Magyar P, *et al.*
Lancet, 2006; **368**: 744–753

Steroid–formoterol combinations are proving very successful.

This study compared budesonide–formoterol inhalers to as-needed formoterol or terbutaline. It looked at their use as relievers and their ability to reduce exacerbations. In 289 centres across 20 countries, 2294 patients were randomised.
- The budesonide–formoterol combination prolonged the time to a first severe exacerbation compared to the simple relievers, decreased symptom scores and increased peak flow and FEV_1 with fewer inhalations.
- Formoterol reduced severe exacerbations more than terbutaline.

The budesonide–formoterol combination is recommended as first line for moderate to severe asthma, being more efficacious than a long-acting beta agonist and a short-acting beta agonist used on their own for relief.

We now know that both of the ingredients individually result in improved asthma control.

RESPIRATORY

Using a combination inhaler (budesonide plus formoterol) as rescue therapy improves asthma control

Barnes PJ
BMJ, 2007; **335:** 513

The author puts the case strongly for the adoption of budesonide–formoterol combination inhalers as relievers, replacing the traditional use of a short-acting beta agonist in those with mild, moderate and severe asthma. Fewer puffs. Fewer admissions.

SMART stands for something else here: Single Inhaler Maintenance and Reliever Therapy. Inhaled formoterol is as fast as salbutamol as a reliever and even more effective. It is even better with the steroid built in, as compliance seems to improve, heading off exacerbations as they are brewing up. The fluticasone/salmeterol inhaler cannot be used as rescue therapy due to the slower onset of action of salmeterol.

Future products will cash in by combining formoterol with other steroids. But costs overall are likely to fall with this approach. It is simple and effectiveness has been shown even in children.

ONGOING MANAGEMENT

A randomized clinical trial of peak flow versus symptom monitoring in older adults with asthma

Buist AS, Vollmer WM, Wilson SR, *et al.*
Am J Respir Crit Care Med, 2006; **174:** 1077–1087

This study looked at nearly 300 adults, average age 66 years, with moderate to severe asthma. They kept a daily diary of symptoms and half of them also used peak flow measurements daily or as needed to adjust their treatment themselves. After 2 years there was no advantage of using peak flow over symptom monitoring alone in terms of lung function, use of services or quality of life.

The commentary in *Evidence-Based Medicine* (2007; **12:** 49) suggests the patients may not be as severe as claimed and the use of PFR may not be optimal. They seemed to have looked at personal bests and chosen a cut-off point of 60%, which may be a little too arbitrary for patients with different variability of PFR.

However, the conclusion seems to be that symptom-based action plans seem to be sufficient for most elderly patients.

Accessibility, clinical effectiveness, and practice costs of providing a telephone option for routine asthma reviews: phase IV controlled implementation study

Pinnock H, Adlem L, Gaskin S, *et al.*
Br J Gen Pract, 2007; **57:** 714–722

A large UK general practice with 1809 asthma patients compared telephone review of its asthma patients with face-to-face review and concluded:
- a routine asthma review was achieved in 66% of patients in the telephone-option group compared with 55% in the face-to-face-only group
- no detriment in morbidity resulted

- enablement and confidence in asthma management were greater in the telephone-option versus the face-to-face-only group
- the cost per telephone review was around 20% lower than the face-to-face-only service
- routinely offering telephone reviews is a practical and cost-effective way to increase asthma review rates

RESPIRATORY

CHRONIC OBSTRUCTIVE PULMONARY DISEASE

The Challenge

COPD is one of the commonest causes of death in the UK and is largely a disease of vulnerable smokers. Admissions for acute exacerbations have increased by 50% in the last decade and sit at around 90 000 admissions per year. An average stay of 11 days means a million bed days a year in the UK. Annual NHS costs attributable to COPD have been estimated at around £1 billion.

COPD has been significantly underdiagnosed in the past. It is diagnosed if the patient has an FEV_1 of less than 70% of predicted normal and an FEV_1/FVC ratio of less than 70%, with less than 15% reversibility. Spirometry improves detection rates of COPD and its use is promoted in the current GP contract.

Only smoking cessation and oxygen have been shown to alter the natural history of the disease. However, pulmonary rehabilitation is effective in the short to medium term in improving exercise tolerance, smoking cessation, symptoms and quality of life. Its role is firmly established and advocated, as are recommendations for the availability of ambulatory oxygen. Unfortunately suitable rehabilitation programmes are by no means universally available. As a result, physicians continue to prescribe expensive pharmacotherapy that is considerably less effective for a disease that by definition is resistant to drug treatment. In addition the ongoing fears over the use of long acting beta agonists add to the complexity of treatment.

We should focus our efforts on interventions that really work like smoking cessation, as well as making sure we do not mistake asthma for COPD.

What we know already:

- The 2004 NICE guidelines, unlike other guidelines, make no recommendation to measure the post-bronchodilator change in spirometry to assist in identifying reversibility. It uses symptoms to guide treatment rather than a percentage drop in FEV_1.
- Beta agonist inhalers – both short and long acting and particularly in combination with a steroid – modestly improve lung function and symptoms.
- Meta-analysis shows that inhaled corticosteroids taken for more than 2 years reduce the progression of airflow limitation. Benefits, however, are small at only 7.7 ml/year of FEV_1 gained. More severe patients benefit more.
- Salmeterol can give symptomatic and physiological improvements in severe COPD despite 'non-reversibility' on spirometry.
- Prevention of exacerbations of COPD is a major target. Analysis indicates that use of a budesonide/formoterol inhaler has a NNT to prevent one such exacerbation of only 2.
- There is an absence of high quality data to support the use of theophylline or amino-phylline to treat exacerbations of COPD for either symptoms or lung function.
- A Dutch study worked-up over 400 patients with a diagnosis of COPD but without a diagnosis of heart failure and found that as many as 20% had previously unrecognised heart failure. None had right-sided heart failure.

- Hospital at home with nursing support may not be appropriate for everybody but is as safe as hospital care in terms of end points of re-admission and death. Costs can be saved by reducing the number of extended hospital stays.
- Health professionals do not discuss prognosis with COPD patients as openly as with cancer patients. Recognition of the serious nature of the disease needs to be reflected in our communication.

Guidelines

National clinical guideline on management of chronic obstructive pulmonary disease in adults in primary and secondary care. National Collaborating Centre for Chronic Conditions for NICE. *Thorax*, 2004; **59**(suppl 1): 1–232.

Global strategy for the diagnosis, management, and prevention of chronic obstructive pulmonary disease. GOLD – Global Initiative for Chronic Obstructive Lung Disease. World Health Organization, 2007. These guidelines now refer to COPD as 'preventable and treatable' in order to present a positive outlook and stimulate effective programmes.

Recent Papers

Developing COPD: a 25 year follow up study of the general population
Løkke A, Lange P, Scharling H *et al*.
Thorax, 2006; **61**: 935–939

This extensive study analysed information and lung function tests from over 8000 men and women aged over 30 years to determine the 25-year absolute risk of developing COPD in the general population.
- The percentage of men with normal lung function ranged from 96% of never smokers to 59% of continuous smokers.
- They estimate that COPD goes undiagnosed in 80% of those with the condition.
- More than one-third of those with COPD were still smoking.
- Sufferers were more likely to be older, manual workers, male and more socio-economically deprived.
- The 25-year incidence of moderate and severe COPD was 20.7% and 3.6%, respectively.
- Deaths from COPD constituted 3.7% of all deaths and, as expected, there were almost no COPD deaths during the first 10 years of follow up.
- COPD is becoming as common in women as in men. Although women may be slightly more susceptible to tobacco, men smoke more to make up for this difference.
- Absolute risk is an easier concept to convey to patients and at around 25% the absolute risk of developing COPD among continuous smokers is larger than previously estimated.

CLINICAL ISSUES

RESPIRATORY

SPIROMETRY

A randomized controlled trial on office spirometry in asthma and COPD in standard general practice
Lusuardi M, De Benedetto F, Paggiaro P *et al*.
Chest, 2006; **129**: 844–852

The charmingly named SPACE program – Spirometry in Asthma and COPD: a Comparative Evaluation – was a 9 month prospective Italian study that failed to demonstrate that spirometry can help GPs identify asthma and COPD earlier.

Evaluation of possible cases was made with and without spirometry by 570 trained GPs. Specialists were blinded while checking the diagnoses but found no improvement in accuracy where spirometry had been used.

High initial ratings by the GPs in terms of feasibility and usefulness tailed off dramatically and one-quarter failed to respond to the study by the end.

An accompanying editorial suggests the method is best offered only to smokers with dyspnoea on exertion. Clearly, work is needed on the model of clinical back-up that best supports the role of spirometry in primary care.

Effect of primary care spirometry on the diagnosis and management of COPD
Walker PP, Mitchell P, Diamantea F *et al.*
Eur Respir J, 2006; **28**: 945–952

This study offered an open access service to a primary care area in the UK between 1999 and 2003 in which over 1500 patients were referred for spirometry and reversibility testing.
- 53% had pre-bronchodilator airflow obstruction.
- 19% of subjects responded fully to reversibility testing.
- Half of those in whom obstruction persisted received a diagnosis of COPD.
- COPD was significantly undertreated prior to spirometry.
- Testing led to considerable increases in prescribing of anti-cholinergics, beta agonists and inhaled steroids.

This well-organised service is a good model of how spirometry can be useful in uncovering COPD, improving treatment and avoiding misdiagnosis by using reversibility testing.

Primary care spirometry: test quality and the feasibility and usefulness of specialist reporting
White P, Wong W, Fleming T, Gray B
Br J Gen Pract, 2007; **57**: 701–705

Now that spirometry is a requirement in primary care, are we any good at it? Well, no. Not yet.

This study in large practices in London found that there were lots of clinically relevant disagreements when interpreting the results when compared to specialist reports.

Differences in opinion about the quality of the data, the diagnosis and the severity of the condition occurred in one-third of tests.

We know spirometry is feasible in terms of doing it, but now we need to do it adequately.

Room for improvement then.

MANAGEMENT

Long acting ß$_2$ adrenoceptor agonists are effective in poorly reversible chronic obstructive pulmonary disease. *Evidence-Based Medicine,* 2007; **12**: 12
The following paper is reviewed
Long-acting beta-2 agonists for poorly reversible chronic obstructive pulmonary disease
Appleton S, Poole P, Smith B, *et al.*
Cochrane Database Syst Rev, 2006

> This Cochrane review took in 23 RCTs and 6061 patients. It compared inhaled salmeterol or formoterol with placebo in patients with moderately severe but stable COPD (without asthma). Subjects qualified for the study by virtue of poor reversibility to a dose of a short acting beta-2 agonist.
>
> Salmeterol and formoterol reduced exacerbations in these patients and improved both lung function (FEV$_1$ and FVC) and quality of life. The gains were small but statistically significant, but what about the fear of mortality with such drugs?

Anticholinergics but not ß$_2$ agonists reduce exacerbations requiring hospital admission and respiratory deaths in COPD. *Evidence-Based Medicine,* 2007; **12**: 13
The following paper is reviewed
Meta-analysis: anticholinergics, but not beta-agonists, reduce severe exacerbations and respiratory mortality in COPD
Salpeter SR, Buckley NS, Salpeter EE
J Gen Intern Med, 2006; **21**: 1011–1019

> Anticholinergics such as ipratropium and tiotropium may be better than beta agonists such as salmeterol, formoterol and albuterol at reducing exacerbations of COPD. According to this meta-analysis of 22 RCTs and over 15 000 subjects, beta agonists as a group also increase the risk of respiratory death.
>
> Combining short and long acting anticholinergics in one study may muddy the waters when trying to draw conclusions. The commentary on the two papers above reveals concerns about the rigidity of the conclusions when mortality was not designed as a primary end point and numbers were small.
>
> Anticholinergics even seemed to increase survival but both these conclusions are premature without better data. Evidence is currently too weak to say definitively which group of drugs works better than the other or confirm the mortality worries. Combination therapies, however, do provide hope for the future.

Salmeterol and fluticasone propionate and survival in chronic obstructive pulmonary disease
Calverley PM, Anderson JA, Celli B, *et al.*
N Engl J Med, 2007; **356:** 775–789

The TORCH investigators (TOwards a Revolution in COPD Health) have a large (*n*=6112) ongoing trial looking at the use of a long acting beta agonist, an inhaled steroid, both or neither.

Results over 3 years confirm the symptomatic benefit of the medicines but still cannot say for certain if they actually save lives. Combination therapy seems to do so but just misses statistical significance by a whisper.

Encouragingly, at least none of the approaches increase mortality in this study and plenty of other outcome measures improved. Those given an inhaled steroid – fluticasone – alone or in combination, however, had a small but significant increase in risk of pneumonia.

LONG-TERM CARE

Oxygen treatment at home
Gibson GJ
BMJ, 2006; **332:** 191–192

Long-term oxygen for hypoxaemic COPD improves survival. This paper refers to the February 2006 changes in the supplying of oxygen to patients in England and Wales.

Although GPs can still prescribe oxygen, this is likely to be more for emergency and palliative care purposes.

More detailed assessment of new candidates for oxygen at home and ambulatory oxygen will be coordinated by hospital respiratory and paediatric services, in liaison with companies that service regional NHS contracts.

Those suitable for ambulatory oxygen are usually those well-motivated patients who desaturate on exertion and demonstrate improvement when breathing oxygen during exercise – estimated as half of those currently receiving long-term oxygen therapy on the NHS.

The intention is for the changes to be cost-neutral, with the costs of the increased staffing required for these more detailed evaluations hopefully offset by savings in inappropriate prescribing. It will be tricky, however, to get those who have had oxygen inappropriately prescribed to understand that shortage of breath does not necessarily mean shortage of oxygen, but this rationalisation should provide an improved service. Children, for example, need frequent reassessments as they grow and many will probably benefit from ambulatory oxygen.

RESPIRATORY INFECTION AND ANTIBIOTICS

The Challenge

Most prescribing of antibiotics takes place in primary care. In Western countries, withholding antibiotics for minor complaints such as otitis media, rhinitis, conjunctivitis and sore throat can be considered harmless as complications such as rheumatic fever, mastoiditis and quinsy have become rare. Clinical guidelines advise against the routine use of antibiotics and for a while it seemed the message was getting through. Prescribing rates by GPs in the UK declined by 45% between 1994 and 2000. Halving the prescribing of antibiotics to children did not lead to an increase in hospital admissions for peritonsillar abscess or rheumatic fever.

In qualitative interviews, GPs have taken the credit for these reductions in prescribing. Most know that antibiotics are generally unnecessary. They claim to have responded to research, local advice and published reports that advised reductions in antibiotic prescribing. They were still more likely to prescribe for sicker and more deprived patients and justified this because of concerns about complications. They all felt their decision-making was "rational and systematic, informed by personal clinical experience and research evidence and influenced by advice from policy makers and local microbiologists". They are mostly comfortable with their decisions and happy they were not prescribing just to maintain the doctor–patient relationship.

However, this is a bit hard to swallow and at the very least a leap of faith because prescribing of antibiotics has actually been increasing in recent years. In 2000, antibiotics were still prescribed to two-thirds of patients presenting with respiratory infection, including over 90% of those with chest infection, 80% with ear infections, and 60% with sore throat. In fact it turns out that the main factor leading to reduced antibiotic prescribing prior to 2000 was a considerable reduction in the burden of disease rather than more targeted prescribing.

Why do we still do it? We know the possible benefits of antibiotics are generally minimal. Antibiotics have not been shown to be useful routinely in infections such as pharyngitis, otitis media, rhinitis, and sinusitis. Neither do they improve the course of most uncomplicated lower respiratory infections. Marginal benefits on rare long-term complications do not translate into cost-effectiveness in the UK population.

There is also plenty of downside in terms of side effects, costs, issues of resistance and the unfortunate medicalisation of self-limiting illness.

Navigating these consultations and re-educating patients and parents is a time-consuming job. The tired or lazy GP might resort to his prescription pad quickly. Clinical examination is certainly unreliable for differentiating between viral and bacterial infection yet we still have GPs diagnosing 'Strep throat' with a glance.

What is going wrong? The evidence suggests that GPs may perceive more pressure to prescribe than actually exists and by reducing prescribing we prevent future requests for consultation. Maybe we can blame the patients? But the evidence actually tells us that patients seem willing to tolerate a fair level of symptoms in order to avoid antibiotics. They are even keener to avoid their children having antibiotics.

In condoning the overuse of antibiotics, primary care has contributed to a huge problem. Patients have tended not to be aware or concerned about antibiotic resistance. The pace and development of new antibiotics have not kept up with the growth in antibiotic resistance and we may be approaching the end of the antibiotic era.

CLINICAL ISSUES

RESPIRATORY

Delayed prescribing is a useful additional tool in the consultation which may help bridge the expectation gap. It may help to avoid 'uncomfortable resolutions' to the consultation although the barrier to receiving the drugs could come over as 'untrusting and paternalistic'. Some GPs worry it makes them look incompetent, but studies have shown that after 3 days, only around 30% of delayed prescriptions are cashed in, with no adverse effects. Qualitative research suggests that once their patients were weaned off the expectation of antibiotics, the need for delayed prescriptions became redundant. This may be a useful intermediate step rather than going 'cold turkey'.

What we know already:

- Four out of ten people believe that antibiotics are effective in viral conditions.
- Simple prediction tools using clinical measures such as temperature, presence of exudates, enlarged cervical lymph nodes and absence of cough are imperfect but can help predict ß haemolytic streptococcal pharyngitis in combination with knowledge of local prevalence.
- Expected recovery from cough is consistently overestimated by clinicians. At 2 weeks, one in four has not recovered and one in eight may have a complication – such as rash or painful ears. Informing patients will align expectations.
- Cough syrup medicated with dextromorphan or diphenhydramine is no better than sugar water in suppressing night-time cough in children. Misunderstandings that these linctuses can shorten or 'cure' a respiratory illness persist. They promote reflex salivation as well as secretion of airway mucus and cure no better than placebo.
- Recent exposure to antibiotics can be strongly related to resistance within the same individual.
- Meta-analysis suggests that exposure to at least one course of antibiotics in the first year of life may predispose to asthma later in childhood with more courses possibly increasing the risk. More work is needed to verify this.
- A re-emergence of susceptibility to older semi-retired 'forgotten' antibiotics may give us another weapon in our antibacterial strategy. However, we may find that the bacteria 'recover' rapidly by reactivation of resistance-encoding genes.
- Human metapneumovirus (hMPV), first isolated in 2001, is an important new virus in young children. Over a 25 year period, 20% of children, mean age 12 months, with a lower respiratory infection tested positive for hMPV. It usually presented as bronchiolitis, but also as croup and exacerbations of asthma.

Guidance

UK Antimicrobial resistance strategy and action plan. *Dept of Health, 2000.*
This report describes how surveillance, prudent use of antimicrobials and infection control are the key elements to controlling resistance and maintaining the effectiveness of antibiotics.

Recent Papers

ANTIBIOTIC RESISTANCE

Effect of antibiotic prescribing on antibiotic resistance in individual children in primary care: prospective cohort study
Chung A, Perera R, Brueggemann AB, *et al.*
BMJ, 2007; **335:** 429

Resistance in an individual is directly measurable after a single course of anti-biotics.

The elements of resistance are mobile elements than can moves like plasmids between bacteria.

This study of 199 children under 12 years found that a course of amoxicillin doubled the chance of recovering one of these elements from the child's throat 2 weeks later, and caused resistance to ampicillin. A gene encoding lactamase had been transferred to *Haemophilus.*

Normalisation occurred by 12 weeks but the process is sufficient to sustain a high level of antibiotic resistance in the population and make it endemic in UK children.

The relationship between prescribing and resistance is complex. It has appeared to be weak in the UK as it depends of patterns of antibiotic use, interactions between bacterium and drug, and the stage of resistance that the particularly country is in. Denmark and Sweden have higher rates of prescribing but lower resistance whereas Finland has lower prescribing but higher resistance.

Prescribing in young children is high and, after recent improvements, may be rising again.

If a second course of antibiotics is required within 3 months it may be sensible to choose a beta lactamase producing strain rather than a further course of amoxicillin.

Prescribing antibiotics in primary care
Del Mar C
BMJ, 2007; **335:** 407–408

This editorial warns that antibiotic resistance will eventually appear for every new antibiotic we develop. The resource should be thought of like oil, a non-renewable resource to be carefully husbanded, claims the author.

Unfortunately we cannot stop people cashing it in for short term gain so the community may suffer.

Evidence based medicine has taught us that antibiotics are minimally effective against a host of infections, even those usually caused by bacteria such as acute otitis media, and the message is finally beginning to permeate. Tools such as delayed prescription help. Also, we now realise that resistance affects individuals, as well as populations so the prescribing may become easier to resist.

Future research may even be able to estimate whether people dying of infection died because of a prescription for trivia in the past.

RESPIRATORY

Or perhaps our model of 'attack by bacterium' needs refining. Bacteria-containing foods sell well. Perhaps we should look closer at what may just be an imbalance with our symbiotic friends.

All this stuff may help convince us to only use antibiotics when we really need them.

Avoiding antibacterial overuse in primary care
Drug Therap Bull, 2007; **45:** 25–29

This is an excellent review of the realities of prescribing antibiotics appropriately. The aim is cost-effectiveness to maximise therapeutic benefit while minimising drug-related toxicity. Unfortunately doctors get in the way of this and so do patients.

- Approaches such as delayed prescription help reduce use of antibacterials with no difference in outcomes.
- Generally, the modest benefits of antibiotics are counter-balanced by side effects.
- Short courses have been shown to be as effective as longer courses in several conditions and more research like this is useful.
- Clinical predictors and point of care tests which help to identify those in whom antibiotics would not work are also very desirable.

DELAYED PRESCRIPTIONS

Delayed prescribing of antibiotics for upper respiratory tract infection
Little P
BMJ, 2005; **331:** 301–302

Widespread adoption of delayed prescribing since 1997 may explain the reduction in the proportion of prescriptions delivered to the pharmacist in recent years.

Asking the patient to return for the prescription means few ending up taking antibiotics but given the higher reconsultation rates, this is not clearly preferable. This editorial explains that we cannot turn our back on antibiotics for uncomplicated respiratory infections. After all, there are expectations and occasionally complications. Delayed prescriptions are a compromise that seem to re-educate patients gently. Don't leave it any longer than 72 hours to recheck an otitis media for the need for antibiotics and you should be fine.

CHEST INFECTION

Protective effect of antibiotics against serious complications of common respiratory tract infections: retrospective cohort study with the UK General Practice Research Database
Petersen I, Johnson AM, Islam A, *et al.*
BMJ, 2007; **335**: 982

This large cohort study looked at the risk of complications in over 3 million respiratory infections in UK general practice. The data were taken from 162 practices between 1991 and 2001. They use the term chest infection to cover acute bronchitis where antibiotics are not routinely recommended and pneumonia where antibiotics are recommended.

Serious complications were viewed as mastoiditis after otitis media, quinsy after sore throat and pneumonia after respiratory infection.

- Antibiotics reduced the complications with a NNT of 4000 overall.
- Community-acquired pneumonia is a life-threatening condition. Risk of this in the month after a diagnosis of chest infection was high in the elderly. Antibiotics protected against this substantially.
- NNT was relatively modest at 39 in the over 65s and the same in smokers and those with COPD and cardiac disease.
- GPs should not base their prescribing on the risk of rare, serious complications. It is now unlikely that a study large enough to measure these effects will ever be conducted.
- Research should focus on algorithms and technologies to enable confident distinction between bronchitis and early pneumonia.

The study has certain design limitations. The term 'chest infection' will probably be used to include bronchitis and pneumonia although this study excluded cases coded as pneumonia at presentation. They accept that the term acute bronchitis was rarely coded and that, without X ray, it is clinically indistinguishable from pneumonia. This misclassification could have overestimated the risk of pneumonia after chest infection. The term pneumonia may even have been used to justify the use of antibiotics.

The design of the study does not allow analysis of length of illness, cough, days off work or fever.

Antibiotics for respiratory tract infections in primary care
Coenen S, Goossens H
BMJ, 2007; **335**: 946–947

An accompanying editorial reminds us that the non-randomised nature of the study above means that patients with more severe disease will be more likely to be treated with antibiotics. Study randomisation eliminates confounding but generally lacks sufficient power to study rare events and participants may not be representative of those seen in practice.

In industrialised countries the rarity of complications means that most infections can be managed by watchful waiting.

For lower respiratory infections we cannot be confident about who will benefit from antibiotics and who will not. Further research into microbiologically based diagnosis is ongoing.

CLINICAL ISSUES

RESPIRATORY

Management of community acquired pneumonia
Bjerre LM
BMJ, 2007; **335:** 1004–1005

Although mainly referring to hospital treatment, this editorial draws attention to the controversial area of the need to cover atypical pathogens in diagnosis of community acquired pneumonia. Levels can reach 28% in Europe, making drugs that have atypical coverage (macrolides, tetracycline, fluroquinolones) more appealing.

Use of these drugs reduces total mortality and improves the level of clinical stability at 1 week. Perhaps a switch to these antibiotics would be appropriate in pneumonia patients who have not responded to first line antibiotics in a few days.

Community acquired pneumonia in primary care
Goossens H, Little P
BMJ, 2006; **332:** 1045–1046

This editorial highlights the lack of evidence which could help us target antibiotics towards high risk patients.

There is a lack of adequately powered studies giving us good prediction rules for adverse outcomes in community-acquired pneumonia. Doctors still use their own arbitrary criteria and seldom have the advantage of a chest X-ray or microbiology. Times may change. Rapid nucleic acid detection assays and amplification techniques are showing promise as diagnostic tools in LRTI and molecular diagnostics is expected to boom in the next decade. When we get rapid answers at an affordable price we will no longer have to rely on nineteenth century methods and can hope to be able to combat resistance and preserve our remaining antibiotics.

Information leaflet and antibiotic prescribing strategies for acute lower respiratory tract infection. A randomized controlled trial
Little P, Rumsby K, Kelly J *et al.*
JAMA, 2005; **293:** 3029–3035

This UK study included over 800 adults and children with cough and at least one other symptom referable to the lower respiratory tract (coloured sputum, chest pain, dyspnoea, or wheezing). Asthma and COPD were excluded. The authors found:
- antibiotics provided little or no benefit for patients with cough and lower respiratory tract symptoms, including fever and green sputum
- cough lasted about 3 weeks in most patients regardless of treatment method, and for at least a month in 25%
- providing a verbal explanation about the expected course is required for patient satisfaction
- the duration of 'moderately bad' symptoms was shorter in the immediate antibiotic group, but only by one day
- elderly patients were less likely to benefit from antibiotics

- results for vulnerable subgroups and those with green sputum were no more convincing

---

Comparison of first-line with second-line antibiotics for acute exacerbations of chronic bronchitis
Dimopoulos G, Siempos II, Korbila IP
Chest, 2007; **132**: 447–455

Aware of increasing antibiotic resistance, this study compared first line antibiotics (such as amoxicillin, trimethoprim, and doxycycline) and second line antibiotic regimes (such as macrolides, quinolones, co-amoxiclav, and second and third generation cephalosporins) in exacerbations of chronic bronchitis.

Although not taking into account age or lung function, meta-analysis of 12 RCTs concluded that first line antibiotics were associated with lower treatment success (but not less safety) than second line antibiotics. Mortality was unaffected.

COUGH

Whooping cough in school age children with persistent cough: prospective cohort study in primary care
Harnden APR, Bruggemann AB, Mayon-White R *et al.*
BMJ, 2006; **333**: 174–177
and
Whooping cough in general practice
Butler C, Francis N, Dinant G
BMJ, 2006; **333**: 159–160

This article and accompanying editorial describes the underdiagnosis of *Bordetella* infection in school-age children of 5–16 years.

Precisely diagnosing the cause of persistent cough is difficult for GPs. Children often end up with empirical prescriptions for asthma inhalers or getting an unneeded chest X-ray.

GPs rarely diagnose or consider pertussis in these children, but in this cohort of 172 children in the UK who had a persistent cough lasting more than 2 weeks (and who consented to a blood test for serology and kept a cough diary), 37% had evidence of a recent *Bordetella* pertussis infection even though 85% of these had been fully immunised as children. Cough persisted for a median of 16 weeks.

Doctors do now recognise that acute cough persists longer than previously thought, irrespective of treatment, and ideally would be able to provide a confident diagnosis.

Unfortunately, laboratory testing is currently not considered very practical nor clinically important as there is little evidence that prescribing erythromycin reduces symptoms or prevents transmission.

GPs will need to think about this diagnosis even in immunised children and stop thinking of it just as a condition of very young children who whoop. New non-invasive salivary tests may help.

Now that we have a pre-school booster for pertussis, the reservoir of infection

RESPIRATORY

may reduce but perhaps we also need a booster in adolescents, as they have in the US.

Prednisolone versus dexamethasone in croup: a randomised equivalence trial
Sparrow A, Geelhoed G
Arch Dis Childhood, 2006; **91**: 580–583

Oral dexamethasone is used to treat croup but sometimes doctors substitute prednisolone. This Australian study of 133 children with an average age of 37 months compared single doses of equivalent potency in children with mild to moderate croup and suggests that this is not a legitimate thing to do.

Some 29% of the prednisolone group needed further medical care compared to just 7% of the dexamethasone group, probably due to its longer half-life. More doses of prednisolone may be needed if using this drug.

RELATED INFECTIONS

Sinusitis

Antibiotics and topical nasal steroid for treatment of acute maxillary sinusitis
Williamson IG, Rumsby K, Benge S, *et al.*
JAMA, 2007; **298**: 2487–2496

More than 90% of patients within the UK and US still receive antibiotics for sinusitis. This randomised study of 240 adults found that neither amoxicillin at a dose of 500 mg three times a day nor intranasal budesonide were likely to give any relief.

The end point measured was symptoms at 10 days and these remained in around one-third. Even a combination of the two drugs was no better than placebo.

The strictness of the inclusion criteria for this study – purulent nasal discharge and pain – means than in the real world of general practice such an approach is likely to be even less valuable.

Rhinitis

Are antibiotics effective for acute purulent rhinitis? Systematic review and meta-analysis of placebo controlled randomised trials
Arroll B, Kenealy T
BMJ, 2006; **333**: 279

Some GPs prescribe for a purulent nasal discharge – a familiar feature of a common cold. This review showed that although a small benefit is possible, the number needed to treat overlapped the number needed to harm – usually in terms of gastrointestinal effects. As most patients get better anyway antibiotics should not be first line treatment.

Conjunctivitis

Topical chloramphenicol was not effective in children with acute infective conjunctivitis.
Evidence-Based Medicine, 2006; **11**: 18
The following paper is reviewed
Chloramphenicol treatment for acute infective conjunctivitis in children in primary care: a randomised double-blind placebo-controlled trial
Rose PW, Harnden A, Brueggemann AB *et al.*
Lancet, 2005; **366**: 37–43

> This study of 326 children in 12 primary care practices in Oxfordshire found that whether or not chloramphenicol drops or placebo drops were used, there was no difference in cure rates at 7 days for conjunctivitis. This is especially important as the study was done in primary care, unlike the specialist clinics that produced studies that did show benefit. Perhaps disease in this group was milder but more relevant to the sort of patients seen by GPs. Although a self-limiting disease, pressure often comes from nurseries that prevent children with red eyes from attending.

A randomised controlled trial of management strategies for acute infective conjunctivitis in general practice
Everitt HA, Little PS, Smith PWF
BMJ, 2006; **333**: 321

> A study of over 300 adults and children with infective conjunctivitis were treated with immediate chloramphenicol, no antibiotics or delayed treatment. They found delayed prescribing to be a cost-effective strategy as it reduced antibiotic use (by around half compared to immediate antibiotics) and reduces medicalisation (as fewer intended to consult for the same thing in the future). Duration and severity of symptoms were reduced to a similar degree as in the immediate group and 30% of those who were allotted to the 'no antibiotics' group came back later and got them anyway.
>
> It might be right to prescribe when early symptoms are severe and when social issues such as day care for children are highlighted, but chloramphenicol is now available over the counter in the UK so primary care strategies may be sidelined.

Otitis

Wait-and-see prescription for the treatment of acute otitis media: a randomized controlled trial
Spiro DM, Tay K, Arnold DH *et al.*
JAMA, 2006; **296**: 1235–1241

> Delayed prescriptions may also take off in the US. Children with otitis media had similar short and medium term outcomes whether or not they were given antibiotics immediately or with a delayed prescription. Use of antibiotics reduced from 87% to 37% with no differences in ear pain, fever or use of analgesics. More parents said they would do without next time.

Children <2 years of age with bilateral acute otitis media and children with otorrhoea benefit most from antibiotics. *Evidence-Based Medicine*, 2007; **12:** 47
The following paper is reviewed
Antibiotics for acute otitis media: a meta-analysis with individual patient data
Rovers MM, Glasziou P, Appelman CL, *et al.*
Lancet, 2006; **368:** 1429–1435

In this meta-analysis of six randomised trials and 1643 children under 2 years old, bilateral acute otitis media and ear discharge responded beneficially to antibiotics. This may be a group in which we can justify the benefit of antibiotics, but as a rule we overuse them in children.

The rare problem of mastoid infection was reassuringly absent from the control group. But the common problems of diarrhoea, rash, increased antibiotic resistance and increases in re-attendance would usually outweigh any benefits.

THE WHEEZY CHILD

Commonly used pharmacological treatments for bronchiolitis in children do not seem to be effective. *Evidence-Based Medicine*, 2004; **9:** 141
The following paper is reviewed
Pharmacologic treatment of bronchiolitis in infants and children: a systematic review
King VJ, Viswanathan M, Bordley WC *et al.*
Arch Pediatr Adolesc Med, 2004; **158:** 127–137

In children with bronchiolitis, little consensus exists about optimal management strategies although medicines such as bronchodilators and corticosteroids are commonly used. This systematic review set out to look at the effectiveness of commonly used treatments for bronchiolitis in infants and children and reviewed 44 studies of the most common interventions – epinephrine, β-2-agonist bronchodilators, corticosteroids and ribavirin.

The only positive effects that seemed to be shown were possibly a temporary relief of symptoms immediately after a bronchodilator nebuliser. It is postulated that these short-term benefits might improve feeding and reduce restlessness and therefore be appealing but results are inconsistent at best. Inhaled budesonide even seemed to prolong symptoms. There was generally an impressive absence of good quality evidence to support a routine role for any of these drugs in bronchiolitis. No convincing effects on hospital admissions or length of stay were illustrated.

A sufficiently large, well-designed pragmatic trial of the commonly used interventions for bronchiolitis is called for.

Corticosteroids do not reduce hospital length of stay or respiratory distress in infantile acute viral bronchiolitis. *Evidence-Based Medicine*, 2005; **10**: 20

The following review is presented

Glucocorticoids for acute viral bronchiolitis in infants and young children

Patel H, Platt R, Lozano JM *et al.*

Cochrane Database Syst Rev, 2004

A Cochrane review of 13 RCTs in infants and young children with acute viral bronchiolitis proclaimed that systemic corticosteroids are no better than placebo for respiratory distress or shortening hospital stays. Neither is any drug, according to Cochrane reviews. Most infants are only admitted to hospital due to inability to predict which children will have apnoea or respiratory failure.

CLINICAL ISSUES

RESPIRATORY

INFLUENZA

The Challenge

Over 3000 deaths occur each year from influenza-related causes. Two interventions can lessen the impact of influenza – immunisation with inactivated vaccines and treatment and prophylaxis with antivirals.

Vaccination reduces admissions, mortality and morbidity in high-risk groups and health policies target high-risk individuals. Annual vaccination accelerates reductions in the risk of death year on year.

Mortality being a rare end-point, it has been difficult to prove the effectiveness of influenza vaccine on mortality directly in a large population, but meta-analysis of observational studies estimates the effectiveness of influenza vaccine regarding all cause mortality at 68%. During a flu outbreak, all cause mortality, predominantly respiratory, was lower in those who had received the vaccine than in those who had not, and in vaccinated people mortality was so low that it escaped association with the higher levels of circulating influenza completely.

Research in US nursing homes found that control of an outbreak depends on how quickly it is recognised and the extent of antiviral use.

Influenza is also an important cause of acute respiratory illness in young children. Attack rates among preschool children often exceed 40% in epidemic years. Common childhood complications including febrile convulsions, otitis media, bronchiolitis, and croup, and lead to heavy prescribing of antibiotics. There is growing opinion in the UK that we should follow the US model and vaccinate children against influenza.

What we know already:

- Fears over immunising COPD patients are unfounded. Although an increase in prescriptions for oral steroids given on the day of influenza vaccination has been observed, there is no increased risk of adverse outcomes.
- Older antivirals, such as amantadine and rimantadine, are limited by rapid emergence of resistance, lack of effectiveness against influenza B, and central nervous system side-effects.
- Neuraminidase inhibitors are recommended in identified outbreaks of influenza in the community and are effective prophylaxis, resulting in a relative reduction of 70–90% in the odds of developing flu.
- For treatment of flu, systematic review shows that zanamivir or oseltamivir reduce duration of symptoms by between 0.4 and 1.0 days. Given within 48 hours, they provide around 30–40% relative reduction in the odds of complications requiring antibiotics.
- Most of the elderly have difficulty using inhalers of zanamivir, particularly loading and priming Diskhalers. This limits their use of this delivery system.
- Near patient testing has shown a sensitivity of 44% and a specificity of 97% in children. Being good at ruling in influenza might assist optimal management, improve surveillance of flu, and satisfy parents denied antibiotics. However, the test cannot rule out influenza.

- A study of symptomatology and spirometry in 700 asthmatic children concluded that influenza vaccination had a moderately beneficial effect on quality of life in influenza-positive weeks of illness.

Recent Papers

IN THE ELDERLY

Effectiveness of an influenza vaccine programme for care home staff to prevent death, morbidity, and health service use among residents: cluster randomised controlled trial.
Hayward AC, Harling R, Wetten S, *et al*.
BMJ, 2006; **333:** 1241
and
Influenza in elderly people in care homes
Jordan RE, Hawker JI
BMJ, 2006; **333:** 1229–1230

The effect of vaccinating all elderly residents of care homes is modest. This trial (also reviewed in *Evidence-Based Medicine*, 2007; **12:** 81) looked at vaccinating staff, as well as residents, at UK nursing homes during two consecutive influenza seasons. Most UK care homes do not vaccinate their staff but over the two seasons of this trial in 44 private care homes, half the homes were offered influenza vaccination and half were not.

Staff vaccination levels were still not great at around 30–40% and influenza activity was low in one of the years and still not particularly high in the other year. Still, levels of illness were significantly lower in intervention homes even though there were already high levels of vaccination in residents.

Benefits were equivalent to preventing 5 deaths, 2 admissions to hospital, 7 GP consultations and 9 influenza-like cases per 100 residents during the period of influenza activity.

Interestingly, in the second year studied when influenza rates were substantially lower than average, no significant differences were found.

The most pessimistic scenario means that vaccination of healthcare workers costs as little as £274 per life year gained showing that it is the correct policy. There would be fringe benefits in the workers in reducing their risk of influenza and employers may well benefit with reduced absenteeism.

Staff do not seem to much fancy the idea of the vaccination, so educational campaigns and perhaps bribes may be in order.

CLINICAL ISSUES

RESPIRATORY

IN ASTHMA

Influenza vaccination in patients with asthma: why is the uptake so low?
Keenan H, Campbell J, Evans P
Br J Gen Pract, 2007; **57:** 359–363

Despite known susceptibility to influenza, annual uptake of vaccination in asthmatics is only 40% and has not increased much in recent years. A questionnnaire set out to elicit the reasons why. Two-thirds responded.

Those vaccinated had a greater belief in its efficacy and in medical advice. They felt more susceptible to complications, were older and were less fearful of side-effects. No other sociodemographic factors were implicated.

IN CHILDREN

The underrecognized burden of influenza in young children
Poehling KA, Edwards KM, Weinberg GA *et al*.
N Engl J Med, 2006; **355:** 31–40

US authorities recommend a yearly influenza vaccination for toddlers between the age of 6 months and 2 years based on high levels of hospitalisation for influenza. This study demonstrates that the burden of influenza is actually very much higher in the community – by a factor between 10 and 250 times.

The commonest symptoms were fever (95%), cough (96%) and runny nose (96%). Doctors recognised the illness in only 28% of inpatients and 17% of outpatients. This may be a missed opportunity if we want to prevent complications and outbreaks.

ARTHRITIS AND NSAIDs

The Challenge

Musculoskeletal conditions account for up to 20% of all general practitioner consultations. Around 5% require referral for a specialist opinion.

Rheumatoid arthritis (RA) is a persistent chronic disease affecting 1% of adults and is associated with progressive joint damage, disability and increased mortality. Standard symptomatic treatment has done little to alter disease progression, but the underlying disease process can be affected by drugs known as disease modifying antirheumatic drugs (DMARDs) that block or reduce the concentration of cytokines. Methotrexate, for example, has been shown to reduce the progression of radiologically evident joint damage and improve long term disability. Prompt early treatment with anti-tumour necrosis factor drugs minimises long-term disability.

Rheumatoid arthritis patients show evidence of the presence of minor levels of inflammation for up to 10 years prior to clinical presentation, making it possible to screen for a disease that is becoming virtually preventable. Primary carers now need to consider early referral in all new cases to minimise lifelong incapacity.

Osteoarthritis (OA) is the most common form of arthritis and accounts for 11% of all sick days and £1.2 billion of annual expenditure. It is the major cause of disability in the elderly, most commonly affecting the knee. Prevalence is rising with the changing demographic. Treatment guidelines for knee osteoarthritis recommend starting pain relief with paracetamol and later substituting with NSAIDs, but in the UK only 15% of patients use paracetamol while 50% use NSAIDs regularly. NSAIDs are riskier. They have a 2–4% annual incidence of serious gastrointestinal ulcer and complications – four times higher than in non-users. They also cause fluid retention and worsen renal function. A review of current evidence has not indicated any convincing evidence that coxibs are a 'safer' class of NSAID.

Another group of medicines that always seems to struggle to reclaim their place in our hearts is our old friend, the topical NSAID. There has been minimal evidence to support the long-term value of topical NSAIDs in osteoarthritis but they are finding favour again in some new research.

It is still frequently debated whether glucosamine and chondroitin have any real value in treatment of osteoarthritis.

Surgical treatments are the last option but it does not help evidence-based analysis when researchers of non-drug treatments for rheumatoid and osteoarthritis fail to report side effects more than half the time. This impairs the ability to judge the benefit–harm balance for options such as surgery, lavage, exercise and psychotherapy when comparing efficacy to drug treatments.

What we know already:

- Imaging with MRI and high resolution ultrasonography can facilitate definitive diagnosis of characteristic features of RA at a early stage.
- Aggressive triple therapy with combinations of three DMARDs (methotrexate, sulfasalazine, hydroxychloroquine) for the first 2 years of early RA is better than just using one DMARD on its own. Long-term radiology improves for at least 5 years in peripheral joints.

- Adding other DMARDs in after 2 years of monotherapy does not make up the difference when the window of opportunity has been lost.
- Combining methotrexate with infliximab – anti-TNF (tumour necrosis factor) alpha monoclonal antibody – provides greater clinical, radiographic, and functional benefits than methotrexate alone.
- A Glasgow study showed the superiority of intensive outpatient management of RA using antirheumatic drugs and intra-articular steroid injections. Regular review of joints led to very substantial improvements in disease activity, radiographic change, physical function, and quality of life at no additional cost.
- Clinical criteria for OA include age >50 years, morning stiffness for <30 minutes, crepitus, bony tenderness, bony enlargement, and no palpable warmth.
- Increased use of careful examination with clinical criteria helps diagnose OA with a sensitivity of 84% and specificity of 89% for acute knee pain, and with less reliance on imaging. X-ray showing the presence of osteophytes with at least one factor from age >50 years, crepitus, or stiffness of 30 minutes, increased diagnostic sensitivity to 91% with a specificity of 86%.
- Although NSAIDs are slightly better than paracetamol for reducing OA-related pain or pain at rest, the downside is not outweighed when symptoms are mild.
- Adverse cardiovascular safety profiles have limited use of COX-2 inhibitors (Rofecoxib was withdrawn from the market in 2004 due to concerns of increased mortality from heart failure; Lumiracoxib was withdrawn in 2007 following reports of suspected adverse liver reactions).
- The risk of serious NSAID gastropathy has declined sharply in recent years. In a US report, 24% of this was accredited to lower doses of NSAIDs, 18% was thanks to proton-pump inhibitors and 14% due to the use of less toxic NSAIDs.
- Systematic review of topical rubefacients containing salicylates shows a dearth of high quality trials; on the whole proof of good efficacy was in short supply, with them generally faring no better than placebo.
- Taking some NSAIDs for more then 2 years appears to reduce the risk of Alzheimer's disease but may be ineffective in established disease and is not a recommended indication.

Recent Papers

RHEUMATOID ARTHRITIS

Diagnosis

Anti–cyclic citrullinated peptide antibody is a more specific test for rheumatoid arthritis than rheumatoid factor. *Evidence-Based Medicine*, 2007; **12**: 183.
The following paper is reviewed
Meta-analysis: diagnostic accuracy of anti-cyclic citrullinated peptide antibody and rheumatoid factor for rheumatoid arthritis
Nishimura K, Sugiyama D, Kogata Y, *et al*.
Ann Intern Med, 2007; **146**: 797–808

> Diagnosis of RA is difficult. It is primarily a clinical diagnosis supported by serum positivity for rheumatoid factor. However, RF can be positive in other conditions such as Sjögren's syndrome and old age. In addition, RF-negative cases are abundant and measurement is not standardised.
>
> With all this uncertainty, how then can we diagnose RA early enough to install the new aggressive therapies that work so well?
>
> It is a good time for a new diagnostic tool. This meta-analysis shows that anti-cyclic citrullinated peptide antibody (anti-CCP) is more specific and just as sensitive as RF for diagnosis of RA. It is also better at predicting the severity of progression. Testing both parameters together in the context of clinical presentation will assist in diagnostic workup. Tests can both still be negative in up to one-third of patients with RA, and here serial monitoring may help.

A clinical prediction guide predicted progression to rheumatoid arthritis in undifferentiated arthritis. *Evidence-Based Medicine*, 2007; **12**: 154.
The following paper is reviewed
A prediction rule for disease outcome in patients with recent-onset undifferentiated arthritis: how to guide individual treatment decisions
van der Helm-Van Mil AH, le Cessie S, van Dongen H, *et al*.
Arthritis Rheum, 2007; **56**: 433–440

> Defining a score based on gender, number and symmetry of affected joints, morning stiffness, CRP level, RF positivity and anti-CCP positivity, these authors were able to predict most of the patients who would progress from undifferentiated arthritis to RA.
>
> Of patients with a score under 6, only 6% developed RA. With a score of over 7, 100% progressed to RA.
>
> This is just the sort of tool to kick-start early diagnosis in day-to-day practice in those who present with swollen joints.

MUSCULOSKELETAL

Medication

Treating rheumatoid arthritis
Emery P, Kvien TK
BMJ, 2007; **335**: 56–57

Treatment for RA has come on in leaps and bounds recently. DMARDs have aimed to induce remission and many regimens have found success. Experiments with stepping up, stepping down and giving three anti-rheumatic DMARDs at the same time have all found success in reducing disease activity, improving function, radiographic changes and quality of life. Only a few have achieved remission, however.

This editorial tells us that drugs that antagonise TNF are particularly impressive and should perhaps be used earlier. They were not initially expected to have much of an effect on symptoms but have actually been shown to give long-lasting protection against bone damage. Those that have anti-TNF early get better results faster with least toxicity. Those who started on methotrexate with an inadequate response benefit little from switching to other conventional DMARDs and should switch straight to anti-TNF.

The most effective treatment for RA is a combination of anti-TNF and methotrexate but will such a widespread use be cost-effective? Research is underway.

Aggressively treating to targets for disease activity scores mean that remission can be achieved in about 40% of patients. Early detection is crucial and facilitated by a high acute phase response, anti-RF, anti-CCP and sensitive imaging.

Patients with suspected rheumatoid arthritis should be referred early to rheumatology
Hyrich KL
BMJ, 2008; **336**: 215–216

Further support for the ever earlier use of DMARDs comes from this argument.

Patients with RA need these drugs as soon as possible. As things stand, most do not receive them within 3 months of onset, even though we know the outcomes are so much better when they do. The strongest predictor of a good outcome is shorter disease duration at start of treatment.

The PROMPT trial found that methotrexate also delayed RA and slowed joint damage in those with undifferentiated polyarthritis, especially if anti-CCP was present. It appears the early benefit may be unique and these medications have a chance of actually switching off the disease.

A large proportion of the delay comes before even presenting to primary care and asking doctors to recognise a disease with no specific criteria is asking a lot. Treatment with NSAIDs could mask and delay the diagnosis. Anti-CCP and better imaging will help.

However, Hyrich argues that a bit of over-diagnosis is a healthy option as the overall benefits would outweigh the risks of drug toxicity in those without RA. A fast-tracked referral to a rheumatologist is a priority. Before the results of the RF test come back!

Prednisolone plus a disease modifying antirheumatic drug improved outcomes in early rheumatoid arthritis. *Evidence-Based Medicine*, 2006; **11**: 79
The following paper is reviewed
Low-dose prednisolone in addition to the initial disease-modifying antirheumatic drug in patients with early active rheumatoid arthritis reduces joint destruction and increases the remission rate: a two-year randomized trial
Svensson B, Boonen A, Albertsson K *et al.*
Arthritis Rheum, 2005; **52**: 3360–3370

This Swedish study of 259 patients who were starting treatment with a DMARD (usually methotrexate or sulphasalazine) for the first time were also given either 7.5 mg of prednisolone or placebo. Radiographic joint damage and functional disability decreased more with prednisolone with no increase in adverse events.

The study was not blinded and only had 2 years follow up but was well executed. The 5% of patients with highly active disease and 115 with osteoporosis were excluded – a reminder that steroids are not ideal for all.

Concerns remain over the aggravation of cardiovascular risk factors by prednisolone and intensive anti-osteoporotic treatment is warranted. Although in this study most patients were treated with a single DMARD, this is increasingly unlikely to be the case in real life with more intensive drug combinations yielding positive results.

Mortality in patients with rheumatoid arthritis treated with low-dose oral glucocorticoids. A population-based cohort study
Sihvonen S, Korpela M, Mustonen J *et al.*
J Rheumatol, 2006; **33**: 1740–1746

Mortality increases where low-dose oral glucocorticoids are used for more than 10 years in rheumatoid arthritis patients. The risk of mortality increased by 14% for each year and by 69% over 10 years compared to those not on steroids. The main reason was cardiovascular death but there were also more deaths due to infections and intestinal perforations due to amyloidosis.

Long-term management

Patient initiated outpatient follow up in rheumatoid arthritis: six year randomised controlled trial
Hewlett S, Kirwan J, Pollock J *et al.*
BMJ, 2005; **330**: 171

This study offered over 200 patients with rheumatoid arthritis direct access to hospital rheumatologists on demand to replace the flabby system of regular planned hospital review that accounts for three-quarters of the workload of a rheumatologist. Clinical and psychological outcomes were almost identical compared to those receiving regular planned hospital review. Satisfaction and confidence in the system were significantly higher throughout the 6 years of the study. Direct access patients needed 38% fewer hospital appointments. The number of GP visits for arthritis was unaffected. The authors offer this as a new model of chronic disease management.

MUSCULOSKELETAL

OSTEOARTHRITIS

Treatment

Osteoarthritis of the knee in primary care
Dieppe P
BMJ, 2008; **336:** 105–106

According to NICE guidance, five interventions are 'core treatments' for osteoarthritis: paracetamol, education, exercises, weight loss and topical NSAIDs. Another 14 interventions range from safe to potentially harmful, such as oral NSAIDs and surgery.

Commenting on the study above, patients who chose ibuprofen were less likely to have adverse events than those randomised to it. This seems to confirm that patients given options make sensible rational choices which may improve efficacy and reduce toxicity. Patients, after all, know their own body, don't they?

Topical NSAIDs seem confirmed as a viable and safe alternative to oral NSAIDs for OA of the knee even if they only activate a placebo effect. In its guidance from February 2008 (Osteoarthritis: the care and management of osteoarthritis in adults), NICE suggests that using them constitutes a cost-effective intervention.

Glucosamine and chondroitin sulphate did not improve pain in osteoarthritis of the knee.
Evidence-Based Medicine, 2006; **11**: 115
The following paper is reviewed
Glucosamine, chondroitin sulfate, and the two in combination for painful knee osteoarthritis
Clegg DO, Reda DJ, Harris CL *et al.*
N Engl J Med, 2006; **354**: 795–808

The latest randomised placebo-controlled trial adds to growing opinion that these supplements have little effect on symptoms of osteoarthritis of the knee.

The end point of GAIT (Glucosamine/chondroitin Arthritis Intervention Trial) was a 20% decrease in the WOMAC pain scale in 1583 patients over the age of 40 years. Response to placebo was as high as 60% and the authors conclude that the effects of treatment are unlikely to be clinically important for most patients.

Patients whose pain was moderate or severe may experience some relief but the study was underpowered to verify this.

Chondroitin for osteoarthritis of the knee or hip
Reichenbach S, Sterchi R, Scherer M, *et al.*
Ann Intern Med, 2007; **146:** 580–590

People sometimes take chondroitin to supposedly prevent pain or damage in OA. Although pretty harmless, this meta-analysis of large-scale, methodologically sound trials indicates that the symptomatic benefit of chondroitin is barely noticeable.

Use of chondroitin in routine clinical practice should therefore be discouraged.

Do coxibs and traditional non-steroidal anti-inflammatory drugs increase the risk of atherothrombosis? Meta-analysis of randomised trials

Kearney PM, Baigent C, Godwin J *et al.*
BMJ, 2006; **332**: 1302–1305

This meta-analysis of 138 published and unpublished trials with 145 000 patients set out to look at three areas: the magnitude of the excess vascular risk associated with COX-2 inhibitors, the risk associated with traditional NSAIDs and the influence of concurrent aspirin.

- Selective COX-2 inhibitors were associated with a highly significant 1.4-fold increase in vascular death largely due to a twofold increase in myocardial infarction.
- This will cause about three extra myocardial infarctions per 1000 patients per year (which could double if everyone who discontinued prescribed COX-2 drugs were fully concordant).
- Determination of whether this was a dose-related effect or indeed differed among users and non-users of aspirin (which chiefly inhibits COX-1 at low doses) was not possible.
- Hazards were not confined to long-term use.
- High doses of traditional NSAIDs (ibuprofen 800 mg t.d.s. and diclofenac 75 mg b.d.) were associated with a similar excess risk of vascular events.
- There was no excess risk associated with high dose naproxen (500 mg b.d.) although there were insufficient data to determine whether it actually protected against cardiovascular effects.

The authors conclude that as numbers of events are relatively small, very large randomised trials will be needed to fill in the gaps.

Life without COX 2 inhibitors

Shaughnessy AF, Gordon AE
BMJ, 2006; **332**: 1287–1288

COX-2 inhibitors were trumpeted as the saviours of safe pain-relief. Now their armour is tarnished and the outpourings of grief continue, how long should we mourn?

As COX-2 inhibitors increase the incidence of myocardial infarction, we should take another look at our alternatives.

Although they rose to prominence on the back of research showing less ulceration, ulceration is neither intrinsically harmful nor a surrogate marker for harm associated with NSAIDs. In addition, gastroscopy findings such as these do not correspond to serious adverse effects and moreover their presence is not related to symptoms of dyspepsia.

Little difference has been shown between COX-2 and the older NSAIDs here. We still have other evidence that provides some insight and options.

- Misoprostol as co-treatment is effective in older people who need NSAIDs.
- Histamine-2 blockers and proton pump inhibitors are not consistently effective protectors and should not be used routinely except by those who develop a peptic ulcer.

CLINICAL ISSUES

MUSCULOSKELETAL

- Topical NSAIDs are safer than oral NSAIDs for osteoarthritis of the knee.
- Paracetamol should be offered first before resorting to other analgesics.
- Opioids can be added later.
- Glucosamine and non-drug options such as therapeutic taping, exercise, and acupuncture are useful in some.

Nonsteroidal anti-inflammatory drugs and risk of first hospital admission for heart failure in the general population
Huerta C, Varas-Lorenzo C, Castellsague J *et al.*
Heart, 2006; **92**: 1610–1615

This study looked at the association of NSAIDs with nearly 1400 admissions for a first episode of heart failure using the UK General Practice Database.

After controlling for other factors, the risk of a first admission for heart failure following NSAID use was 1.3. The main independent risk factor for admission was a prior clinical diagnosis of heart failure which had a relative risk of 7.3.

The usual aetiological factors such as hypertension, diabetes, renal failure and anaemia as well as obesity, smoking and alcohol use added to the increased risk of hospitalisation. Dose or duration did not appear relevant.

The research supports epidemiological studies that NSAIDs trigger heart failure in susceptible patients even if they have not previously been noted to have heart failure.

Advice to use topical or oral ibuprofen for chronic knee pain in older people: randomised controlled trial and patient preference study
Underwood M, Ashby D, Cross P, *et al.* for the TOIB study team
BMJ, 2008; **336:** 138–142

As both topical and oral NSAIDs have shown some short term relief, why not factor in patient preference? In this study, patients with an average age of 64 years could choose their favourite arm of the trial or choose to be randomised. By necessity, the trial was not blinded.

The options were to receive a recommendation to use either an oral NSAID, preferably ibuprofen, or a topical NSAID for knee pain. Those in the non-randomised arm made a free choice. More people wanted to make their own choice and nearly three times more of them chose topical therapy over tablets.

Outcomes were equivalent in both groups in the long term (1 year) in terms of benefit and harm, whether or not they were randomised or chose the treatment themselves.

The results are highly relevant to general practice, claim the authors, as patient choice was built into the study. These choices are likely to be influenced by many factors including past experiences of NSAIDs and pain at other sites.

BACK PAIN

The Challenge

Low back pain accounts for 13% of sickness absences in the UK and poses a major socioeconomic burden. It costs the NHS £1 billion annually and affects 17 million people in the UK alone. Those aged 35–55 years are affected most often and up to 7% of acute episodes of low back pain develop into chronic pain.

Evidence tells us that exacerbation of low back pain decreases rapidly in the first month and most patients can return to work. Further improvements occur up to 3 months, but plateau over the next 9 months. Recovery seems not to be as complete as previously advertised. Pain and disability from residual symptoms persist at low levels and most people have a recurrence within 12 months.

Some features worsen prognosis such as catastrophisation (excessively negative orientation towards pain) and kinesiophobia (fear of movement and injury), both of which predict chronic disability. Counselling on prognosis has been shown to reassure patients and improve functional outcomes.

Some suggest looking for psychological factors at the initial visit. Primary care is well placed to dole out a brief intervention to check for the patient's ideas about the cause of pain, fear-avoidance beliefs and behaviour, family reactions and occupational factors. Unfortunately, one intervention that tried this sort of approach and then offered information, reassurance and advice in a 20 minute session made no impact on disability, recovery or sick leave.

In fact little evidence exists for the routine use of many interventions and they consume a substantial amount of healthcare resources. Even a training strategy supporting stricter adherence to the RCGP guidelines for back pain only managed to increase use of physiotherapy and back pain units. There was no change in use of X-rays, sick notes, prescribed drugs or secondary care referrals and the value was minimal.

It is becoming clearer that back pain and neck pain share similarities as multifaceted problems requiring multiple approaches. Neck pain accounts for 15% of all soft tissue problems in general practice and is a common reason for referral to a physiotherapist. Unfortunately NHS physiotherapy is expensive and adds little to an advice sheet. Some doubt it is a responsible use of resources. Reinforcing advice to patients to stay active seems to be the best way to go while they will undoubtedly seek out other treatments when we 'fail' them.

What we know already:

- Overall, 1% of people presenting with back pain have a neoplasm, 4% have compression fractures and 1–3% have a prolapsed disc.
- Imaging is not routinely required for back pain of <6 weeks duration without a high suspicion of systemic disease or progressive neurological deficit.
- MRI is the most sensitive and specific imaging method for systemic disease. MRI and CT are similarly accurate for degenerative conditions with neurological impairment. Plain X-ray is commonly used but of limited value.
- Red flags such as bilateral or alternating leg symptoms, neurological disturbance, sphincter disturbance and history of malignancy help to identify those who need investigation.

MUSCULOSKELETAL

- Pain which was worse in the leg than the back has been shown to have a sensitivity/specificity of 82%/54% at predicting nerve root compression as confirmed on MRI scan. Pain worse on coughing, sneezing, or straining had figures of 50%/67%.
- Age over 45 years, smoking, more than one neurological sign and high levels of distress were associated with non-recovery at 3 months.
- Physiotherapists in the NHS treat 1.3 million people for low back pain annually, but there is only weak evidence for the effectiveness of many of their methods.
- Patients randomised to physiotherapy using methods such as low velocity spinal joint mobilisation techniques, lumbar spine mobility exercises and abdominal strengthening did report some improvements in mental health and physical function compared to a control group. But there was no objective evidence that it made any actual difference over and above a simple assessment session and advice from a physiotherapist to remain active.
- The TEAMS experiment improved a poorly resourced musculoskeletal service in Wales using GPs with special interests (GPwSIs) and physiotherapists. Referrals more than doubled, revealing the unmet burden of need, duplicate referrals to different resources were abolished and the need for surgery was unchanged.

Recent Papers

LOW BACK PAIN

Predicting persistent disabling low back pain in general practice: a prospective cohort study
Jones GT, Johnson RE, Wiles N *et al.*
Br J Gen Pract, 2006; **56**: 334–341

Good coping strategies such as staying active reduce disabling low back pain. Passive strategies include relying on others for help with the daily tasks and feeling as though they cannot do anything to improve the pain. This study of 922 people with back pain found a threefold increase in persistent disabling pain in those with these high levels of negative coping strategies.

After controlling for severity of symptoms, those who reported a high passive coping score were still at 50% increased risk of a poor outcome.

Assessment of diclofenac or spinal manipulative therapy, or both, in addition to recommended first-line treatment for acute low back pain
Hancock MJ, Maher CG, Latimer J, *et al.*
Lancet, 2007; **370:** 1638–1643

This trial randomised 240 patients with acute low back pain who had been given advice and paracetamol as an initial treatment.

Treatment options were diclofenac 50 mg bd, physiotherapy using spinal manipulation, neither, or both. Each intervention had a placebo alternative and treatment lasted up to 4 weeks.
- Neither diclofenac nor spinal manipulation therapy speeded up the recovery.

- Time to the first pain-free day was a median of 2 weeks regardless of therapy with one or both treatments.
- 10% had adverse effects but these were equally common in the placebo groups.

This paper strongly supports advising patients with low back pain to mobilise as much as they can, use regular paracetamol and avoid other NSAIDs and physiotherapy.

Opioid treatment for chronic back pain: prevalence, efficacy, and association with addiction
Martell BA, O'Connor PG, Kerns RD, *et al.*
Ann Intern Med, 2007; **146**: 116–127

Opioids are often prescribed for back pain but this meta-analysis found little evidence that they are effective. There was a trend towards some relief in the short term but it did not reach significance and there was no evidence on how to identify the characteristics of those that benefit, if indeed such a group exists.

A significant minority of patients with back pain are at risk of substance use disorder and show aberrant medication-taking behaviour.

PHYSICAL THERAPIES

Spinal manipulative therapy is not better than standard treatments for low back pain.
Evidence-Based Medicine, 2004; **9**: 171
The following article is reviewed
Spinal manipulative therapy for low back pain
Assendelft WJ, Morton SC, Yu EI *et al.*
Cochrane Database Syst Rev, 2004

This Cochrane review quantifies the evidence for spinal manipulative therapy (SMT) in low back pain by comparing different treatment strategies.

They looked at 39 studies with comparisons to sham therapies. The modest short and long-term improvements in low back pain did not differ significantly from three other interventions: GP care/analgesics, physical therapy/exercise, or back school.

The presence of a beneficial effect for SMT is unproven rather than disproven. Small benefits may yet be a cost-effective weapon against the epidemic but at present there is insufficient evidence for routine use.

United Kingdom back pain exercise and manipulation (UK BEAM) randomised trial: effectiveness of physical treatments for back pain in primary care
UK BEAM Trial Team
BMJ, 2004; **329**: 1377

This is a large study of 181 general practices in the Medical Research Council General Practice Research Framework taken in 63 community settings around 14 centres across the United Kingdom. Some 1334 patients with back pain were randomised to different physical treatments for back pain: a class-based exercise programme ('Back to Fitness'), a package of treatment by a spinal manipulator (chiropractor, osteopath or physiotherapist), or both.

MUSCULOSKELETAL

The control group is 'best care' in general practice, placebos being very hard to come by in this area:

- spinal manipulation showed a small to moderate benefit at 3 months and a small benefit at 12 months
- exercise alone improved back function by a small margin at 3 months but not at 12 months
- combined manipulation followed by exercise classes showed a moderate benefit at 3 months and a small benefit at 12 months

An accompanying economic paper showed that manipulation alone is probably the best value for money of these options. The authors argue that the sick leave saved would more than compensate for the chiropractic costs and argue for a major expansion of this role within the NHS. In the meantime they suggest hiring from the private sector.

Physiotherapy for neck and back pain
Harvey N, Cooper C
BMJ, 2005; **330**: 53–54

This editorial summarises that it is clear that back pain and neck pain share a tendency towards intractability. Biopsychosocial approaches will be necessary to manage this rather than concentrating on physical symptoms alone.

Trials in this area are often hampered by too much diversity – of treatments, of therapists and of approach. Perhaps it is not surprising that they fail to show how one specific intervention improves disability when the psychosocial component to chronicity is so great.

Research into subgroups of patients is needed to tell us who responds best to what. Broad-based public health interventions must work alongside these measures to alter public beliefs about back pain and reduce its medicalisation. Otherwise we might stay in the quagmire we are in at the moment.

SURGERY

Surgery for disc disease
Gibson JNA
BMJ, 2007; **335**: 949

This editorial looks at the role of surgery for acute disc prolapse and degenerative disease. The three most common conditions for which spinal surgery is performed are disc herniation, degenerative spondylolisthesis and spinal stenosis.

Quoting a Cochrane review, discectomy for carefully selected people with sciatica can provide faster relief at 1 year but without longer term advantage or harm. Outcomes at 1 year are similar if surgery is earlier at around 2 weeks compared to later around 19 weeks, but recovery was faster in the earlier group. Early surgery seems to show advantages for all locations of herniation.

The recent research supports early referral by the GP of patients with sciatica who are 'failing non-operative treatment'. A larger evidence base for advances in minimal intervention surgery is now needed.

HRT

The Challenge

In 2002, the WHI (Women's Health Initiative) investigators reported that there was no justification for women continuing to use HRT as preventative therapy because the risk of stroke, DVT and breast cancer outweighed the benefits. Panic ensued and women around the world suffered a great deal of alarm and distress. Many suddenly stopped their HRT without medical consultation, in some cases with adverse consequences. Prescriptions for HRT halved.

What went wrong? Early studies on HRT had fallen prey to misleading biases. Widespread discussion in the media and high levels of lay awareness, along with anecdotal evidence, allowed the errors to prosper. The absence of high quality evidence and uncertainty amongst doctors further authorised the abuse of HRT. Ever larger numbers of prescriptions flourished. Hopefully we will learn that prescriptions for large populations require large good quality trials to justify them. Observational studies are unreliable and mass markets have massive commercial vested interests which can exploit and successfully market uncertainty with illegitimate conviction.

Long-term HRT, including oestrogen-only therapy, is no longer recommended for the prevention of heart disease or osteoporosis. It is only to be used in the lowest effective dose for the shortest possible period to relieve troublesome symptoms.

The 'critical window' or 'timing' hypothesis refers to the remaining suggestion that oestrogen might have cardioprotective and neuroprotective effects in younger menopausal woman. The risk–benefit equation may be different from that seen in the older women in the WHI study. The theory is that it perhaps works better before the vasculature has been compromised.

What we know already:

- Although HRT is effective in treating osteoporosis, benefits should be weighed against harm and the risk–benefit ratio is unfavourable even for those at the highest risk of fracture.
- The HABITS Study (hormonal replacement therapy after breast cancer – is it safe?) was a randomised comparison stopped early when it determined HRT should not be prescribed in patients with a previous breast cancer due to unacceptable risk of new breast cancer events.
- Women in leadership roles may find symptoms of menopause crippling and seek pharmaceutical options.
- Paroxetine reduces flushes compared with placebo. Clonidine and gabapentin reduced hot flushes a little but both had unpleasant side effects and long-term safety was unresolved. These therapies may have some use in highly symptomatic women who cannot take oestrogen.
- The legacy of the HRT fiasco has been estimated in the US alone as an extra 1400 cases of breast cancer, 1200 cases of heart disease and 1400 cases of stroke against 860 fewer hip fractures and 1000 fewer cases of colorectal cancer.

Important trials

Million Women Study

The Million Women Study was an observational study set up to investigate the effects of specific types of HRT on incident and fatal breast cancer.

Number of participants: 1 084 110 UK women
Age range: 50–64 years
Launched: 1996
Follow up: 4.1 years

Key results

- Current users of HRT at recruitment were more likely than never-users to develop breast cancer and die from it.
- False positive recall was significantly increased in current users (with an increase of 64%) and past users of HRT. The effect decreased with time but was still significant 5 years after stopping HRT.
- Breast cancer incidence was significantly increased for unopposed oestrogen, tibolone, and greatest of all, in combined oestrogen–progestagen preparations.
- There was little difference between specific oestrogens and progestagens or between continuous and sequential regimens.
- Past users were not at an increased risk of incident or fatal breast cancer.
- 10 years' use of HRT was estimated to result in 5 additional breast cancers per 1000 users of unopposed oestrogen and 19 additional cancers per 1000 users of combination HRT.
- Use of HRT by women over 50 in the UK has resulted in an estimated 20 000 extra breast cancers, 15 000 associated with combination therapy.
- Use of HRT was estimated to have been responsible for around 20% of the false positive recall in the NHS breast screening programme, or around 14 000 cases per year.

References
BMJ, 2004; **328**: 1291–1292.
Lancet, 2003; **362**: 419–427.

WHI – Women's Health Initiative

This was a massive and important trial in 40 US clinical centres involving a randomised placebo-controlled trial which used conjugated equine oestrogen and medroxyprogesterone acetate (MPA), as well as looking at an unopposed oestrogen arm post-hysterectomy.

Number of participants: 16 608 post-menopausal women
Age: 50–79 years, mean age 63 years
Launched: 1995
Follow up: extended to 6.8 years

Important because?
It dismantled most of the arguments for the apparent benefits of HRT. Differences in the baseline variables in areas such as cardiovascular risk had not been apparent in previous observational studies and allowed dangerous conclusions.

What happened?
The conjugated oestrogen and progestagen arm was stopped prematurely in 2002, at an average follow-up of 5.2 years, when benefits were exceeded by risks of breast cancer, stroke, and deep vein thrombosis. Publication of the results led to a dramatic fall in the use of HRT.

The oestrogen only arm continued until February 2004 when an increased stroke incidence was found.

Key results

General observations:
- high rates of discontinuation (42%) suggest that adverse effects may be underestimated
- risks increased with age suggesting the risk–benefit profile may be better in younger women

Breast cancer:
- combined HRT increased invasive breast cancers by 15% in those taking HRT for less than 5 years and by 53% after more than 5 years
- every 10 000 women on combined HRT yields 8 more cases of invasive breast cancer per year
- no increase in breast cancer death was seen (but the study did stop early)
- the final arm of the study – unopposed oestrogen – caused no increases in breast cancer in 6.8 years; this is reassuring for hysterectomy patients. There was even a trend towards a reduction in breast cancers that just missed statistical significance.
- the oestrogen group required more follow-up in terms of more mammograms at shorter intervals and, compared to those on placebo, had a hazard ratio of 0.67

Cardiac effects:
- increased risk of coronary heart disease events in the first year of HRT
- no beneficial cardiac effect during longer follow up
- the unopposed oestrogen arm showed no cardiac complications (in fact a 9% non-significant reduction); a protective effect in those aged 50–59 years has been proposed – good news for those who need the use it peri-menopausally

Stroke:
- increase in incidence of ischaemic (not haemorrhagic) stroke (this agrees with a previous meta-analysis and the known prothrombotic effects of HRT)
- unopposed oestrogen also increased incidence of stroke by 39%

Osteoporosis:
- combined HRT reduced fractures but only in women whose calcium intake was at least 1200 mg/day
- a global model assessing treatment effects on all outcomes, found there was no net benefit to HRT even in women at high risk of fractures
- unopposed oestrogen reduced incidence of total osteoporotic fractures by 30%

Colorectal cancer:
- six fewer colorectal cancers per 10 000 women per year; the mechanism is unclear
- no differences demonstrated in the oestrogen only arm

Cognitive:
WHIMS – The WHI Memory Study – was an ancillary study, with a follow-up of 4 years, measuring incidence of dementia and global cognitive function annually using the Modified Mini-Mental State Examination.
- It indicated that combined HRT caused a twofold increase in probable dementia which was not influenced by duration of treatment and was possibly related to small cerebral thromboses.
- Unopposed oestrogen does not improve and may increase risk of dementia or cognitive impairment.

HRT

Urinary:
- recent analysis shows that post-menopausal women using either oestrogen alone or combined therapy have increased incidence and severity of both stress and urge urinary incontinence – the door on the concept of HRT to treat incontinence is beginning to close

Questions for future research:
- is the increased risk of breast cancer related to all progestagens or just MPA?
- is the neutral breast effect related to equine oestrogens or is this translatable to all oestrogens?
- is the risk of stroke (and DVT) more of a risk with oral than with transdermal oestrogen?
- what are the advantages of using lower doses of oestrogen?
- what is the role for the local use of vaginal uterine preparations?

References
Evidence-Based Medicine, 2003; **8**: 170–171, 172.
Evidence-Based Medicine, 2004; **9:** 52, 82, 184.
Evidence-Based Medicine, 2005; **10:** 121.
NEJM, 2003; **348**: 1839–1854.
JAMA, 2004; **291**: 1701–1712 , 2947–2968, 3005–3007.
JAMA, 2006; **295**: 1647–1657.

HERS – Heart and oEstrogen/progestagen Replacement Study

This was another important trial in 20 US outpatient and community centres which randomised conjugated oestrogen and medroxyprogesterone against placebo.

Number of participants: 2763 postmenopausal women with established heart disease
Age: under 80 years, mean age 67 years
Follow up: 4.1 and, for **HERS-2**, 6.8 years

Cardiac
- This study was the first to challenge the suggested cardioprotective effects of HRT, showing no difference in coronary heart disease events up to 6.8 years.
- There were, however, more coronary events in the first year of HRT than placebo and fewer in years 3–5, implying an 'uncovering' of susceptibility to cardiac disease.

Stroke
- Non-significant 9% increase in stroke and transient ischaemic attacks. Significance may have been prevented by high rate of aspirin use (80%) in the HERS patients, all of whom had heart disease.

Breast cancer
- Similar increases to the WHI study.

Colorectal cancer
- Similar decreases to the WHI study.

Cognitive
- No benefit of combined therapy on global cognitive function after 4 years of treatment.

Other
- Increased risks for biliary tract surgery and venous thromboembolism.
- Rates of fracture or mortality did not differ.

Reference
Evidence-Based Medicine, 2003; **8**: 12, 13.

Conclusions from the major trials

- The harms of oestrogen plus progestagen exceed benefits in those without menopausal symptoms.
- HRT remains a suitable option for women with bothersome menopausal symptoms particularly if also needing osteoporosis protection.
- Women should be counselled and understand that there are some risks.
- Need for treatment should be regularly reassessed, perhaps every 6 months, aiming to use the lowest effective dose for the shortest possible period.
- Use of HRT to prevent cognitive decline is not recommended.
- We should not assume that different formulations or lower doses of HRT will avoid all the risks observed in WHI.
- We can reassure women on oestrogen-only after hysterectomy of no increased cardiac or breast cancer risk for at least 6.8 years. Risks of stroke may not apply until they reach normal post-menopausal age.
- Long-term users of combined HRT over 5 years double their risk of invasive breast cancer, regardless of the pattern of progesterone use. There are additional risks over 15 years. It seems HRT must contain progesterone to promote breast cancer.

Recent Papers

PRESCRIBING HRT

Hormone therapy for younger women may not increase CHD risk during 5–7 years follow-up, but stroke risk was increased independent of age. *Evidence-Based Medicine*, 2007; **12:** 137
The following paper is reviewed
Postmenopausal hormone therapy and risk of cardiovascular disease by age and years since menopause
Rossouw JE, Prentice RL, Manson JE, *et al.*
JAMA, 2007; **297:** 1465–1477

The WHI investigators produced this further analysis which allays some fears caused by their devastating headlines in 2002.

In symptomatic peri-menopausal women, pooled data from the two WHI trials looked at 8832 women under 60. No statistically significant increase in stroke or any other adverse outcome was found and total mortality was reduced.

This supports a body of work that states that women under 60 years taking HRT for less than 5 years are not at increased risk of breast cancer, heart attack or stroke. Another survey has found that less than 10% of women stay on HRT longer than 5 years.

We can return with confidence to the short term use of peri-menopausal HRT to improve quality of life where vasomotor symptoms are significant.

HRT

Symptom experience after discontinuing use of estrogen plus progestin
Ockene JK, Barad DH, Cochrane BB, *et al.*
JAMA, 2005; **294:** 183–193

So we advise women with menopausal symptoms who want HRT to take the smallest effective dose for the shortest possible time. But what happens when they stop?

According to those that stopped taking combined therapy when the WHI trial was terminated, more than half get withdrawal symptoms. Those who had originally suffered with vasomotor or pain/stiffness symptoms get them again. (This was much less in those who had been taking placebos during the trial period and in those who had started HRT without symptomatology.)

THE TIMING HYPOTHESIS

Hormone replacement therapy comes full circle
Roberts H
BMJ, 2007; **335:** 219–220

An accompanying editorial reminds us that there is a trend in the subgroup analysis for a reduction in cardiovascular risk in women under 60 years on HRT. There is uncertainty, however, whether this will turn out to be statistically significant. Even if it is, the benefit is unlikely to progress with age and all the time the risk of stroke is increased in those on HRT.

The best case scenario is having to treat 1000 women each year to prevent one cardiovascular event. It is not a strategy for cardiovascular disease prevention. Stick to treating severe menopausal symptoms. At that age you can use HRT for a few years if you must due to the low absolute risk of cardiovascular problems in that age group.

Postmenopausal hormone therapy
Grady D, Barrett-Connor E
BMJ, 2007; **334:** 860–861

This editorial refers to US guidance from the North American Menopause Society. Nevertheless, it makes some good points.

HRT is a highly effective treatment for hot flushes and vaginal atrophy and should be used for the shortest possible time to control troublesome menopausal symptoms. Increased risk of breast cancer, stroke, DVT and dementia are harms serious enough to avoid the use of HRT to prevent disease.

The 'timing hypothesis' is what has given the debate a new lease of life. It refers to subgroup analysis of data from the two WHI trials that showed no clear difference in the risk of heart disease within 10 years of menopause. There could even be a reduced risk in these women whereas those taking it in their seventies definitely had an increased coronary risk.

The data are not rock solid and it could be a coincidence. However, the timing hypothesis may never be directly confirmed or refuted as the numbers of cardiac events in peri-menopausal women is so small. It would involve randomising a huge number of women to HRT or placebo for a decade.

Main morbidities recorded in the women's international study of long duration oestrogen after menopause (WISDOM): a randomised controlled trial of hormone replacement therapy in postmenopausal women
Vickers MR, MacLennan AH, Lawton B, *et al.*
BMJ, 2007; **335:** 239

When the WHI trial released results noting increased risks of stroke, embolism and breast cancer, then this large study – WISDOM – was stopped early. The trial is on the same lines but importantly reflects a population representative of the general population of women in the UK.

Starting HRT an average of 15 years after the menopause increased cardiovascular and thromboembolic risk. The abbreviated follow up period limits other conclusions about other conditions although there was a trend for fracture prevention.

The trial ended up being too brief to examine the 'timing hypothesis' to see if oestrogen shortly after menopause is actually cardioprotective. A long term trial in this younger group is still needed to prove this but would be a very difficult sell.

They conclude that HRT offers no overall disease prevention benefit and there is some risk.

CLINICAL ISSUES

HRT

OSTEOPOROSIS

The Challenge

About 1.2 million women in the UK have osteoporosis but most remain undiagnosed. One-third of women over 50 sustain a fracture, and fractures related to osteoporosis cost the NHS an estimated £1.7 billion annually. Osteoporotic fractures are expected to increase exponentially worldwide. Of the 200 000 osteoporotic fractures each year in Britain, most are fractures of the hip, radius and spine caused by falls. Women with fragility fractures often do not start treatment for osteoporosis. Debate exists on how much age-related decline in bone density is actually related to the risk of fracture in the elderly.

GP visits for osteoporosis have increased with the availability of new therapeutic options but there is still a low level of awareness among postmenopausal women. Current recommendations advise GPs to identify women at high risk of osteoporosis using clinical risk factors. Risk factor-positive patients were defined as having at least one of the factors in the Royal College of Physicians' 1999 guidelines such as: BMI <19 kg/m^2, height loss >2 inches, maternal hip fracture, menopause or hysterectomy <45 years, fracture after age 50, and secondary amenorrhoea >1 year. Those at risk can be offered bone density screening prior to starting anti-resorptive treatment. Unfortunately risk factor enquiry is a poor predictor. Only 1 in 5 has osteoporosis and one-third of affected women are not identified.

There remains a distinct concern about the cardiovascular safety of calcium supplementation particularly in older post-menopausal women. High calcium intakes are favourably associated with an increase of HDL to LDL cholesterol and suggestions had been made regarding a benefit to the cardiovascular system. However, this is starting to look like a red herring and it seems calcium actually increases cardiovascular risk.

Evidence surrounding the separate or combined use of daily calcium and vitamin D supplements has been conflicting and confusing to say the least. Results may depend on how deficient the population tested is, but often those data are unknown. Vitamin D supplementation has an important secondary effect in reducing falls by reversing muscle weakness in deficient people.

What we know already:

- Heel ultrasound scanning alone has nearly twice the specificity as just using risk factors. Adding ultrasound to risk factor assessment improved sensitivity by 22% and reduced specificity by 4%, identifying 90% of the women with osteoporosis.
- Dual energy X ray absorptiometry (DEXA) is the gold standard diagnostic investigation for osteoporosis but is costly and availability varies.
- Cochrane review indicates that calcium supplementation and vitamin D supplementation alone may separately have a small positive effect on bone mineral density but do not clearly independently reduce risk of fractures in the elderly.
- Combined calcium and vitamin D supplements have been shown to reduce the risk of hip fractures in elderly institutionalised women who are deficient in calcium and vitamin D. The combination can be recommended for frail older people confined to long term care institutions.

- High dose vitamin D supplementation in the elderly may be a promising strategy but the necessity for calcium is still unclear.
- Posting a capsule containing a large dose (100 000 IU) of vitamin D_3 to people aged 65–85 living in the community once every 4 months for 5 years reduced the risk of a first fracture by 22%. Findings were similar in men and women with no adverse effects. To prevent one fracture, the NNT would be 250. It's simple and safe and at less than £1 a year, it is feasible as a population strategy.
- Treatment with alendronate daily for 10 years increases bone mineral density at the lumbar spine by 14%, at the trochanter by 10%, and at the femoral neck by 5%. The drug was well tolerated but discontinuation resulted in a gradual loss of effect.

Guidelines

New NICE guidance (2007) recommends calcium and vitamin D supplementation for post-menopausal women on osteoporosis treatment unless clinicians are confident they have adequate intake. Bisphosphonates are recommended for women over 70 years with specified risk factors. Raloxifene is not recommended for primary prevention but strontium ranelate can be used for those intolerant of bisphosphonates (www.nice.org.uk).

Recent Papers

SCREENING

Absolute risk please
Godlee F
BMJ, 2008; **336**: 19 Jan

The *BMJ* editor warns against the over-medicalisation of another precursor condition – in this case "pre-osteoporosis", otherwise known as osteopenia. Here, bone densities are slightly below normal. Some consider these women to be "at risk of being at risk".

But impressive sounding relative risk reductions after treatment with various regimes mask much smaller reductions where the data are quoted in terms of absolute risk.

The fact that by far the greater risk of fracture comes from falls rather than osteoporosis may mean that this is where we should really be focusing our attention, but success in this area may be less impressive than previously thought.

High-trauma fractures and low bone mineral density in older women and men
Mackey DC, Lui L-Y, Cawthon PM, *et al.*
JAMA, 2007; **298**: 2381–2388

Older women with low impact fractures are investigated for osteoporosis but we do not tend to scan those who break a wrist in a car accident. This study found that high trauma fractures were also associated with osteoporosis and were pre-

OSTEOPOROSIS

dictive of future fractures in both men and women. The authors suggest assessing these patients for osteoporosis too.

CALCIUM AND VITAMIN D

Calcium did not prevent fractures in elderly women. *Evidence-Based Medicine*, 2006; **11**: 149
The following article is reviewed
Effects of calcium supplementation on clinical fracture and bone structure: results of a 5-year, double-blind, placebo-controlled trial in elderly women
Prince RL, Devine A, Dhaliwal SS *et al.*
Arch Intern Med, 2006; **166**: 869–875

What is the effect of calcium supplementation alone in a population of unselected elderly women?

- Nearly 1500 women over 70 years (average age 75) and not taking any medication were given calcium carbonate 600 mg twice daily, or placebo.
- There were 297 osteoporotic fractures over the 5 years of this Australian study.
- There was no fewer fractures due to calcium based on intention to treat (the preferred method of reporting data such as this, i.e. regardless of compliance).
- However, the non–ITT analysis showed that in the 57% who were compliant (more than 80% of tablets taken as prescribed), calcium did reduce fractures overall.

The commentary reminds us that non-ITT analysis can undermine the purpose of randomisation. Non-compliant women may be older, weaker and slower.

The study is also uncertain that there were sufficiently high levels of vitamin D in the population for optimum skeletal calcium handling.

However, the trial was large and well-designed and it will remind us to remind our patients on calcium to keep taking the tablets.

Vascular events in healthy older women receiving calcium supplementation: randomised controlled trial
Bolland MJ, Barber PA, Doughty RN, *et al.*
BMJ, 2008; **336:** 262–266

This study looked at the complex area of calcium supplementation. A lot has been written on its effect on bone mineral density, but we still do not know if all that calcium ends up lining our arteries and killing us by the back door. Some of the largest studies do not even mention vascular events and no randomised trials (including this one) have been primarily designed to assess the effect. It had been hoped that calcium supplements might reduce vascular events but this further analysis suggests the opposite.

This RCT in 1471 postmenopausal women in New Zealand, mean age 74 years, had previously confirmed improvements in bone density. They have now confirmed that calcium supplements were associated with an increase in cardiovascular events, more so when compliance was high. It is uncertain to what degree this finding is countered by the benefits on bone.

The effect was of borderline significance for the composite end-point of stroke, MI, and sudden death (*P* value around 0.05). A closer examination is needed before a widespread promotion of calcium supplements can take place.

Although this study is small, it is consistent with other studies. Secondary analysis of the Women's Health Initiative showed a trend towards adverse cardiovascular effects in those with low calcium intake who took supplements. A less bioavailable formulation of calcium was used and compliance was lower and this group was heavier, younger (average age of 62 years), and 50% were taking HRT.

Cardiovascular risks of calcium supplements in women
Jones G, Winzenberg T
BMJ, 2008; **336**: 226–227

This editorial summarises the current data on the role of calcium. Calcium has not generally been thought to be harmful aside from a little constipation and the odd kidney stone. Indeed as lipid profiles improve, hopes have been high for calcium as a cardioprotective agent. The study by Bolland *et al.* (previous summary) refutes this, so until better data arrive, monotherapy in the elderly with calcium does not seem to be justified unless perhaps calcium intake is very low. It may turn out to be safer in younger women but the large time for which it would have to be taken puts a question mark over it.

Although calcium and vitamin D have been shown to reduce the risk of hip fracture in elderly institutionalised women who are deficient, a recent meta-analysis failed to confirm this in the community. Adherence may not have been so rigid in real life and we know regular dosage is very important for calcium to successfully reduce fractures. A benefit of 12% reduction is possible (*Lancet*, 2007; **370**: 657–666).

However, the number needed to harm for 5 years outweighs the number needed to treat for benefit by a considerable margin. The current data suggest that net benefits would only occur in those women at a very high risk of fracture.

On the other hand, bisphosphonates are only effective with co-administration of calcium and vitamin D so in this case supplementation should continue.

Calcium plus vitamin D supplementation and the risk of fractures
Jackson RD, LaCroix AZ, Gass M *et al.*
N Engl J Med, 2006; **354**: 669–683

A report based on 36 282 women enrolled in the Women's Health Initiative also showed the effect of calcium and vitamin D supplements in healthy women between 50 and 79 years based on intention to treat.

It identified:
- increased hip bone density after 7 years of follow up
- no difference in the number of hip or total fractures
- a significant increase in renal calculi

OSTEOPOROSIS

Effect of vitamin D on falls: a meta-analysis
Bischoff-Ferrari HA, Dawson-Hughes B, Willett WC *et al.*
JAMA, 2004; **291**: 1999–2006

This meta-analysis of five randomised controlled trials was also reviewed in *Evidence-Based Medicine* (2004; **9**: 169). It concluded that:

- a daily supplement of vitamin D reduced falls in older people by around 20%
- the effect was independent of calcium use
- the number needed to treat was only 15
- benefit has been shown to begin within 2–3 months
- the mechanism is unknown but it may be that vitamin D enhances muscular strength with muscle cell growth
- vitamin D might now be considered for routine use in older people but optimal dose and type of vitamin D is unknown

---

Recent developments in vitamin D deficiency and muscle weakness among elderly people
Venning G
BMJ, 2005; **330**: 524–526

There are previously unsuspected high levels of prevalence of vitamin D deficiency in elderly people. This is associated with muscle weakness, body sway, and a tendency to falls and fractures.

According to this clinical review, supplementation of 800 IU of vitamin D daily (or an equivalent, such as 100 000 IU every 4 months) is needed to have an effect on falls. Treating elderly housebound people with this should be seriously considered.

Effect of cholecalciferol plus calcium on falling in ambulatory older men and women
Bischoff-Ferrari HA, Orav EJ, Dawson-Hughes B *et al.*
Arch Intern Med, 2006; **166**: 424–430

Does calcium/vitamin D supplementation reduce the risk of falling in the elderly?

This placebo-controlled 3 year randomised controlled trial studied 199 men and 246 women and found the following.

- Combined supplementation reduced the odds of falling in ambulatory older women by 46%.
- Benefit was more evident in less active women with a 65% reduction in falls.
- There was no such benefit recorded in men regardless of their physical activity level.

BISPHOSPHONATES

Continuing alendronate for an additional 5 years maintained bone mineral density in postmenopausal women. *Evidence-Based Medicine*, 2007; **12:** 70.
The following paper is reviewed
Effects of continuing or stopping alendronate after 5 years of treatment: the Fracture Intervention Trial Long-term Extension (FLEX): a randomized trial
Black DM, Schwartz AV, Ensrud KE, *et al.*
JAMA, 2006; **296:** 2927–2938

How long do you continue bisphosphonates for?

The FLEX trial assessed over 1000 women with a mean age 73 years and 97% white. Continuing alendronate for a further 5 years beyond the original 5 years maintained bone mineral density. Those taking placebo lost a little bone density, but overall fractures did not increase, implying that 5 years treatment may usually be enough in post-menopausal women with low bone mineral density.

Those with known risk factors placing them at high risk (such as previous vertebral fracture) may still benefit from longer treatment. Remeasuring bone density could help guide treatment.

RALOXIFENE

The effect of raloxifene after discontinuation of long-term alendronate treatment of postmenopausal osteoporosis
Michalská D, Stepan JJ, Basson BR *et al.*
J Clin Endocrinol Metab, 2006; **91:** 870–877

This randomised study shows that those that have to stop taking alendronate can successfully switch to raloxifene and keep most of the benefit in terms of bone mineral density at the lumbar spine compared with taking a placebo. All of the patients were taking supplemental calcium and vitamin D.

OSTEOPOROSIS

OLDER PEOPLE

The Challenge

By 2025, almost one-quarter of the population of Europe will be over 65. By 2050, there will be a threefold increase in the number of people aged 60 or older to 2 billion. Elderly people at home and in care homes provide an increasing workload for the GP and arrangements for delivering care to the elderly have been haphazard. Insufficient use of beneficial drugs, overuse of unnecessary drugs and poor monitoring of chronic disease are commonplace, and yet attempts at screening to detect problems early has limited value too.

Dementia has become a pressing challenge, with 5% of those aged over 65 and one-fifth of those over 80 having some degree of dementia. The number will double over the next 30 years. Inadequate detection, referral and management of dementia have long been recognised in primary care. The Alzheimer's Society says that more than half of those who have the disease will never receive a formal diagnosis. Unfortunately it rarely presents with clear, well demarcated symptoms. Diagnosis is confusing and there is little training of primary care teams. Tools to aid diagnosis are often not culturally sensitive and community services are often not well coordinated.

And do we have anything to treat it with when we find it? Debate continues over the benefits of cholinesterase inhibitors, but some studies have claimed they produce small improvements in cognitive and global assessments in Alzheimer's disease. Doctors at the very least need to play their part by responding to concerns about changes in memory and behaviour. They need to make comprehensive assessments to find the cause while focussing on what can be done and not worrying about a cure.

Falls are also a major case of disability. They may lead to loss of function, anxiety, depression, impaired rehabilitation, increased length of hospital stay, and inability to return to previous residence, thus contributing to NHS costs of around £1 billion a year.

In the UK, approximately 30% of people over 65 years and 50% over 80 years will fall in a given year. Hip fracture is the commonest reason for admission to an orthopaedic ward and often results in death or permanent disability. By 2050, there will be 4.5 million hip fractures in the elderly so prevention will be crucial.

Prevention of falls and injuries has been a major focus of research. Diverse risk factors have been identified such as balance problems, muscle weakness, use of medication, and environmental hazards, and they all increase the risk of falls. Several types of intervention have been shown in randomised controlled trials to be effective. Risk factor intervention with muscle strengthening, balance training and withdrawal of psychotropic medications are all considered to be likely to be beneficial in prevention.

Falls clinics have sprung up to provide individualised multifactorial interventions but are costly and labour intensive. Most falls seem related to the effects of illness and ageing and many falls prevention programmes have been poorly focussed. The optimum configuration is elusive.

Who will look after us in our old age? Informal caregivers provide an enormous service to society but receive little training for their role and their needs are often sidelined. Nearly 6 million people are informal carers. Only around half of them are in good health. Data from the UK census suggests that of those over 65 years, more than a million (12%) were informal carers, roughly evenly split between men and women. The oldest age group – the over 85s – still contained 44 000 carers. Even 1.4% of children between 5 and 15 years provided informal care. This is a large burden for children and pensioners. Paid employees would be in violation of the European Working Time Directive.

How are we at the end of life care? There is agreement on the need to target symptoms and maintain quality of life but uncertainty about the most effective models of palliative care. There may be unmet needs in terms of symptom control in patients who are dying but who have not been identified as terminal. Cancer patients are more likely to have had the end of their life identified as such, making them more likely to have had palliative medication. We give less palliative attention to end-stage cardiorespiratory illness, for example, which is equally deadly and has similar demands in terms of co-morbidity and number of consultations.

Many chronic diseases such as COPD and cardiac failure could benefit from doctors identifying a need for end-of-life care by asking themselves a simple question – "Would I be surprised if my patient were to die in the next 12 months?". GPs with their patient-centred holistic approach in the community, and hopefully patient trust, are ideally placed for this. Training GPs with a special interest in palliative care could be one way to enhance collaborative care. Unfortunately out-of-hours services are even less well set up to facilitate dying at home than they were before.

What we know already:

- Assessing five priority domains of unmet need can add "SPICE" to later life: Senses (vision and hearing); Physical ability (mobility and falls); Incontinence; Cognition; Emotional distress (depression and anxiety).
- A trial with over 30 000 responders in UK general practice, showed that screening over 75s with a brief multidimensional assessment with suitable follow-up by nurse or referral, makes no difference to outcomes in terms of mortality or admission rates.
- Decision support software improved rates of detection of dementia and is now incorporated into the popular EMIS practice system where it is available to 5000 practices in the UK as a simple, practical tool.
- A census of private nursing homes showed the very high dependency need of the residents. More than 50% of residents had dementia, stroke or other neurodegenerative disease, 78% had at least one form of mental impairment, 76% of residents required assistance with their mobility or were immobile, and 71% were incontinent. Some 27% of the population were immobile, confused and incontinent.
- The mean age of hip fracture in women is 81 years; the expected additional life for an 80 year old will be 8.7 years so there is plenty of time to benefit from prophylactic measures.
- Rapid muscle loss mainly from the legs induced by bed rest in the elderly probably contributes to the functional decline that older people suffer when in hospital.
- Unsponsored randomised trials have so far failed to confirm benefits for donepezil and it seems that neither carer nor patients can tell the difference between that and a placebo.
- Rates of diabetes, anaemia, thyroid dysfunction, hypertension and atrial fibrillation in the over 85s have been shown to be surprisingly high.
- A Danish study showed that home visits made by GPs and, to a lesser extent community nurses, in the final 3 months of a patient's life were inversely associated with dying in hospital regardless of the nature of the disease.
- Since April 2006, Quality and Outcomes Framework points have been awarded for holding a palliative care register and reviewing those patients on the register at a multidisciplinary team meeting at least three-monthly.

Guidelines

The National Service Framework for Older People (2001) aims to provide a high standard of care regardless of age. Resources are being targeted towards increased numbers of elderly care specialists and associated nurses and therapists as well as operations such as cataracts and joint replacements.

Since its inception, one-third of older people needing intensive daily help now receive this in their own homes rather than in residential care; delayed discharge from acute beds has reduced by two-thirds; and services for stroke and falls continue to improve.

A New Ambition for Old Age: Next steps in implementing the national service framework. London: Department of Health, 2006 (www.dh.gov.uk).

This document emphasises three themes – dignity in care, joined up care, and healthy ageing. Improvements of services in appropriate environments, stronger commissioning arrangements and dealing with any remnants of age discrimination will build on the success of the NSF.

Recent Papers

SCREENING

Health risk appraisal in older people 1: are older people living alone an 'at-risk' group?
Kharicha K, Iliffe S, Harari D, *et al.*
Br J Gen Pract, 2007; **57**: 271–276

Population screening of old people has failed in the UK.

We now aim to target at-risk groups, so why not target older people living alone?

This study in 860 people over 65 years who were living alone, reported higher levels of disease and disability with constellations of pathologies. They also had higher risk of falling. A lot of this was attributable to older age, lower education and female sex.

Health risk appraisal in older people 2: the implications for clinicians and commissioners of social isolation risk in older people
Iliffe S, Kharicha K, Harari D, *et al.*
Br J Gen Pract, 2007; **57**: 277–282

More than 15% of the older age group is at risk of social isolation, estimates this study. However, this group does not seem to have the help-seeking behaviour which would make them heavier users of medical resources. So while targeting and screening this group might give an opportunity for ameliorating the problems found, there is no evidence that this intervention would lead to cost savings in the future.

Some screening tests for dementia in older people are accurate and practical for use in primary care. *Evidence-Based Medicine,* 2007; **12:** 182
The following paper is reviewed
Does this patient have dementia?
Holsinger T, Deveau J, Boustani M, *et al.*
JAMA, 2007; **297:** 2391–2404

> This study compared a number of screening tests for dementia.
>
> The Mini Mental State Examination (MMSE) is the standard instrument but many other tests examine cognition and memory. They concluded that they can vary in diagnostic accuracy and some take up to 45 minutes to complete, further limiting their usefulness. However, MMSE is useful for both ruling in and for ruling out dementia. It is less useful if the patients has visual problems or is less familiar to the tester.
>
> They mention a shorter tool that was also useful – the Memory Impairment Screen – but conclude that physicians should aim to know one tool well and start to use it.

Dementia screening in primary care: is it time?
Brayne C, Fox C, Boustani M
JAMA 2007; **298:** 2409–2411

> This paper summarises the argument against screening and why we should still focus on investigating people based on clinical suspicion.
> - There are no reliable tests to diagnose or predict dementia in asymptomatic people.
> - No biomarkers are available.
> - Cognitive tests misclassify a lot of people.
> - Imaging is expensive and impractical.
> - There are no treatments that convincingly halt dementia or reverse it when found.
> - People have limited desire for screening. The impact on their independence may adversely affect their health as well as their life insurance.

DEMENTIA

Cholinesterase inhibitors in mild cognitive impairment: a systematic review of randomised trials
Raschetti R, Albanese E, Vanacore N, Maggini M
PLoS Med, 2007; **4:** e338

> We have no clear definition of what exactly defines mild cognitive impairment or how much this condition is a precursor for dementia.
>
> This review trial of cholinesterase inhibitors – donepezil, rivastigmine, and galantamine – found eight trials. None of the drugs helped delay or ease the effects of dementia, establishing they have no preventative role in this group of people. This is in addition to the questionable benefits in those who already have dementia. Side effects were common.

Cholinesterase inhibitors may be effective in Alzheimer's disease. *Evidence-Based Medicine,* 2006; **11**: 23

The following paper is reviewed

Cholinesterase inhibitors for patients with Alzheimer's disease: systematic review of randomised clinical trials.

Kaduszkiewicz H, Zimmermann T, Beck-Bornholdt HP, *et al.*

BMJ, 2005; **331**: 321–327

NICE sanctions the use of cholinesterase inhibitors in mild to moderate Alzheimer's disease. The consensus at the moment is that they probably have a small beneficial effect on cognition and perhaps behaviour in some patients, but the clinical significance seems arguable. Clinicians often argue that they work in a subset of 10–20% which cannot be identified in advance and so all should be treated.

This systematic review looked at the current evidence surrounding use of cholinesterase inhibitors (donepezil, rivastigmine, or galantamine) in Alzheimer's disease.

The authors found 12 placebo-controlled randomised trials that examined clinical outcomes and identified many areas of poor methodology and possible bias in the published studies. They do nothing to change that consensus.

Good evidence is lacking on treating Alzheimer's disease with these costly drugs. How to identify responders, how long to treat and cost-effectiveness are as elusive as ever.

Non-degenerative mild cognitive impairment in elderly people and use of anticholinergic drugs: longitudinal cohort study

Ancelin ML, Artero S, Portet F *et al.*

BMJ, 2006; **332**: 455–459

This valuable study, in 372 people aged over 60 years in 63 general practices in France, looked at use of anticholinergics and their impact on cognition.

As doctors try to spot signs of dementia early, we will need to think how many subtle effects can be explained by drugs.

Polypharmacy is common in the elderly and many drugs have anticholinergic effects including antiemetics, antispasmodics, bronchodilators, antiarrhythmics, antihistamines, analgesics, antihypertensives, antiparkinsonian agents, steroids, ulcer drugs, and psychotropic drugs.

In this study, nearly 10% of subjects used at least one of these drugs for extended periods. Eighty per cent of continuous users were classed as cognitively impaired compared with 35% of non-users. They performed poorly in reaction time, attention, narrative memory, visuospatial construction and language tasks, but not on tasks of reasoning, recall of lists or implicit memory. The patients whose impairment could be explained by the medication were no more likely to deteriorate into dementia.

The ageing brain is easier to poison – the blood–brain barrier is leakier, metabolism is slower and drug elimination is impaired. Use of many non-prescription compounds can further muddy the waters. Doctors need to start associating cognitive dysfunction with anticholinergic toxicity.

RESIDENTIAL CARE

Case management for elderly people in the community
Black DA
BMJ, 2007; **334**: 3–4
and
Impact of case management (Evercare) on frail elderly patients: controlled before and after analysis of quantitative outcome data
Gravelle H, Dusheiko M, Sheaff R *et al.*
BMJ, 2007; **334**: 31

A UK pilot study looking at case management for frail elderly people, trailblazed a role for the community matron. The Evercare model piloted this in 10 PCTs following US research that nurse practitioners could save money by reducing the number of admissions of long-stay nursing home residents to hospital.

The Department of Health invested enthusiastically, combining elements of nurse-led assessment and intensive case management, only this was in the community not in a nursing home setting. During the study period they found the following:

- there were no significant effects on rates of admission, use of emergency departments or mortality for this high-risk population
- people seemed to like the additional services, but this type of intervention by nurse practitioners is not supported by evidence
- there was criticism about the failure to produce a properly controlled study before this investment took place; public funds had largely been spent on travel, consultancy fees and going on courses

Nurse practitioners seem not to be able to replace a proven intervention such as a comprehensive geriatric assessment as an inpatient, which has been shown to reduce mortality, institutionalisation, and improve function.

Effect of family style mealtimes on quality of life, physical performance, and body weight of nursing home residents: cluster randomised controlled trial
Nijs K, de Graaf C, Kok F *et al.*
BMJ, 2006; **332**: 1180–1184

This Dutch study encouraged family style mealtimes (being served in a group at a dressed dinner table with a choice of food and a member of staff at the table) for nursing home residents, average age 77 years. Although the study was impossible to blind, they found that this simple social interaction maintained quality of life, physical performance and body weight in preference to similar nutritional content eaten from trays. This more convivial approach provides a sense of ambience, structure, security and meaning in a more stimulating environment to ease the psychosocial elements of 'the anorexia of ageing.'

OLDER PEOPLE

MEDICATION

Preventive health care in elderly people needs rethinking
Mangin D, Sweeney K, Heath I
BMJ, 2007; **335**: 285–287

This paper argues that many modern treatments, rather than adding years to life, simply change the method of our death, without involving us actively in the decision. Immunisations and antibiotics have helped the richer countries combat infectious disease. Those saved from these epidemics have had the opportunity to die from an epidemic of cardiovascular disease. As we improve targets for coronary heart disease, what do we die of next as our bodies come to the end of their finite life?

The supposedly proven effects of many medicines may not always apply to those who have already exceeded an above average lifespan. Sensitive arguments over ageism fuel the extension of single disease perspectives to age groups which may not typically benefit.

Statistics can betray us too. The NNT works less well in chronic conditions where co-existing conditions increase the absolute risk of dying. They may magnify a single intervention while the benefit in years of life may be negligible. For example, pravastatin in the PROSPER trial did not benefit any outcome in elderly women (aged 70–82) implying that mortality and morbidity from other causes must have increased. Indeed a new diagnosis of cancer – a potential substitute death – was significantly more likely. They call this a "contemporary phenomenon that is historically unprecedented".

The problem is not the data. It is the conclusions we pull from them. We should stop extrapolating data from the young and applying them directly to the old until we can prove it leads to longer or better lives.

Many patients fear their mode of death more than death itself and preventative treatments do not relieve suffering directly, so we must be cautious in the claims we make for them. Certainly, the drug companies will not object and targets and financial incentives may further muddy the waters.

Sedative hypnotics in older people: meta-analysis of risks and benefits
Glass J, Lanctôt KL, Herrmann N *et al.*
BMJ, 2005; **331**: 1169

More than 10 million prescriptions for hypnotics are dispensed each year in England – 80% are for people over 65 years.

In people over 60, sedative hypnotics do improve the quality of sleep but only in a small way and not enough to outweigh the disadvantages, according to this meta-analysis of 24 RCTs and 2400 participants which looked at any pharmacological agent used for at least five days.

The NNT for improved sleep quality was 13 and the number needed to harm for any adverse event was 6. This ratio indicates that an adverse event is roughly twice as likely as enhanced quality of sleep. Those particularly at risk of falls or who already have cognitive impairment will not get a net benefit. Non-pharmacological therapies such as CBT have been shown to be just as good for insomnia in older people.

Effect of New York State regulatory action on benzodiazepine prescribing and hip fracture rates
Wagner AK, Ross-Degnan D, Gurwitz JH, *et al.*
Ann Intern Med, 2007; **146:** 96–103

>Tighter controls of benzodiazepine use led to a halving of prescribing in the elderly in New York.
>
>This would be expected to reduce the likelihood of falls and be reflected in hip fractures. No such luck. The authors are not sure why this "natural experiment" did not work, unless benzodiazepines do not increase the risk of hip fracture as assumed.

PALLIATIVE CARE

Good end-of-life care according to patients and their GPs
Borgsteede SD, Graafland-Riedstra C, Deliens L *et al.*
Br J Gen Pract, 2006; **56**: 20–26

>This study interviewed GPs and their patients who had a life expectancy of less than 6 months due to cancer, COPD or heart failure.
>
>Feelings of both doctors and carers were comparable. Areas consistently thought to be important were continuity of care and availability of GPs for home visits outside of traditional hours, as well as professional competence and cooperation with other members of the care team. The more modern, slightly fractured ways of delivering primary care such as part-time jobs and restricted home visits may threaten these valued aspects.

Palliative care in the community
Munday D, Dale J
BMJ, 2007; **334**: 809–810

>In primary care more people die in hospital than at home but that does not reflect patient preference.
>
>The Gold Standards Framework has a reputation as a good model of community palliative care for the end of life (www.goldstandardsframework.nhs.uk). It provides guidance through workshops, local expertise and documentation. Patients are identified systematically and given a lead GP and community nurse, and a multidisciplinary team. It applies for all end of life care not just cancer and is endorsed by NICE and the RCGP.
>
>Variations in commitment do happen and the administrative burden is seen as a drawback, but the approach is undoubtedly valued. It will need to be properly resourced.

CLINICAL ISSUES

OLDER PEOPLE

INFORMAL CARERS

Who will care for the oldest people in our ageing society?
Robine J-M, Michel J-P, Herrmann FR
BMJ, 2007; **334:** 570–571

The number of informal carers for the frail elderly is set for a steep decline. Mostly this has been considered in the past in terms of a three age model: the young, those of working age, and the elderly. The changes in the population structure have made these authors propose a fourth age group by splitting the elderly group into the younger retired people and the oldest people. They propose looking at the ratio of 50–74 year olds to those over 85 years to better anticipate future planning of care.

Women have historically had a key role to play but changes in working practices and migration are changing this. The oldest might prefer to pay for formal care rather than rely on family support. Home modifications, safety technology and personal helper robots may facilitate this.

Caring for the oldest old
MacAuley D, Morris ZS
BMJ, 2007; **334:** 546–547

This editorial also refers to the needs of the "oldest old".

Is the reality of old age a longer disease-free life or of a longer life with more than one chronic condition? That depends on how lucky we are. Coronary heart disease is dropping and cancer is increasing. As they become 'managed conditions', the WHO estimates a doubling of chronic disease in the over 65s by 2030.

Informal carers carry a huge unsung burden and we need millions more. But will the next generation be willing to help? Are they even in the neighbourhood? Women traditionally have carried the brunt of the care load but would modern women still be prepared to help with their changing aspirations and expectations.

Two alternatives remain – neglect or formal care.

FALLS

Preventing falls in elderly people living in hospitals and care homes
Cameron ID, Kurrle S
BMJ, 2007; **334:** 53
and
Strategies to prevent falls and fractures in hospitals and care homes and effect of cognitive impairment: systematic review and meta-analyses
Oliver D, Connelly JB, Victor CR *et al.*
BMJ, 2007; **334:** 82

This meta-analysis and accompanying editorial describes the certainty and uncertainty surrounding prevention of falls.

- The best outcome of falls to measure is the number of falls prevented rather than reductions in the overall number of fallers.

- Multifaceted interventions in hospital significantly reduce falls but not fallers or fractures.
- Evidence was inconclusive for multifaceted interventions in those cared for in the community in care homes.
- No single intervention other than hip protectors (including calcium/vitamin D or exercise) improved outcomes.
- Hip protectors significantly reduce hip fractures in care homes but not numbers of falls (there were too few studies on fallers).
- There was no evidence that presence of dementia or cognitive impairment influences the effect of any interventions.

There were many gaps in the evidence partly because of the variety of approaches used. But it seems widespread adoption of injury prevention strategies are of uncertain value in the different environment and type of patients we get in the community.

The cornerstones of care remain adequate supervision, encouragement of mobility, individually tailored aids, a safe environment, sensible prescribing, and early treatment of medical complications. Future studies into a standardised multifactorial intervention should involve these elements.

Multifactorial assessment and targeted intervention for preventing falls and injuries among older people in community and emergency care settings: systematic review and meta-analysis
Gates S, Fisher JD, Cooke MW, *et al.*
BMJ, 2008; **336:** 130–133

Another meta-analysis found little evidence to show that multifactorial intervention programmes are effective in reducing the numbers of fallers or fall-related injuries when they are targeted on community or emergency settings.

Research needs to focus on showing a benefit on fall-related morbidity such as the rate of peripheral fractures – a robust parameter not measured in any of the trials. They concluded differently from a previous Cochrane review by virtue of inclusion of further studies and increased the direct relevance to primary care settings. The quality of evidence available was still not high and was open to bias.

These multifactorial interventions have seemed like an attractive idea. The lack of much evidence, of much of a benefit, and the fact that they must cost a fortune makes them pretty dubious.

Effectiveness of hip protectors for preventing hip fractures in elderly people: systematic review
Parker MJ, Gillespie WJ, Gillespie LD
BMJ, 2006; **332:** 571–573
and
Hip protectors to prevent femoral fracture
de Rooij SE
BMJ, 2006; **332:** 559–560

This update of a previous systematic review included further studies and ended up revising its original conclusions that hip protectors seem to reduce hip fracture.

Selection bias, publication bias or design and reporting flaws were examined in the context of new evidence. Hip protectors are uncomfortable and unattractive and poor compliance itself also presents huge problems of analysis as well as of interpretation.

Also, different hip protectors may have different effectiveness.

The bottom line is that when people are randomised as individuals rather than in clusters, hip protectors were found to be ineffective for those living at home.

Whether or not they work in institutionalised care is questionable.

The accompanying editorial describes that, in the light of this evidence, these devices should not be widely used until studies show benefit. Hip protectors may yet show some value in specific subgroups of the elderly – perhaps highly motivated people at high risk of fracture where use is backed up by encouragement from nursing staff.

MEDICALLY UNEXPLAINED PHYSICAL SYMPTOMS

The Challenge

Medically unexplained conditions are poorly understood and thought to represent complex adaptive systems related to biological, psychological, and social factors. GPs feel that about one-fifth of patients who consult them have physical symptoms not explained by a disease process. These symptoms generally do not conveniently cluster into well-defined distinct syndromes and many patients receive a lot of largely ineffective investigations and treatments in primary care.

Chronic fatigue syndrome, also known as myalgic encephalomyelitis, and increasingly by the shorthand CFS/ME, is such an illness of unknown nature and cause. Its very existence has been questioned down the years (by up to 50% of GPs) leading to a breakdown in communication between doctors and the public. It is probably relatively common in the UK, but uncertainties surrounding its diagnosis and management have limited our understanding and probably even contributed to a worsening of the impact of symptoms. It does not help that parental labelling of children with 'ME' bears no correlation with definitions of chronic fatigue syndrome.

Doctors have a tendency to negatively stereotype patients with chronic fatigue syndrome and yet not patients with other unexplained conditions such as irritable bowel syndrome. Research says that the lack of a precise bodily location which would allow a plausible pathological mechanism contributes to this. Reclassification and relabelling of CFS/ME over time have not helped; the variety of names reflecting the hope that such labels can impose some certainty where little exists. And the perception that patients might be using the sick role to skive creates conflict between doctor and patient. These barriers to effective clinical management explain why doctors feel less comfortable and more hopeless dealing with chronic fatigue syndrome rather than IBS.

How we communicate with these patients with any sort of diagnostic certainty within a limited time window is a huge challenge. Developing trust and discussing misconceptions will be a good start while we focus on symptom relief and walk the tightrope of the labelling trap.

What we know already:

- Chronic fatigue is severe fatigue causing functional impairment lasting longer than 6 months. Chronic fatigue syndrome on the other hand is less common and has a more complex definition.
- In a UK survey of 1000 GPs, half did not feel confident with making a diagnosis of CFS/ME and 41% did not feel confident with the treatment options.
- Systematic review shows that CBT improves pain, disability, and depression in chronic back pain and probably has positive effects in CFS.
- Treating co-existent anxiety / depression may help alleviate physical symptoms.
- A Birmingham survey estimated IBS prevalence at 10.5–7% of men and 14% of women. Over half had consulted their general practitioner within the previous 6 months and 16% had been referred to hospital.

- Less than half of those reporting symptoms of IBS according to the well-validated Rome II criteria had received a diagnosis of IBS.
- Patients with moderate or severe IBS who were taking, but were resistant to, mebeverine, have shown benefit on the severity of symptoms at 6 months and this may be a useful intervention for some that can be performed in primary care.

Recent Papers

CHRONIC FATIGUE

What causes chronic fatigue syndrome?
White PD
BMJ, 2004; **329**: 928–929

Chronic fatigue syndrome, also known as myalgic encephalomyelitis, and increasingly by the shorthand CFS/ME, is an illness of unknown nature and cause, but its existence is generally accepted.

Markers of predisposition for the conditon are being female, having a premorbid mood disorder, and increased use of their GP for up to 15 years prior to diagnosis. Although there may be viral triggers, there is no evidence of ongoing infection. Cortisol levels tend to be low but this may be due to sedentary activity and there is no recognised biological marker for the condition. The heterogeneity of the group makes research tricky.

A paper in the same issue as this editorial (*BMJ,* 2004; **329**: 941) examined the British birth cohort from 1970 and found that 10 year olds whose mothers reported that they 'never or hardly ever' played sport in their spare time had twice the risk of CFS in adulthood.

Other risk factors for children were a limiting long-standing physical condition in childhood and higher social class (remember the term 'yuppie flu'?). However, in contrast to previous studies, there was no associated incidence of CFS/ME with maternal or childhood psychological problems, birth weight, obesity, school absence/ability, and parental illness.

Inactivity increases the perception of effort during exercise – this awareness is a phenomenon called interoception. This can be reprogrammed with graded exercise therapy which along with cognitive behavioural therapy has been shown to be effective.

Chronic fatigue syndrome or myalgic encephalomyelitis
White P, Murphy M, Moss J, *et al.*
BMJ, 2007; **335:** 411–412

The reluctance of doctors to make a diagnosis of CFS/ME and the many misunderstandings about the condition have resulted in recent NICE guidelines to help navigate the uncertainties.

We are reminded that it serves no purpose to disbelieve the patients who may be severely disabled by the condition, and that prolonged malaise and fatigue are the characteristic features. The diagnosis is clinical – no diagnostic tests are available.

The recent NICE guidelines involve an array of healthcare professions and remind us to exclude alternative diagnoses, negotiate a management programme and provide access to the most proven treatments – CBT and graded exercise therapy.

Worries that a study found that graded exercise therapy was harmful in 50% have been countered by the claim that it was performed with inadequate advice and backup, claim these authors.

Primary Care Trusts are required to provide services locally and GPs need to be confident in making a diagnosis and providing initial management and referral.

Although there is at least agreement within the Royal Colleges that the condition exists as an independent diagnosis, services and funding have failed to keep up.

Diagnosis and management of chronic fatigue syndrome or myalgic encephalomyelitis (or encephalopathy): summary of NICE guidance
Baker R, Shaw EJ
BMJ, 2007; **335:** 446–448

The NICE guidelines spell out the ideal approach to take which starts with acknowledging the reality and impact of the condition as well as providing information in a supportive collaborative relationship.

Diagnosis is made with a suitable index of suspicion in relation to a persisting or recurrent presentation over a 4 month period characterised by post-exertional malaise or fatigue. Red flag symptoms such as significant weight loss and focal neurology suggest more sinister diagnoses. A battery of blood tests is advised to exclude other conditions.

The treatment plan should outline appropriate use of rest and exercise as well as avoidance of unproven pharmaceuticals, dietary supplements and complementary therapies, unless used within a self-management plan. Speed of referral depends on severity of symptoms.

Ideally the programme is individualised and overseen by a single named professional with emphasis on CBT and graded exercise therapy.

Concerns remain over the lack of availability of the resources to implement these recommendations.

Evidence remains weak for the "proven interventions" claims the ME Association. The huge expense of CBT is estimated at £1500 for 12–16 one-on-one sessions and could be prescribed to 200 000 people. In addition, the harms demonstrated by the graded exercise are discouraging.

There is uncertainty over where the £300 million funding will come from, casting doubt over the value of the NICE recommendations (*BMJ*, 2007; **335:** 528).

MEDICALLY UNEXPLAINED PHYSICAL SYMPTOMS

The management of children with chronic fatigue syndrome-like illness in primary care: a cross-sectional study
Saidi G, Haines L
Br J Gen Pract, 2006; **56**: 43–47

Little is known about the characteristics of children with CFS/ME who present to primary care. This survey identified around 100 patients from 62 practices aged 5–19 years who consulted their GP with severe fatigue lasting over 3 months and who filled in questionnaires which were considered by a clinical panel to meet CFS criteria.

- 73% were girls, 94% were white, mean age was 12.9 years, and median illness duration was 3.3 years.
- GPs had principal responsibility for 62%.
- A diagnosis of CFS/ME was made in 55%, one-third of these within 6 months.
- Half had illness of moderate severity.
- Paediatric referrals were made in 82% and psychiatric referrals in 46% (median time of 2 and 13 months respectively).
- Advice was given on setting activity goals, pacing, rest and graded exercise.

GPs look after the majority of these patients and seem to be successful in fairly rapid diagnosis and appropriate interventions. Cases were milder than in tertiary care but similar in characteristics.

THE DOCTOR–PATIENT RELATIONSHIP

Do patients with unexplained physical symptoms pressurise general practitioners for somatic treatment? A qualitative study
Ring A, Dowrick C, Humphris G *et al.*
BMJ, 2004; **328**: 1057

This paper examined how patients with unexplained symptoms might pressure their GP for somatic management. Analysing audiotapes of consultations in practices in Merseyside, they found 36 relevant consultations where the doctor agreed that symptoms had existed for at least 3 months, caused significant distress (to the patient) and could not be explained by a recognisable physical disease.

- Abdominal symptoms, headache and limb pain were the most common complaints.
- All but two received somatic treatments.
- Most received a prescription although few asked for one.
- No patient asked for investigation or referral but nearly half received this.
- Reasons for this are usually attributed to pressure from patients.

Patients seem to convey the need for a response while curtailing the doctor's ability to deliver it, putting pressure on GPs in subtle ways by:

- conveying their suffering with graphic and emotive language
- emphasising social effects of symptoms
- describing complex symptom patterns
- negating a doctor's attempts at explanation

- refering to other individuals, e.g. family, as testimony to the severity of symptoms
- using biomedical explanations

The authors state that this research does not support the assumption that patients with unexplained symptoms pressure GPs for symptomatic treatments. This may reflect the need to maintain a long-term relationship. Doctors may respond with symptomatic treatments if they mistake patients' needs, if they lack another solution or if they just feel too helpless.

But if the game is softball in general practice, it is hardball in hospital outpatients. Research in secondary care, where patients may only get one shot at the consultation, shows that treatments are explicitly requested, consequences of the doctor's failure to supply them are trumpeted, and blame is put on doctors for worsening their lot.

Voiced but unheard agendas: qualitative analysis of the psychosocial cues that patients with unexplained symptoms present to general practitioners
Salmon P, Dowrick CF, Ring A *et al.*
Br J Gen Pract, 2004; **54**: 171–176
and
Normalisation of unexplained symptoms by general practitioners: a functional typology
Dowrick CF, Ring A, Humphris G M *et al.*
Br J Gen Pract, 2004; **54**: 165–170

This research examined audiotapes of 36 consultations to see whether patients who are considered to have medically unexplained symptoms give opportunities to GPs discuss psychological issues. All but two presented these opportunities. Patients perceived emotional and social problems as symptoms of mood disorder or stress and asked questions about symptoms with explicit concern, cautious reference to more serious possibilities, and even suggestions that disease may be absent.

By missing these cues to tackle elements of their problem with a new perspective, unnecessary symptomatic interventions were used.

Dangers still persist if normalisation – simple empty reassurance – is used without making this relevant to patients' concerns. The patients were much more likely to accept an effective narrative that linked their physical symptoms with psychological factors.

CLINICAL ISSUES

MEDICALLY UNEXPLAINED PHYSICAL SYMPTOMS

DEPRESSION

The Challenge

Depressive disorder is a major health problem in primary care. Costs reach around £9 billion in England each year and reductions in quality of life are comparable to those seen in major chronic diseases. In fact, depressive disorders often accompany many chronically morbid disorders. Physical conditions such as visual impairment, malignancy and neurological illness are strongly linked with suicide in the elderly.

The National Service Framework (NSF) for mental health was released in September 1999 to improve quality and structure of mental health services. It has seven standards focusing on mental health promotion and addresses standards for primary care, prevention of suicides and the problems of carers.

Nine out of ten depressed patients are treated solely in primary care but only 40% are diagnosed on the first consultation. Review increases pick-up rates but up to half of these disorders remain undetected, including for one in six who has severe symptoms of depression.

Many studies have used pleasingly brief screening tools claiming respectable specificities and sensitivities for screening in low prevalence settings. One such example is a two question screen asking "During the last month have you often been bothered by feeling down, depressed, or hopeless?" followed by "During the past month have you often been bothered by little interest or pleasure doing things?". A positive screen is a yes to either question. In this example, adding a third question improves diagnosis: "Is this something with which you would like help?". But of course no test is ideal.

Fortunately, half resolve without treatment. The danger of missing depression may therefore have been overstated in the past, but undertreatment is still identified as a major problem.

Depression in primary care may even have a different aetiology and natural history from cases in secondary care. Research on these milder levels of depression and dysthymia is sparse. In fact, many of the conclusions about effectiveness of therapies seem to come down to which studies you believe.

Depression can be devastating to a young person's academic and social development and can adversely affect family relationships. But optimal treatment for depression in adolescents is not clear cut. Adolescent depression carries a high risk of recurrence, chronicity and suicide.

Selective serotonin reuptake inhibitors (SSRIs) are used in treatment, although there are concerns regarding both efficacy and the raised risk of suicide. Systematic review shows that fluoxetine may be the only antidepressant to do more good than harm, but there are dangers in interpreting marginally positive results. The placebo response and adverse effects are enhanced in children and assumptions of efficacy should not be extrapolated to children based on adult studies. Access to unpublished data is critical to avoid 'evidence-biased medicine'.

The idea that parasuicide and suicide involves different populations is not supported by the evidence and 3–5% of those who self-harm commit suicide within 10 years. Up to 15% of those with unipolar depression eventually commit suicide.

Maybe psychotherapy is the answer... but hang on. Demand for services is great but its legitimacy has never been more in question. Psychotherapy is not formally recognised as a profession and treatments delivered behind closed doors are a lottery for patients. Evidence on cost-effectiveness is patchy at best. The prickly attitudes of some have not helped open the door to government money and interventions are in danger of appearing to be a private luxury for the wealthy. The therapist may be the most important factor in treatment rather than the type of therapy chosen, but even so relapse rates still look high. A glut of recent work on cognitive behavioural therapy has made a big splash but, as the evidence trickles in, is its bubble about to burst?

What we know already:

- Suicidal thoughts seem to occur at similar levels in males and females (around 13–15%) but less than one in five go to their GP about this. Men appear to need higher levels of morbidity in order to seek help or confide in someone. This may increase their risk of crisis and suicide.
- The Hampshire Depression Project educated GPs on the use of a clinical-practice guideline. It failed to increase diagnosis or treatment of depression, implying that the problem is more complex than researchers may have thought.
- Screening for depression is not improved by routinely administered questionnaires prior to consultation.
- Effective treatments include medication, psychological techniques, exercise and self-help materials.
- There is no significant difference in efficacy between SSRIs and tricyclics, but withdrawal from treatment is more common with tricyclics.
- In children, fluoxetine has a favourable risk–benefit balance as things stand but even that will only be of use to around one in ten cases.
- The largest independent treatment trial for adolescent depression found that combined CBT and fluoxetine was the best option for moderate to severe depression in adolescents.
- GPs can be effective in CBT after an extensive instruction programme. However, brief training for GPs does not improve patient outcomes but does increase referral rates.
- The internet has been show to be a feasible and powerful tool to deliver psycho-education and CBT to patients in the community, with low dropout rates.
- Resources associated with threefold increases in levels of NHS antidepressant prescribing in England between 1991 and 2002 could have employed 7700 therapists (26 per PCT) to deliver six sessions of CBT to 1.5 million patients – more than one-third of adults with depression or mixed anxiety depression. This alternative might actually float.
- Outcomes improve with enhancement of follow-up by telephone or direct contact with primary care and mental health workers. Some psychotherapies may simply have a compliance-enhancing effect.
- Suicide rates are higher in those who have a history of parasuicide by a factor of at least 40 – an effect that persists for at least 2 years.
- A Swedish study in nearly a million 18 year old men showed a strong inverse association between intelligence test scores and risk of suicide, perhaps reflecting the importance of cognitive and problem-solving ability to work through life's crisis points.
- In one study, giving CBT to people who attempted suicide reduced the recurrence rate by 50% but there was no difference in suicidal ideation, just presumably the ability to deal with it and ride out the crisis.
- At 8.2 per 100 000 people, the suicide rate in England in 2003–5 was the lowest on record.
- Evidence suggests that asking about suicidal ideation or behaviour in teenagers does not create distress or increase suicidal ideation.

DEPRESSION

Recent Papers

GENERAL

NICE guidelines for the management of depression
Middleton H, Shaw I, Hull S *et al.*
BMJ, 2005; **330**: 267–268

The NICE guidelines advocate a stepped care approach, clarifying guidance on treatment of moderate to severe depression with SSRIs as the first choice of medication. They support the use of CBT but no other psychodynamic psycho-therapies.

The advice for mild depression will not be much help in uncertain decisions when a particular case may or may not benefit from medication, but this reflects the evidence available.

These milder presentations may be subthreshold disorders where doctors allow the medicalisation of unhappiness in order to legitimise the engagement, when all that people may really need in these times of growing social isolation is some support.

DETECTING DEPRESSION

Should we screen for depression?
Gilbody S, Sheldon T, Wessely S
BMJ, 2006; **332**: 1027–1030

GPs are increasingly being required to screen patients for depression as part of their enhanced services.

NICE recommends targeting those at high risk but screening programmes need to ensure they do more good than harm and in the case of depression this is far from clear.

A variety of screening questionnaires have been used but practices rarely keep using them once the trial is over. A prevalence of under 10% makes even a test with good sensitivity and specificity have a positive predictive value of under 50%, leading to a lot of unnecessary follow-up. In addition, there is little to suggest that patients appreciate this sort of screening very much.

Although drugs and psychological interventions are effective, they are less so in cases of mild depression – perhaps the very depression that GPs see most often. Even prescribing of drugs can be somewhat *ad hoc*, with drugs not continued for as long as they should be.

Evidence is therefore scant that screening improves outcomes.

It would seem to be a 'no-brainer' to screen those at high risk such as those with physical illnesses or alcohol problems, but there are no studies that evaluated this strategy. With a lack of randomised data on the harms of screening (stigma, medicalisation, discrimination by insurance companies, etc.), the authors do not recommend even this approach.

Screening has a role when good collaborative care systems are in place, for example, in diabetics already attending a review process on a regular basis.

Population strategies will only be effective when our efforts minimise the chronic long-term effects of this relapsing condition rather than uncover more minor morbidity that may have got better without interference.

Although screening for depression does not yet meet the criteria of the National Screening Committee, this fact seems to have been bypassed by the enormous size of the problem and the availability of antidepressants.

Is depression overdiagnosed? Yes
Parker G
BMJ, 2007; **335:** 328

This head to head *BMJ* argument looks at the steep rise in the diagnosis of depression in recent years.

Parker believes it is overdiagnosed and, given that it is normal to feel depressed at times, we are probably medicalising sadness. The ubiquitous nature of depressed mood states means that a low threshold for diagnosis makes normal emotional states an illness.

We have struggled for years to find a reliable model which is valid for diagnosing depressive disease. Many criteria used have low reliability.

Curiously, prevalence paradoxically seems to fall with age, implying that people surveyed might forget about episodes of major depression in their lives. This could mean the episodes are less important.

Minor states of dysthymia have been expanded to the even less severe 'subclinical depression'. Is any sort of distress a disease?

With the approach to treatment taken by many psychiatrists, the false positives that we overdiagnose will be treated with inappropriate treatments known to cause harm.

Is depression overdiagnosed? No
Hickie I
BMJ, 2007; **335:** 329

Hickie argues that diagnosis has other benefits – reduced stigma, fewer problems with insurance, and tells us we have now abandoned the terms 'stress' and 'nervous breakdown' (have we?). He tells us that most doctors can differentiate normal sadness and distress (can we?).

DEPRESSION

He expresses concern that evidence is less strong in those under 18 years old but sees no problem with the label of depression. Receiving a diagnosis of a life-threatening condition is a good thing, he explains. Early diagnosis provides opportunities for interventions before patterns become engrained.

However, he agrees that a new clinical model combing interventions and staging is desperately needed.

Do ultra-short screening instruments accurately detect depression in primary care? A pooled analysis and meta-analysis of 22 studies
Mitchell AJ, Coyne JC
Br J Gen Pract, 2007; **57:** 144–151

This study compared questionnaires which screen for depression using one, two or three questions.

A one-question test identified only 3 out of 10 making it unacceptable.

The two or three question tests identified 8 out of 10, but false positives were high – only 4 out of 10 were actually depressed. So they may help us rule out the diagnosis of depression, but screening directed at a population depends on the availability of local resources to deal with the positives.

Managing depression in primary care
Tylee A, Jones R
BMJ, 2005; **330:** 800–801

Primary care is still the 'right place' for most depression to be treated but it is easy to criticise primary care for its role in depression and the concerns over SSRIs have not helped. There are many reasons why we fail to pick up the diagnosis:
- patients may attribute symptoms wrongly
- patients insufficiently active in seeking care, feeling undeserving of the doctor's time and uncertain whether the problems were legitimate
- presentation of physical rather than psychological symptoms
- patients may attend too infrequently
- GPs may have negative attitudes towards mental health problems and may lack time or consulting skills

ANTIDEPRESSANTS

A qualitative study exploring how GPs decide to prescribe antidepressants
Hyde J, Calnan M, Prior L *et al.*
Br J Gen Pract, 2005; **55:** 755–762

A qualitative study of 27 Bristol GPs found that:
- GPs balance clinical and social criteria in the decision to employ antidepressants
- the preferred strategy is 'wait and see', but antidepressants are used appropriately earlier in illness that is perceived as severe, classic or persisting
- decisions depend on time constraints, lack of alternative psychological services options, cost of prescribing, and perceived attitude of patients
- this suggests the 'watchful waiting' guidance of NICE will be well received

Efficacy of antidepressants in adults
Moncrieff J, Kirsch I
BMJ, 2005; **331**: 155–157

This controversial but fascinating paper suggests that, after all, antidepressants have no clinically meaningful benefit.

The NICE meta-analysis of placebo-controlled trials, they argue, identifies differences in symptoms so small as to be unlikely to be clinical important. This is consistent with other meta-analyses performed.

Lack of consensus on what an important difference is does not help. Statistical aberrations such as publication bias and methodological aberrations such as poor blinding may explain the small levels of apparent superiority seen.

In addition they argue that the claim that antidepressants work better for severe rather than mild depression is far from proven.

The paper calls for a re-evaluation of our entire approach to treating depression and a need to address the now raised expectations of society.

Efficacy and safety of second-generation antidepressants in the treatment of major depressive disorder
Hansen RA, Gartlehner G, Lohr KN *et al.*
Ann Intern Med, 2005; **143**: 415–426

Reviewing 46 head-to-head randomised, controlled trials comparing one second-generation antidepressant with another, this systematic review found no major differences in the numbers of adults with major depression who responded to any particular drug. Adverse events varied in nature but not incidence.

Almost all (96%) of these trials were sponsored by the pharmaceutical industry or had financial ties to the industry. Sponsorship was associated with a 5% advantage for the sponsor's drug over the comparator drug, and publication bias obscured the evidence even further.

Venlafaxine for major depression
Cipriani A, Geddes JR, Barbui C
BMJ, 2007; **334:** 215–216

This editorial summarises many of the problems surrounding the interpretation of the evidence regarding antidepressants.

Observational analysis showed that venlafaxine was more likely than fluoxetine, dothiepin or citalopram, to be associated with suicide. However, making allowances for the many confounding factors reduces, and could eventually negate, the risk. The research group chose to compare only certain antidepressants and could have chosen harder outcomes measures by not including unsuccessful attempts at suicide.

Methodological problems are rife. Observational studies rarely show cause. Randomised trials can give very different results based on accuracy of reporting rare events such as suicide.

Currently though, the observational evidence is that antidepressant use in

DEPRESSION

suicidal patients is associated with increased suicide and venlafaxine may be the most implicated. It should not be used as first line in major depression, say these authors.

POSTNATAL DEPRESSION

Psychosocial and psychological interventions for prevention of postnatal depression: systematic review
Dennis C
BMJ, 2005; **331**: 15

Postnatal depression is a major health issue. Sufferers are likely to experience future depression and endure impaired maternal–infant interactions. Psychological and psychosocial risk factors such as life stress, marital conflict, self esteem, and lack of social support have been identified.

This systematic review of 15 trials, however, did not find that any diverse interventions in these areas in the form of classes, debriefings and interpersonal psychotherapy, reduced the number who went on to develop postnatal depression. Targeting of at-risk women may be more effective.

MANAGEMENT PROGRAMMES

Long term outcomes from the IMPACT randomised trial for depressed elderly patients in primary care
Hunkeler EM, Katon W, Tang L *et al.*
BMJ, 2006; **332**: 259–263

Few studies deal specifically with the needs of elderly depressed patients.

The IMPACT trial – Improving Mood Promoting Access to Collaborative Treatment – involved 1801 patients, mean age 71 years, who met the DSM-IV criteria for major depression or dysthymia. The trial has already reported benefits in outcome over a year with a management programme involving a depression care manager (a nurse or psychologist), who personalises and supports a treatment plan which may use drugs and psychological modalities in liaison with a psychiatrist and a primary care physician.

The intervention group used more drugs and more psychotherapy, raising the suggestion that the case worker may just have removed some barriers to accessing care.

However, this further study extends the original findings.

One year after IMPACT resources were withdrawn, the active engagement of these elderly and often reluctant patients was still paying dividends in terms of less depression, healthier lives and better physical functioning.

The particular care manager may be an important factor as it was still not possible to determine which part of the package led to the enduring benefits.

Collaborative care for depression
Simon G
BMJ, 2006; **332**: 249–250
and
Depression should be managed like a chronic disease
Scott J
BMJ, 2006; **332**: 985–986

Undertreatment has resulted from doctors failing to prescribe effectively and from patients failing to take their drugs. Non-specific counselling is not going to solve the problems of case management and even CBT is not for everybody.

Collaborative care models, however, have successfully used structured collaboration between patient, specialist and primary carers combined with evidence-based protocols to actively monitor adherence to treatment and clinical outcomes. These two editorials note that evidence has consistently shown the value and the acceptability of this strategy. IMPACT used such an approach with brief monthly follow-up telephone calls documenting persisting benefit after 2 years – valuable evidence of a successful intervention for such a relapsing and remitting chronic disease.

The research is clear. Now it is time to disseminate the message and graduate from the *ad hoc* management of isolated acute episodes of depression and attend to the maintenance and continuation phases. These chronic disease management models can be as effective in depression as they have been in asthma and hypertension.

Patient involvement in primary care mental health: a focus group study
Lester H, Tait L, England E *et al.*
Br J Gen Pract, 2006; **56**: 415–422

The personal experience of psychiatric patients can enhance the care of others. Patients with serious mental illness in this survey felt that early contact with someone who had been in their shoes would have given them valuable insight into their new diagnosis and the issues they would be facing. The survey of 39 GPs and 45 patients also failed to yield examples of a shared-decision making approach to the consultation. Patients felt that decisions were made by the health professional and felt unable to challenge this due to a lack of information about alternatives.

Daily practicalities such as resource limitations impact on the ability to provide a better service but this may be an excellent area for voluntary patient groups to help out.

CHILDREN

Depression in adolescents
Hazell P
BMJ, 2007; **335**: 106–107

This editorial suggests that adding CBT to the use of SSRIs is unlikely to improve outcomes.

CLINICAL ISSUES

DEPRESSION

The ADAPT trial (adolescent depression antidepressant and psychotherapy trial) recruited a heterogenous group that reflected real world patients well. It compared SSRIs with and without psychological therapy and failed to confirm the benefit of adding CBT to an SSRI for adolescent outpatients referred to UK specialists. This challenges NICE guidance that only combination therapy should be used in adolescents and suggests fluoxetine can be used safely alone (*BMJ*, 2007; **335:** 142).

TADS (treatment for adolescents with depression study) was the original study that displayed the success of combination therapy; in this case showing fluoxetine/CBT working better together than either one alone against depressive symptoms. But it has limited generalisability and recruited half of its participants through advertising. Other studies have failed to confirm such benefits. At best the advantage of adding CBT is likely to be modest in adolescents. Further endpoints such as suicidal thoughts have not been clearly measured.

Contrary to the NICE guidelines, SSRIs seem to be reasonable monotherapy, particularly if CBT is hard to access. It is worth noting that those randomised in the ADAPT trials had frequent reviews and monitoring, so the intervention did not end at the prescription.

Should young people be given antidepressants? No
Timimi S
BMJ, 2007; **335:** 751

His argument goes that medics endorsed use of SSRIs in adolescents before good evidence existed and, now that it does, it has shown them to be no better than placebo and increases suicides.

Fluoxetine escaped with a good report but the data were flawed. Combination therapy was unblinded and may have exaggerated the effect of fluoxetine. Journals have failed in their peer review processes and published incomplete reports on areas of (lack of) significance on primary outcomes measures. Even the ADAPT trial did not have a placebo arm "giving the (false) impression that SSRIs have already been assumed to be more effective than placebo".

Should young people be given antidepressants? Yes
Cotgrove A
BMJ, 2007; **335:** 750

The antithesis goes that to deny these vulnerable groups the possibility of antidepressants would be inappropriate due to their evidence of success as "objective meta-analysis shows benefit over placebo for SSRIs".

The risk of suicide is small and can be reduced by careful monitoring claims the author. The newer research downplays the effect of CBT so what does that leave us with? Even NICE has endorsed their use by specialists.

They note the "worrying methodological errors, publication bias and omissions of evidence" but still claim that "objective review means that tablets have a place".

So I suppose it depends what you choose to believe. But surely the standard of proof to know you are not doing harm to children should be high?

SUICIDE

A qualitative study of help seeking and primary care consultation prior to suicide
Owens C, Lambert H, Donovan J *et al.*
Br J Gen Pract, 2005; **55**: 503–509

A qualitative study found that relatives and friends often played a key role in determining whether or not suicidal individuals sought medical help.

Half the suicides in the study had consulted in the final month of their life and many were persuaded to do so by a relative or friend. Of the others, some had not suggested going to the GP because no-one was aware how serious the situation was.

More attention paid to these lay networks to combine medical and non-medical strategies might prevent suicides.

SSRIs AND SUICIDE

Association between suicide attempts and selective serotonin reuptake inhibitors: systematic review of randomised controlled trials
Fergusson D, Doucette S, Glass KC *et al.*
BMJ, 2005; **330**: 396

This systematic review of 702 published RCTs with 87 650 patients compared SSRIs with either placebo or other active treatments in patients with depression and other clinical conditions.

- There was an almost twofold increase in suicidal attempts in users of SSRIs compared with placebo or other therapeutic interventions other than tricyclics.
- NNT for harm for SSRIs was 684.
- Users of SSRIs had no increase in fatal suicidal attempts compared to placebo.
- No differences were observed when overall suicide attempts were compared between users of SSRIs and tricyclic antidepressants. This conclusion was shared by case-control analysis on nearly 150 000 primary care records with a first prescription of an antidepressant (*BMJ,* 2005; **330**: 389).

Suicide, depression, and antidepressants
Cipriani A, Barbui C, Geddes JR
BMJ, 2005; **330**: 373–374

This editorial gives us some help on the SSRI debate by reminding us that study designs influence the conclusions we can make. These are the insights the authors summarise:

- SSRIs and tricyclics may induce and worsen suicidal ideation and suicide attempts in the early phase of treatment possibly due to agitation and activation
- at this time close follow up and family involvement should be considered
- patients should be advised to avoid sudden discontinuation of therapy

DEPRESSION

- evidence in favour of antidepressants cannot necessarily be extrapolated to mild depression
- in children and adolescents on SSRIs and other antidepressants, evidence of suicidal behaviour and lack of long-term data should discourage routine prescribing

---

The risk of suicide with selective serotonin reuptake inhibitors in the elderly
Juurlink DN, Mamdami MM, Kopp A *et al.*
Am J Psychiatry, 2006; **163**: 813–821

This case control study in 1138 cases in Ontario, also reviewed in the *BMJ* (2006; **332** – 20 May), revisits the question of suicide and SSRIs.

They concluded starting treatment with SSRIs – fluoxetine, fluvoxamine, paroxetine, sertraline and citalopram (venlafaxine was not included) – was associated with a risk of suicide five times higher than any other class of antidepressant. This was predominantly related to violent suicide in young men but only apparent in the first month of treatment.

The absolute risk was still low – estimated as 1 in 3300 for SSRIs and 1 in 16 000 for those on other antidepressants.

Because of the way they matched the cases to controls, the authors feel this is unlikely to be due to doctors giving SSRIs to those more prone to suicide.

The risk of undertreatment is still likely to be much worse than these observations.

DOMESTIC VIOLENCE

The Challenge

Domestic violence (aka intimate partner abuse) includes emotional, sexual, and financial intimidation as well as physical violence. A quarter of women in the UK report being assaulted by an intimate partner and many do not know how to get help.

It is a major public health problem affecting all parts of society including children and same-sex couples as well as many vulnerable groups such as the elderly or disabled. It is estimated that half a million elderly people in the UK are being abused at any one time, usually by family members.

Certainly GPs need to be more vigilant but how do we go about it? We usually wait for specific clues to help identify cases. But rates of disclosure of abuse without direct questioning are known to be poor, and routine enquiry may be the only pragmatic way of getting to the truth. Only a minority of health professionals are in favour of screening for domestic violence, but simple enquiry seems to have a high level of acceptability among women. Even though a minority do not like the idea, domestically abused women identify doctors as the people they would most like to talk to about their situation. The frequent contact they have with health services makes them the best place for such enquiry.

Still, most doctors feel unprepared. Most are afraid of annoying or endangering patients and do not know what they would do with a positive screen. There is limited research on the GP management of partner abuse and studies on interventions are rare. Is there sufficient evidence of a lack of harm from our interventions? Some studies do show positive outcomes from outreach services in terms of reduced violence over time and leaving abusive relationships, but training for health professionals is urgently needed. Protocols that prioritise safety are essential to alleviate concerns about 'opening a can of worms'. They will also ease their ambivalence, frustration and worry at dealing with issues of child protection, legalities and pressure of time.

The consequences of under-delivering in this sensitive area are many. In the short term, they include injury such as fractures and burns, and in the long term there are chronic health problems such as pain syndromes, headaches and mental illness.

The 'unspoken' nature of the abuse means that surveys of prevalence may be doomed to underestimation.

What we know already:

- 80% of abuse victims are women and 30% of the abuse begins in pregnancy.
- Victims have three times the usual consultation rate.
- One in seven men experience physical assault by a current or former partner but incidents in men are likely to involve less fear and injury.
- Children growing up with domestic violence are 30–60% more likely to develop emotional, behavioural, educational and health problems. Children are more likely to repeat these patterns as an adult.
- In a recent study, 1 in 4 Australian women who had suffered depression had suffered intimate partner abuse in the previous year. The association remained after adjusting for other

DOMESTIC VIOLENCE

sociodemographic factors such as poor education, low income, unemployment and being abused as a child.

- The presence of depression may heighten awareness to possible partner abuse and encourage enquiry, and vice versa.
- Systematic review suggests that there is insufficient evidence to justify screening. The most important factor against it is the lack of proof that interventions are successful and not harmful.
- Pathways of referral are still to be defined. Meantime, non-judgemental assistance, Victim Support, emergency shelter and legal advice seem good places to start.

Guidelines

Domestic violence: the general practitioner's role. *RCGP*, 1998.

Domestic violence: a resource manual for health care professionals. *Dept of Health*, 2000.

The WHO multi-country study on women's health and domestic violence against women. *World Health Organization*, 2003 onwards.

Recent Papers

PREVALENCE

Intimate partner violence
Ferris LE
BMJ, 2007; **334**: 706–707

The WHO Multi-country Study on Women's Health and Domestic Violence against Women has released initial results on prevalence and health outcomes based on responses of 24 000 women in 10 countries.

Lifetime prevalence of intimate partner violence in women who had ever had a partner ranged from 30 to 60% at most sites. Research is making advances in terms of recommended practices and women's health clinics. We have started looking at women's acceptance of health screening but we still do not know if universal screening is a good idea, or the best strategies for intervening.

This editorial outlines the many overlapping roles of doctors, such as medical expert, communicator, team collaborator, manager of resources and health advocate. Frameworks such as these should be used for competencies and an international consensus on standards in this area of global concern would be welcome.

CASE IDENTIFICATION

The acceptability of routine inquiry about domestic violence towards women: a survey in three healthcare settings
Boyle A, Jones P
Br J Gen Pract, 2006; **56**: 258–261

This study took place in three general practices, one emergency department and an antenatal clinic. Questionnaires were used to determine the characteristics of women who found inquiry concerning domestic violence unacceptable. Of 2300 women, 63% responded:
- 8.4% of those that responded found inquiry unacceptable
- abuse within a year was strongly associated with finding inquiry unacceptable
- lifetime abuse was not associated with finding inquiry unacceptable

The authors conclude that screening for domestic abuse in this way is acceptable to most women particularly if they have recently been free from abuse.

Utilisation of health care by women who have suffered abuse: a descriptive study on medical records in family practice
Lo Fo Wong S, Wester F, Mol S, *et al.*
Br J Gen Pract, 2007; **57**: 396–400

This study looked at data from sufferers of abuse seen in Dutch primary care between 2001 and 2004. The heavy use of medical services was noted and pain was the most frequently presented health problem.

Women who were victims of abuse consulted twice as often for pain and received up to seven times the amount of prescribed drugs in terms of analgesia, tranquillisers and antidepressants. These findings may help target our enquiries and add to the concept of the 'symptomatic' victim.

MANAGEMENT

General practitioner management of intimate partner abuse and the whole family: qualitative study
Taft A, Broom DH, Legge D
BMJ, 2004; **328**: 618

This study of 28 Australian GPs found that their own stress and difficulty in resolving tensions led to neglect of risks to children, contraindicated practices, unsuccessful attempts at counselling and breaks in confidentiality between the couple.

It illustrated how poor Australian doctors were at their attempts to resolve partner abuse issues. They were confused about when normal conflict became abnormal and seemed to underestimate the number of cases on their books.

The empathetic GPs suffered with non-compliant patients and lack of positive feedback. Feelings of despair and helplessness were common and female GPs got the brunt of it. The GPs on the other end of the spectrum were concerned how much money they were losing due to long consultations.

DOMESTIC VIOLENCE

Responses to the male partners – the abusers coming in for treatment for their depression, pain and alcohol problems – could be hostile. Some entered into raising the issues in a watered down version of amateur counselling despite this model being contraindicated due to the associated risks.

Some, of course, just ignored the problem and most doctors overlooked the impact on children despite the powerful catalyst this can be for change. They did not feel equipped to help and were distrusting of child protection services.

Unfortunately there were few agencies to which to refer patients and little information on whether intervention is beneficial.

Intimate partner abuse cannot be solved by general practice alone but identification and referral plays a critical role in the process.

This study reinforces the need for guidelines for managing the whole family, acting on behalf of children and the need to refer to specialist agencies. Training, supervision and support for the health professionals is needed to cope with the stress of this difficult work.

SCREENING CONCEPTS

The Challenge

Screening has intuitive appeal to doctors and patients. The idea that early diagnosis means definitive gain is seductive and has led to procedures that have sidestepped the usually necessary gold standard of a randomised controlled trial or two. This has been shown to be a mistake on several occasions. Huge controversy still surrounds PSA as a detector of prostate cancer. Breast self-examination and testicular self-examination have both failed due to lack of scientific rigour. They had been advocated on the assumption they could do no harm. They do: more biopsies, more anxiety, same deaths. Public health bodies need to avoid promoting unproven screening procedures when health resources are limited.

Neither may traditional history taking be the best way of detecting disease. The era of doctors formulating their plans from a muddle of questions may be coming to an end. Its effectiveness is, after all, unproven and largely based on habit and ritual. But how many conditions can a GP realistically screen for?

Maybe we should work harder to summon people for healthcare check-ups rather than wait for them to turn up for other reasons and then opportunistically target them. But this intervention only works for those who attend and clinicians practising this need to confine themselves to only those components with strong proof of efficacy.

Clinical prediction rules may be the future. The Mini-Cog, for example, shows promise for detecting dementia but more such tools are needed as we are at the dawn of the 'diagnostic age'. We won't discard our old habits without a fight of course – that wouldn't be any fun at all.

New tests are good though aren't they? And the screening industry loves to sell them to us. But how then do we define what is normal? Our usual method of taking two standard deviations from the mean fails us when there are thousands of measurements. Many will cross into the 'abnormal' 5% threshold and the only question becomes exactly how abnormal is each of us! That may not be terribly helpful and our ignorance of the natural history of many diseases exposes our good intentions.

There are many candidates of diseases to screen for and the list will grow with new evidence-based diagnostics. However, things are rarely as straightforward as they seem when it comes to adopting widespread screening protocols.

And what are the consequences of over-screening? The government's advisory committee on the medical aspects of radiation have warned private health clinics to stop offering whole body CT scans to the 'worried well' because they carry too high a radiation risk. A typical CT scan carries a one in 2000 lifetime risk of developing a fatal cancer, but market forces are not too interested in hanging around for a decade to await the results of randomised trials.

What we know already:

- Chest screening with CT detects lung cancers but our ignorance of the natural history of the cancers means we do not know how useful this is. False positives can reach 70% and some may be a case of 'dying with' rather than 'dying from'.
- Whole body CT magnifies these results and most findings are false positives.

CLINICAL ISSUES

SCREENING

- Many investigations and interventions adversely affect quality of life.
- Recognising coeliac disease is difficult in primary care as symptoms can be non-specific or absent, yet estimates of prevalence of undiagnosed and preclinical coeliac disease range from 0.7% to 2.0%.
- New tests help to detect coeliac disease but we still do not know if people with serous positivity but preserved villous structure benefit from treatment. Screening of the general population would be expensive, difficult and probably unacceptable to patients – positives must be confirmed by biopsy.

Recent Papers

INTERPRETATION

Health professionals' and service users' interpretation of screening test results: experimental study

Bramwell R, West H, Salmon P
BMJ, 2006; **333**: 284

Different groups of people draw differently incorrect conclusions when presented with results of screening.

This study looked at the interpretations of people involved in antenatal care – midwives, obstetricians and pregnant women and their companions.

The data were related to the blood test for Down's syndrome that is offered to all pregnant women and actually predicted a 50% probability of Down's.

- 86% of the responses were incorrect.
- The incorrect answers given were mostly very high or very low.
- Obstetricians gave more correct answers but still were right only 43% of the time.
- Pregnant women interpreted correctly in 9%.
- Midwives – the major provider of information – interpreted correctly in 0% of cases.
- Many health professionals were confident in their incorrect answers, displaying a lack of insight into the meaning of crucial information.
- Presentation of the information as frequencies (which is presumed to promote a more natural style of reasoning) rather than percentages improved interpretation but only in obstetricians – to 65%. Almost all the others were still wrong.
- Participation was voluntary so things could be even worse in reality.

Ways of conveying information sorely need updating, with visual aids, for example. They need to be relevant to the academic ability and level of education of patients and others interpreting them.

More and more screening technologies are becoming available and we are making more use of probabilistic information. It is crucial to draw correct conclusions from the information we gather. If we do not, the concept of screening is damaged.

THE CT CONTROVERSY

Computed tomography – an increasing source of radiation exposure
Brenner DJ, Hall EJ
N Engl J Med, 2007; **357:** 2277–2284

It is estimated that more than 62 million CT scans per year are currently obtained in the United States. For most people in this US survey, the risk outweighs the benefits and the recent increase in usage for screening is worrying.

This paper estimates that 1–2% of all cancers are attributable to ionising radiation following enthusiastic use of the CT scanner.

Children are more radiosensitive and have longer to grow their cancer. In the US, 6–11% of scans are performed on children often to diagnose or rule out appendicitis. Scans are used defensively and repeatedly for headaches and blunt trauma. Up to one-third could be replaced with other diagnostic tests or not be done at all.

CT screening for lung cancer: spiraling into confusion?
Black WC, Baron JA
JAMA, 2007; **297:** 995–997
and
Computed tomography screening and lung cancer outcomes
Bach PB, Jett JR, Pastorino U, *et al.*
JAMA, 2007; **297:** 953–961

This study and editorial comments on the use of CT to screen for lung cancer in over 3000 current or former smokers and compares the results to a prediction model.

In the absence of better evidence and RCTs, this is the best evidence so far that such screening does not save lives. It does increase the chance of an invasive procedure such as biopsy, and a resection carries a 5% mortality rate in the US.

Three times as many cancers were detected leading to 10 times as many resections, but there was no impact on mortality.

NEWER CANDIDATES FOR SCREENING

Population screening for coeliac disease in primary care by district nurses using a rapid antibody test: diagnostic accuracy and feasibility study
Korponay-Szabó IR, Szabados K, Pusztai J, *et al.*
BMJ, 2007; **335:** 1244–1247

Up to 90% of children with coeliac disease remain undiagnosed and tend to underachieve academically.

District nurses in Hungary tested 2690 6 year old children with fingerpick antibody testing for antibodies to endomysium and transglutaminase, using a rapid point-of-care detection kit at a routine pre-school check up.

- The test was 78% sensitive and 100% specific for coeliac disease.
- Most patients would be identified at an early age.
- 1.4% had coeliac disease.

SCREENING

- After a gluten-free diet children reported improved growth and haemoglobin levels.
- The test was simple, rapid and cheap and this is a possible direction for large scale screening.

Clinical presentation and incidence of complications in patients with coeliac disease diagnosed by relative screening
Sundar N, Crimmins R, Swift G
Postgrad Med J, 2007; **83:** 273–276

Screening first degree relatives for serology helped to identify new cases and provide opportunity for intervention with a gluten-free diet to resolve iron deficiency. Prevalence among relatives was 13% but there was little morbidity in serologically positive individuals.

Patients were younger than those identified with routine care and fewer had complications such as osteoporosis or anaemia.

Larger studies would be needed to see if this is a useful cost-effective approach.

Coeliac disease in primary care
Jones R
BMJ, 2007; **334:** 704–705

Most cases of coeliac disease go unrecognised and diagnosis is delayed. It is characterised by lifelong intolerance to certain proteins collectively known as gluten. Many may have atypical presentations with no classical symptoms of malabsorption.

However, it also causes iron deficiency anaemia, osteoporosis and short stature and unfavourably affects pregnancy.

Serum testing for antigliadin and endomysial antibodies is available with reasonable sensitivity and specificity. The US recommends using tranglutaminase antibody as a single diagnostic test. Confirmation is with the gold standard test – small intestinal biopsy – but even that can have patchy results, though repeat follow-ups lower the diagnostic uncertainty.

Coeliac disease is more common in first degree relatives and, in addition to investigating those with symptoms, screening with antibody tests in first degree relatives could be considered.

The need to test routinely in those with irritable bowel symptoms, however, is controversial. One UK trial showed the prevalence of coeliac disease in those with IBS to be the same as in the population at large.

Screening for carotid artery stenosis: an update of the evidence for the U.S. Preventive Services Task Force
Wolff T, Guirguis-Blake J, Miller T, *et al.*
Ann Intern Med, 2007; **147:** 854–870

A review of the evidence surrounding routine screening to identify candidates for carotid endarterectomy found that it was likely to do more harm than good.

- Ultrasonography has a sensitivity and specificity above 90%, but is still not accurate enough and the surgery is not safe enough to justify screening.
- No RCTs have looked at how the intervention affects stroke.
- Surgery in carefully selected patients reduces stroke but is unlikely to translate to wider populations.
- Up to 5% of patients have a stroke or die within a month of surgery.

CLINICAL ISSUES

SCREENING

COLORECTAL CANCER

The Challenge

Bowel cancer is second only to lung cancer as a cause of cancer deaths in the UK. Five year survival rates remain below 50%. In 2004 the number of deaths exceeded that from breast and cervical cancer combined – both of which have effective screening programmes. Colorectal cancer evolves slowly from premalignant polyps providing a large window of opportunity for screening as the risk of delays in diagnosis is high.

The government first announced its aim to introduce bowel cancer screening in the NHS Plan in 2000. Screening will be introduced for men and women in their 60s – the first cancer screening programme in England to include men.

Contenders for screening have been immunochemical FOB test, flexible sigmoidoscopy, colonoscopy, virtual colonoscopy and faecal DNA tests, but evidence is strongest for guaic FOB testing.

Pilot trials indicate that FOB testing is the only method yet shown to cut the death rate from colorectal cancer (by around 15–18%). The UK Colorectal Cancer Screening Pilot Group illustrated that FOB screening was practical within the context of the United Kingdom's NHS and could save life at reasonable cost.

Of course the test is not perfect. It may only be about 50% sensitive in a screening context but evidence clearly shows it can have a major impact on mortality from colorectal cancer. Studies showed that FOB testing would detect one or two bowel cancers for every 1000 people screened. An additional three or four people would have pre-cancerous lesions removed. An increase in provision of endoscopy services will be promptly needed.

The bowel cancer screening programme is being rolled out across the UK and it is hoped that it will be fully in place by 2009. The government has decided to limit the target age group to 60–69 years rather than 50–69 which may reduce the overall effectiveness of the programme compared to the pilot studies. It plans to extend the programme to those aged 70–75 years by 2012.

What we know already:

- Rectal bleeding occurs in 40% of patients with colorectal cancer.
- One study of patients with iron deficiency anaemia presenting to their GPs found serious pathology in 30% of those investigated. Gastro-intestinal cancers, principally colorectal, were diagnosed in 11%.
- The high prevalence and resulting low predictive value of symptoms such as rectal bleeding, changes in bowel habit, and abdominal pain means that most affected patients have a very low chance of cancer.
- The UK Colorectal Cancer Screening Pilot Group posted a FOB test kit to participants with instructions to smear on some stool and post it back. Those testing positive for blood were investigated with colonoscopy. Acceptance levels were high and 2 in 100 had positive tests requiring further investigation.
- The positive predictive values of a positive test result were 11% for invasive cancer and 35% for adenoma and the cost of screening was about £5900 per life year saved.

- The US has recommended FOB testing from aged 50 since the 1980s – around 40% of the population complies with this advice but their more unregulated approach often dumps faecal testing in favour of colonoscopy.
- Colonoscopy is increasingly popular and yet we cannot say for certain whether it saves lives. It may not be cost effective and a decent randomised trial is needed.
- Virtual colonoscopy where the bowel is pumped up creating a pneumocolon prior to CT scanning is not yet a consistent enough technique to recommend.
- Aspirin may have a role as a reasonably effective treatment to prevent adenomas in high risk patients. But for most people long term use of aspirin to reduce the incidence of colorectal cancer causes too much of a trade off with haemorrhage to be a viable proposition.

Guidelines

Referral guidelines for suspected cancer. *NICE*, 2005.

Recent Papers

SCREENING METHODS

The UK colorectal cancer screening pilot: results of the second round of screening in England
Weller D, Coleman D, Robertson R, *et al.*
Br J Cancer, 2007; **97**: 1601–1605

This group have been studying the screening programme now for 5 years, screening with FOBs every 2 years in those aged 50–69.

The second round of FOB screening in the English site of the UK Colorectal Cancer Screening Pilot included a total of 127 746 men and women.

- 16% were new invitees not included in the previous round.
- Uptake dipped to 52% returning a screening kit.
- Uptake was lower in men (48%) than women (56%) but increased with age.
- Uptake fell as deprivation increased from 61% in the wealthiest areas to 39% in the poorest.
- There were ethnic variations too with uptake lower in those of Indian origin.
- Tests were positive in 1.8%.
- The cancer detection rate (0.94 per 1000) was lower than in the first round.

Strategies will be required to minimise inequalities in uptake, maintain commitment to 2 yearly screening and to ensure adequate capacity of endoscopy services.

The effects of population-based faecal occult blood test screening upon emergency colorectal cancer admissions in Coventry and north Warwickshire

Goodyear SJ, Leung E, Menon A, *et al.*
Gut, 2008; **57:** 218–222

Over the period that the UK Bowel Cancer Screening Pilot was initiated data between 1999 and 2004 from the largest region screened showed:

- there was a decline in emergency workload with a halving of the relative percentage of bowel cancer admissions that presented as emergencies
- mortality within 30 days of the operation fell from 48% to 13%
- the need for stoma formation decreased

These results show that screening is effective and were likely due to better detection, greater public awareness and quicker referrals. Uptake did, however, decrease in the second round so that will need to be monitored.

Impending or pending? The national bowel cancer screening programme

Atkin WS
BMJ, 2006; **332:** 742

and

Colorectal cancer in primary care

Weller D
BMJ, 2006; **333:** 54–55

These editorials discuss the considerable challenges for primary care in trying to recognise potential cases of colorectal cancer while avoiding unnecessary investigations.

We certainly need to reduce the burden of disease and reverse our low ranking of survival rates. This means diagnosis must be made at an earlier stage – preferably when asymptomatic.

England is introducing bowel cancer screening based on the strong evidence of effectiveness and acceptability of FOB testing, but the rollout has been slower than expected. Although some funding was in place in 2004, a phased rollout is not expected to cover the country until 2010, screening 60–69 year olds – around 3 years later than in France (who currently target those aged 50–74 years).

The reasons are clear. Without enough accredited endoscopists in place for the estimated 30 000 colonoscopies needed, people may wait too long or even end up getting priority over those who already have symptoms.

Recruitment for the screening programme and follow up is to be organised centrally but some of the workload will spill over to primary care and inevitably patients outside of the nominated age group will request screening.

In the future, diagnostic algorithms based on symptoms scores could help us prioritise referral decisions as we learn more about the predictive values of different symptoms in primary care populations. Perhaps even risk tables, like those used to evaluate cardiovascular risk, might turn out to be useful.

Does a negative screening colonoscopy ever need to be repeated?
Brenner H, Chang-Claude J, Seiler CM *et al.*
Gut, 2006; **55**: 1145–1150

Colonoscopy is traditionally repeated every 10 years after an initial negative result.

This research suggests that it need not be repeated for 20 years if at all.

This population-based case-control study was adjusted for confounders and found that a previous negative colonoscopy reduces the risk of a positive finding in the future for at least 20 years, particularly if performed after the age of 55 years.

Increased time interval between colonoscopies increases safety by diminishing complications and the cost-effectiveness of screening.

Positive predictive value of fecal occult blood testing in persons taking warfarin
Bini EJ, Rajapaksa RC, Weinshel EH
Am J Gastroenterol, 2005; **100**: 1586–1592

A useful prospective study over a 5 year period that looked at concerns related to warfarin use during FOB testing concluded:
- warfarin use did not decrease the positive predictive value of FOB testing
- there is therefore no need to discontinue warfarin prior to FOB testing
- positive FOB in patients taking warfarin must not dismissed as a false positive

RISK ASSESMENT

Risk in primary care of colorectal cancer from new onset rectal bleeding: 10 year prospective study
du Toit J, Hamilton W, Barraclough K
BMJ, 2006; **333**: 69–70

This was a study in one general practice of patients aged over 45 years who bled rectally and where one of the GPs was familiar with sigmoidoscopy. Some patients received further investigation with barium enemas or colonoscopy.
- The annual rate of new rectal bleeding in this UK general practice population was 9/1000.
- Only two of the patients with cancer had diarrhoea, showing how negatively predictive it is.
- Over a decade, 265 reported rectal bleeding of which 1 in 10 had colonic neoplasia (5.7% had colorectal cancer and 4.9% had colonic adenoma).

The authors state that this incidence means that regardless of other symptoms, rectal bleeding warrants urgent referral in those over 45.

Predicting colorectal cancer risk in patients with rectal bleeding
Robertson R, Campbell C, Weller D *et al.*
Br J Gen Pract, 2006; **56**: 763–767

This observational study of over 600 patients with rectal bleeding looked at symptoms predictive of colorectal cancer.

Significant predictors included blood mixed with the stool, which had a likelihood ratio of 1.5, and age, particularly if over 70 years. In patients with bleeding not mixed with stool and who had haemorrhoids, a cancer, although less likely, was still present in 2%.

These authors conclude that rectal bleeding in isolation had insufficient diagnostic value to be useful in general practice.

Factors identifying higher risk rectal bleeding in general practice
Ellis BG, Thompson M
Br J Gen Pract, 2005; **55**: 949–955

This study also looked at the predictive and diagnostic value of factors in bowel cancer. Some 319 consecutive patients aged 34 years were studied. A questionnaire asked about symptoms and further investigation was with flexible sigmoidoscopy, followed by review at 18 months.

- 3.4% of this age group had colorectal cancer.
- This increased to 9.2% when rectal bleeding was associated with a change in bowel habit and to 11.1% when peri-anal symptoms were absent.
- 36% of cancer patients had a palpable rectal mass.

PROSTATE CANCER

The Challenge

There are 27 000 new cases of prostate cancer a year in the UK, making it the second most common cancer in men causing almost 10 000 deaths a year. Screening for the disease has been controversial. There is a lack of consensus on treatment and a lack of evidence that intervention affects mortality.

Serum prostate-specific antigen (PSA) has been adopted for case-finding among asymptomatic men and has substantially increased the detection and incidence of prostate cancer, but is far from a perfect candidate as a screening test. There is no cut-off point of PSA with simultaneous high sensitivity and high specificity for screening healthy men for prostate cancer. Rather there is a continuum of prostate cancer risk at all values of PSA.

Widespread testing of PSA leads to overdiagnosis of prostate cancer and there is enormous scope here. One study estimates that around half of prostate cancers would not have come to light in the patient's lifetime in the absence of screening.

Poor communication of the risks of screening means that doctors and patients have still been tempted into PSA testing. In the US, around 60% of men over the age of 50 years are being tested annually. The developer of PSA testing has proclaimed the "PSA era is over" and consigned it to the rubbish bin as a detector of cancer. Unfortunately the prostate screening industry is a juggernaut and makes tens of thousands of Americans impotent each year for no reason.

Trials are ongoing but, in the absence of good evidence, many countries including the UK take a pragmatic stance whereby men over 50 may have a test for PSA if they still want it after an informed discussion with their GP. Men younger than 50 are usually offered the test only if they have a family history of the disease, or are of black ethnicity where risks may be higher. More trials are needed for the full picture, and any benefits that might be shown would have to be balanced against the adverse effects of surgery such as urinary and erectile dysfunction

Ultimately, better markers are needed that reflect the size and grade of prostate cancer.

What we know already:

- The main cause of elevated serum PSA concentration is benign prostatic hyperplasia.
- Looking at over 1300 radical prostatectomies over 20 years, although serum PSA was related to prostate cancer 20 years ago, the only trend relating to PSA value in recent years was prostatic weight.
- In men under 60, PSA (at a cut off of 4 µg/l) fails to identify 8 of every 10 men who later have prostate cancer. In older men 65% of cancers would be missed.
- When prostate cancers are diagnosed, despite a low PSA level of <4.0 µg/l, they are no less clinically significant. Research shows that many of these tumours are high-grade, high-volume and extraprostatic.
- The presence of obesity worsens outcome in men with prostate cancer. They tend to have lower PSA probably due to haemodilution.
- Research has shown a long indolent phase lasting 10–15 years after which survival drops sharply, leading to proposals that we should consider early radical treatment among patients expected to live more than 15 years.

SCREENING

- Radical prostatectomy may reduce deaths from prostate cancer and reduce local and distant progression. However, there is no evidence of an overall reduction in mortality more than watchful waiting.
- In the future, new tests could identify genes such as E2F3 which help to predict aggressiveness of prostate cancer.

Recent Papers

SCREENING

The effectiveness of screening for prostate cancer
Concato J, Wells CK, Horwitz RI *et al*.
Arch Intern Med, 2006; **166**: 38–43

In this case-control study, no mortality benefit was found from prostate screening with PSA, with or without digital rectal examination. The authors say that routine testing should not be endorsed and the focus should be on fully informing the patients about the uncertainty of screening. The risks of unnecessary biopsies, overdiagnosis, sexual dysfunction and urinary incontinence all need to be taken into account. Reductions in overall prostate cancer mortality rates in the US mirror those in countries which have no claim that they routinely screen.

Screening for prostate cancer in younger men
Ilic D, Green S
BMJ, 2007; **335:** 1105–1106

The UK promotes informed decision making while we all await the results of trials that will hopefully resolve some of the confusion surrounding screening.

The diagnostic accuracy of PSA and digital rectal examination are questionable and it is unknown if screening improves survival or quality of life. Poor access to decision aids and educational materials, lack of knowledge and differing attitudes to testing still dominate the argument.

Screening is commonplace despite lack of evidence in many settings. Discussion, which is as informed as possible, is all we have to offer prior to testing until the darkness lifts with better evidence.

Detection of prostate cancer in unselected young men: prospective cohort nested within a randomised controlled trial
Lane JA, Howson J, Donovan JL
BMJ, 2007; **335:** 1139

This study looked at the feasibility of testing for prostate cancer in younger men aged 45–49 years in UK primary care. Previously, studies in the US have indicated that PSA levels in the fourth decade predict prostate cancer.

The testing was generally found to be acceptable, albeit that the 34% uptake was lower than in older men. A threshold of 1.5 µg/ml identified 5 cases of clinically relevant cancer in 442 men. The prevalence of prostate cancer was 2.3% – similar to that in older men.

It is still far from certain whether this means we should head towards widespread screening.

'It's a maybe test': men's experiences of prostate specific antigen testing in primary care
Evans R, Edwards A, Elwyn G, *et al*.
Br J Gen Pract, 2007; **57:** 303–310

A qualitative study of 28 interviews with men in Wales regarding PSA testing and the various possible outcomes showed that the decision was affected by social and media factors, but not that is was particularly patient-led. Uncertainty was present before and after the test and led to a good deal of anxiety and regret as a consequence – a 'maybe test'.

Evidence from 2 low quality screening studies does not show a reduction in death from prostate cancer. *Evidence-Based Medicine*, 2007; **12:** 40
The following paper is reviewed
Screening for prostate cancer
Ilic D, O'Connor D, Green S, *et al.*
Cochrane Database Syst Rev, 2006

Systematic Cochrane review of (just) two RCTs with "significant methodological weaknesses" was unable to show any reduction in mortality in men randomised to screening with PSA, DRE or transrectal ultrasound biopsy. Neither study assessed quality of life, screening costs or measuring harms. But the 4% decline in prostate mortality rates noticed in the US must be due to screening. Mustn't it? Nobody really knows. But three better trials are on the way and should in time give us the answers we need.

- The US Prostate, Lung, Colorectal and Ovary (PLCO) trial randomises 38 000 older men with annual PSA testing for 5 years.
- The European Randomised study of Screening for Prostate Cancer (ERSPC) is an efficacy trial in eight countries with about 200 000 subjects. Results are expected before 2010.
- The unique Prostate Testing for Cancer and Treatment (ProtecT) trial in the UK has a treatment trial nested within a screening trial. Recruitment finishes in 2008 then there is 10–15 years of additional follow up.

Meanwhile it's the same old mantra. Give them the facts and let them decide.

CLINICAL ISSUES

SCREENING

NATURAL HISTORY

Clinical features of prostate cancer before diagnosis: a population-based, case-control study
Hamilton W, Sharp DJ, Peters TJ, Round AP
Br J Gen Pract, 2006; **56:** 756–762

Predictive features of prostate cancer are largely unknown. This study looked at the medical records of over 200 patients relating to the two years prior to diagnosis of prostate cancer. They found eight features which were predictive of prostate cancer.

Coming in with positive predictive values at around 3% were urinary retention, impotence and hesitancy. At around 2% were nocturia and frequency. Abnormal rectal examination deemed benign around 3% and if deemed malignant 12%. More mildly positive associations were haematuria and weight loss.

The authors conclude that most men with prostate cancer present with symptoms and these figures will help guide triage. Lower urinary tract symptoms have a small but real risk of cancer, suggesting that PSA testing in these men is appropriate.

20-year outcomes following conservative management of clinically localized prostate cancer
Albertsen PC, Hanley JA, Fine J
JAMA, 2005; **293:** 2095–2101

This retrospective cohort study used registry data along with histology and hospital records to review the progress of 767 men aged 55–74 years with clinically localized prostate cancer.

They found that men with low-grade prostate cancers have a very small risk of dying from prostate cancer during 20 years of follow-up and that the annual mortality rate from prostate cancer appears to remain stable even 15–20 years from diagnosis. Aggressive treatment for localized low-grade prostate cancer was therefore thought to be inappropriate.

AORTIC ANEURYSM

The Challenge

Between 5 and 10% of men over 65 years may have an aneurysm of which they are unaware. Every year about 6000 men die from a ruptured abdominal aortic aneurysm in England and Wales. Death rates are around 50%. Prevalence seems to be increasing although deaths from other atherosclerotic conditions are reducing.

This is still only about 2% of all deaths in men, but the condition is largely preventable as aortic aneurysms can be detected with a simple ultrasound examination presenting an opportunity for life-saving surgery. Ultrasound screening for aortic aneurysm has been shown to be of value in older men who are fit enough for surgery and who have an aneurysm of more than 5.5cm.

Calls for a national screening programme are getting louder. However, surgical intervention is high-risk, very resource intensive and not many lives will be saved. It is estimated that screening could prevent 14 aneurysm-related deaths in 10 000 patients over 4 years. Follow up scans may need to be large in number for those with moderate sized aneurysms. Critics have doubted that there is an overall benefit of screening on mortality but new research refutes this. The illustration of improved survival means if we get a screening programme right, death from AAA could become a rarity.

Screening results cannot yet be generalised to men outside the 65–74 age group. In older patients, other co-morbid conditions influence surgical outcomes and therefore the benefits for life expectancy.

Nor have any benefits yet been shown for women. There are few trials on women and little prospect of more at the moment so only high risk women with strong cardiovascular risk factors might benefit from screening as far as we know.

The place of medical treatments is to be decided as statins and other treatments are expected to slow the growth of small aneurysms. The possibility of less traumatic surgery – endovascular aneurysm repair – also provides hope for the future.

What we know already:

- The Multicentre Aneurysm Screening Study (MASS) in men aged 65–74 years had an uptake of 80% and successfully reduced mortality from AAA.
- Aneurysms are not as common in women but rupture is more frequent and occurs at a smaller diameter.
- It is increasingly likely that a single ultrasonography scan confers a benefit which may last at least 15 years.
- An Australian study was not able to show a benefit when the invited age range was extended to 65–83 year olds. Many failed to attend and they failed to exclude men who would have been ineligible for surgery had they attended.

Recent Papers

Screening for abdominal aortic aneurysms: single centre randomised controlled trial
Lindholt JS, Juul S, Fasting H *et al.*
BMJ, 2005; **330**: 750

The findings of the MASS trial were reproduced in a group of 12 639 Danish men aged 64–73 years (mean age 68 years), as follows:
- more than three-quarters of the group accepted the invite
- 4% of those screened had abdominal aortic aneurysms
- screening reduced deaths specifically due to abdominal aortic aneurysm (not overall mortality), averting 3 deaths for every 1000 screened (NNT to save one life = 352)
- screening reduced the rate of emergency surgery by 75%
- this was offset by a 3–4-fold increase in the total number of aneurysm operations
- screening a population with high prevalence will be most cost effective

Clearly, screening is effective in a population of men 64–73 years of age. The most effective strategy must now be found.

A sustained mortality benefit from screening for abdominal aortic aneurysm
Kim LG, Scott RA, Ashton HA, Thompson SG for the MASS Study Group
Ann Intern Med, 2007; **146:** 699–706

The Multicentre Aneurysm Screening Study (MASS), is a large UK randomised study looking into the effect of screening for AAA with ultrasound in 67 770 men aged 65–74 years. Those with an aneurysm over 5.5 cm had an operation. Smaller aneurysms were monitored with further scans.

The scanned group had less aneurysm-related mortality and fewer ruptured aneurysms. They originally estimated that screening 710 subjects prevents one death.

The new 7 year results showed that the early mortality benefit of screening with ultrasonography is maintained in the longer term. Importantly they also showed a reduction in mortality from all causes.

The cost effectiveness of screening improves over time and a QALY was estimated at a bargain price of £3830.

Screening for abdominal aortic aneurysm
Greenhalgh R, Powell J
BMJ, 2007; **335**: 732–733

This editorial refers to a 2007 Cochrane review which analysed four RCTs which screened asymptomatic people for AAA. They were Chichester (the only one to include women), Viborg, Western Australia, and MASS (excluding the recent 7 year results). There were 127 891 men and 9342 women participating, aged from 65 to 83 years.
- Mortality related to aneurysm halved but aneurysm surgery doubled.
- Reduction in all cause mortality just missed significance overall.

SCREENING

However, a separate meta-analysis incorporating the new 7 year data from MASS did show a definite reduction in all cause mortality (*BMJ,* 2007; **335:** 899).

MASS estimated that cost effectiveness had improved from £28 400 per life year gained at 4 years (which translates as £36 000 per QALY) down to £12 334 per life year gained after 7 years. It is likely to fall further after 10 years. Peculiarly, the Viborg study estimated only £620 per life year gained. Maybe the economists can explain what happened to the decimal point.

The data support a national screening programme at least for men with some details still to be decided. Not least, what will we do with the aneurysms found?

Operative mortality is 5% electively, but the more expensive endovascular repair lowers this to less than 2%. In-hospital mortality figures boost this to 10% and the value of any programme will be very dependent on the operative results of the hospitals concerned.

Screening for abdominal aortic aneurysms in men
Earnshaw JJ, Shaw E, Whyman MR *et al.*
BMJ, 2004; **328**: 1122–1124

The Gloucestershire aneurysm screening project has been running since 1990. They invite 65 year old men to an ultrasound at their local practice and screen 3000 men a year. A nurse coordinator runs the show and sonographers are paid on a sessional basis. Ten men are examined in an hour and get their results immediately. Men with an aorta > 40 mm in diameter are referred to a vascular surgeon. They are scanned every 6 months and elective repair is considered at 55 mm. Annual recalls with the current year's 65 year old men are offered to those with an aortal diameter of 26–29 mm. The rest are discharged.

After 13 years, mortality and incidence of rupture have fallen. Elective surgery has increased and emergency surgery has reduced. Operative mortality for elective repair has reduced from 6.5 to 4.4%.

The scheme misses the 10% that die from ruptured aneurysms before reaching 65 years but aims to be a cost-effective programme. Costs would increase markedly if an extra scan was given before hitting 65 years but they propose targeting those at high risk, i.e. smokers or those with a family history, hypertension or arterial disease.

Starting a widespread scheme could overwhelm vascular services and would need to be sensitively co-ordinated. But it could also lead to additional opportunities to target men at high cardiovascular risk for disease modifying interventions.

BREAST CANCER

The Challenge

It is generally accepted that breast screening with mammography saves lives and is cost effective at least in women over 50. The NHS Breast Screening Programme for England screened more than 1.6 million women in 2005–6, a 10% increase from the previous year. More than 13 500 cases of breast cancer were diagnosed in women over 50 – an increase of 13% from the previous year.

Mammography is not going to prevent most breast cancer deaths, but for every 400 women screened over a 10 year period, one less woman dies from breast cancer as a result of the NHS screening programme in England. It is estimated that screening with mammography saves 1400 lives per year at a cost of £3000 per year of life saved.

There have been doubts over the risk–benefit profile, fuelled by worries at the number of cancer patients created by mammography, but these doubts are slowly are being dispelled. Agreement is wider than ever that mammography saves lives but concerns of over-diagnosis linger. Over-diagnosis is the detection of lesions diagnosed as cancer that would not progress to symptoms or death and would never have presented to anybody were we not searching for it. These patients only suffer harm from our efforts.

Breast cancer mortality has been falling in recent years but how young can the benefit of screening reach? Evidence of benefit in the 40–49 year age group is weak and oft-debated, but benefit is non-existent in those under 40 where false positives are higher and there is increased potential for radiation carcinogenesis.

Breast self examination had been recommended for 70 years without compelling proof of efficacy. It was a mistake. The huge Shanghai trial looked at its value and found that cancers detected in the trial were the same in number and in stage as the control group. There was a poor consensus on methods and frequency of examination and the anxiety that went with the investigation of all the benign lesions found could have led to delay in finding a further possibly malignant lump.

The current policy of breast awareness has probably added to the confusion but is still very important to avoid delay in presentation of new symptoms.

For those presenting with symptoms, doctors and patients want quick referral to reassure patients that they do not have cancer. Since 1999 we have had a 2 week rule for urgent referral. Newer research indicates that the road to hell is paved with good intentions and that the policy in its current form might have done more harm than good.

What we know already:

- Studies have shown rates on breast cancer mortality falling by 28–65% (median 46%) in recent years.
- Regular breast examination does not reduce breast cancer mortality but may increase harm such as the number of biopsies with benign results.
- The risk of being recalled after mammography for further assessment, without eventual diagnosis of breast cancer – 'false positive recall' – is increased by both HRT and obesity.

- The Million Women Study also found that previous breast surgery and being thin (BMI <25) were negatively associated with the efficiency of mammography. Both increase mammographic density.
- There is no adverse effect on mammography from past oral contraceptive use, family history, parity, smoking, or alcohol consumption.
- A study in nearly 2000 Dutch women with at least a 15% lifetime risk of breast cancer found MRI to be around twice as sensitive as mammography in detecting tumours in high risk women, i.e. it is good at ruling out breast cancer. But it was a little less specific meaning more false positives, so it is not so good for lower risk women.
- Contrary to popular belief, cancer does not run a more benign course in the elderly. A study that looked at the likelihood of metastases found no differences in the over-70s that were attributable to age. Perhaps we should have the same screening options regardless of age.

Guidelines

Screening for breast cancer in England: past and future. *Advisory Committee on Breast Cancer Screening.* February 2006 (www.cancerscreening.org.uk/breastscreen).

Recent Papers

REFERRAL

Referral patterns, cancer diagnoses, and waiting times after introduction of two week wait rule for breast cancer: prospective cohort study
Potter S, Govindarajulu S, Shere M, *et al.*
BMJ, 2007; **335**: 288

Since 1998 the government has had a 2 week fast-track rule for referrals for suspected breast cancer but the success of this policy has been in question.

This large study from Bristol looked at all its referrals to breast clinic between 1999 and 2005. They tell us the 2 week referral policy has failed as the number of cancers detected in this group is low and that the proportion of cancers diagnosed in the less urgent referrals, which may take longer than 30 days in some centres, has increased. This potentially disadvantages patients who are waiting longer not to mention having to weather an extra psychological burden due to delays.

The likeliest reason for this is poor predictive value of the referral guidelines, leading to flooding the clinics with inappropriate referrals while undermining of GPs' clinical assessments. GPs have said that they do over-refer due to media pressures and patient expectations.

SCREENING

MAMMOGRAPHY

Screening for breast cancer
Dixon JM
BMJ, 2006; **332**: 499–500

This editorial claims that the controversy over whether or not breast screening with mammography saves lives should be at an end.

Early data have been criticised as methodologically inferior. For example, previous trials which found no reduction in mortality have been noted by the Advisory Committee on Breast Cancer Screening as, for example, randomising groups rather than individuals. The author also notes the following.

- One in eight women who have cancer on screening would never have had their cancer diagnosed.
- He criticises the concept that some women receive mastectomy for disease that would never have presented anyway as a red herring. Saving lives with earlier diagnosis mean that inevitably women have the opportunity to die of something other than breast cancer.
- The mastectomy rate is lower than in those who present with symptoms. Screening is estimated to spare 1 in 8 breast cancer sufferers from mastectomy through earlier diagnosis. This should help to allay the fears of the sceptics of breast screening.
- False positives will always happen and quality assurance measures need to continue to minimise the anxiety and costs that these cause. Digital mammography may help to reduce the figures.
- During the 17 years of the UK breast screening programme, improvements have been made in terms of improved resolution with higher quality equipment, more views and double reading.
- Interval cancers – those that present between mammograms – need better quality data to ensure that all units are delivering a high quality service.

Rate of over-diagnosis of breast cancer 15 years after end of Malmö mammographic screening trial: follow-up study
Zackrisson S, Andersson I, Janzon L *et al.*
BMJ, 2006; **332**: 689–692

Estimates of the rate of over-diagnosis of breast cancer as a result of mammography have varied from 5 to 50%. A long follow up is necessary to estimate the real magnitude of the effect and the Malmö study had this.

This was a Swedish study that randomised 42 000 individual women aged 45–69. The first cohort was born as early as 1908 and the control groups were never invited for screening.

Fifteen years after the trial ended, they measured a 10% rate of over-diagnosis – detection of cases that would never have come to clinical attention without mammography in the patient's lifetime.

Participation in mammography screening
Schwartz LM, Woloshin S
BMJ, 2007; **335:** 731–732

Breast screening for 40–49 year old women is a controversial area and has been a huge political issue in the US in the past.

The current US policy is to advise that each woman make up her own mind about mammography. This seems to be garnering some acceptance with the public finally perhaps beginning to digest the fact that screening involves harms as well as benefits. Biased advertising from sides with a vested interest rarely dwell on the mixed effects and trade-offs.

Many of the figures we draw on are still controversial and based on averages. Current evidence estimates that for every 1000 women screened over 10 years, one life in younger women will be saved from dying from breast cancer in the US. But recall rates are much lower in the UK and vary between mammographers.

False positives are worrying but this editorial supports the opinion that over-diagnosis is the most important harm from screening. Unfortunately we cannot tell which cancers are over-diagnosed so we treat everybody. These women can only be harmed by surgery, chemotherapy and radiation. This is a strange concept and few women know about it. We never hear these sort of stories as these women are paraded as the successes of screening – their lives were, after all, 'saved'.

Screening mammography in women 40 to 49 years of age: a systematic review for the American College of Physicians
Armstrong K, Moye E, Williams S, *et al.*
Ann Intern Med, 2007; **146:** 516–526
and
Breast cancer screening for women in their 40s: moving from controversy about data to helping individual women
Elmore J, Choe J
Ann Intern Med, 2007; **146:** 529–531

This review and accompanying editorial summarises the current harms of screening in the under 50s.

- Review of 117 studies demonstrated a 7–23% reduction in breast cancer mortality in those aged 40–49 years.
- Of 10 000 women who have annual mammography from age 40, only 6 women benefit through reduced risk of dying from breast cancer.
- Benefits outweighed the risk of death as a result of radiation.
- Screening was associated with an increasing risk of mastectomy.
- Up to half had at least one false positive after 10 mammograms.
- Evidence on the harm to psychological well-being of screening is thin.

CLINICAL ISSUES

SCREENING

Annual mammographic screening beginning at 40 years of age did not significantly reduce breast cancer mortality after 10 years in women. *Evidence-Based Medicine,* 2007; **12:** 71
The following paper is reviewed
Effect of mammographic screening from age 40 years on breast cancer mortality at 10 years' follow-up: a randomised controlled trial
Moss SM, Cuckle H, Evans A, *et al*.
Lancet, 2006; **368:** 2053–2060

This study of nearly 161 000 women was underpowered to meet its effect size of a 20% reduction in breast cancer mortality. But it showed that in women in aged 40–49 years being screened in NHS centres with mammography there was:
- a 17% non-significant reduction in breast cancer mortality
- NNT to prevent one death from breast cancer was 2512 but did not reach significance
- 23% who had a false positive screen over 10 years

Both sides of the argument can use these data to support their position on the debate about screening age.

MRI

Screening with magnetic resonance imaging and mammography of a UK population at high familial risk of breast cancer: a prospective multicentre cohort study (MARIBS)
Leach MO, Boggis CR, Dixon AK *et al*.
Lancet, 2005; **365:** 1769–1778

This study supports the increased sensitivity of MRI for detecting breast cancer in young women aged 35–49 years with a strong family history or a proven genetic predisposition. Of the 35 cancers found, 77% were detected by MRI and 40% by mammography.

MRI was more sensitive, mammography slightly more specific. So MRI will have more false positives at further increased cost and it is still unclear whether this saves lives.

Combining the two procedures may be the most effective method.

MRI for diagnosis of pure ductal carcinoma *in situ*: a prospective observational study
Kuhl CK, Schrading S, Bieling HB
Lancet, 2007; **370:** 485–492

This study of 7300 women referred for breast screening over 5 years found that MRI was more sensitive for detecting ductal carcinoma *in situ* making it more useful for detecting cancer at its earliest stage.
- 56% of ductal cancers were picked up by mammography and 92% by MRI.
- MRI was more sensitive for high grade cancers.
- Almost all the cancers detected by mammography alone were low grade.

The results further challenge the role of mammography as the gold standard for screening and even larger trials are now needed.

INFORMATION

Presentation on websites of possible benefits and harms from screening for breast cancer: cross sectional study

Jørgensen KJ, Gøtzsche PC
BMJ, 2004; **328**: 148

This paper looked at how information is presented on the internet and compared information from advocacy groups, government institutions and consumer organisations.

In the European Union an average of 23% of the population use the internet to find information about health issues. This will surely only increase with time and yet the information available is very mixed.

The authors found that in their searches:

- advocacy groups and governmental organisations chose information that shed a positive light on screening probably because screening programmes depend on high participation rates
- there were potential conflicts of interests. For example, all the advocacy groups accepted industry funding whereas the three consumer organisations acknowledged the risk of bias related to industry funding, and two of them did not accept such funding at all
- research quoted was selective rather than representative and there was widespread omission of adverse effects
- overdiagnosis (around 30% of cases) and overtreatment, the major harms of screening, were under-reported except by the consumer organisations. Only 18% of publications mention false positives and false negatives
- few people appreciate that screening contributes to the rise in incidence of breast cancer
- serious consequences of increased use of unnecessary radiotherapy were infrequently mentioned and even then usually downgraded
- inflated claims of saved mastectomies were not uncommon (the opposite – an increase in mastectomy – seems to occur)
- information was often misleading – women are not told the numbers needed to screen to prevent one death – or erroneous, not reflecting recent findings. The exception again was the consumer sites, which were much more balanced and comprehensive
- positive spin was commonplace – terms like 'psychological distress' are abandoned for the more friendly and less threatening 'anxiety'
- in one study half of those who failed to attend for a second mammogram said it was due to pain experienced previously, despite the process often being said to be painless
- only the consumer sites reliably mentioned that detected cancers may never progress

They concluded that material provided by professional advocacy groups and governmental organisations is 'severely biased in favour of screening' and that few websites live up to accepted GMC standards for informed consent. Requirements for consent need to be particularly strict when dealing with a healthy population. Are we in danger of sacrificing our role as informers in order to be paternalistic and push the NHS agenda?

CLINICAL ISSUES

SCREENING

CERVICAL CANCER

The Challenge

Worldwide, 400 000 women contract cervical cancer annually. It is the second most common malignancy in women after breast cancer.

Screening in the UK began in 1964, but cervical cancer mortality in England and Wales in women under 35 years rose threefold from 1967 to 1987. National screening with a more efficient recall system was launched in 1988 and reversed this rising trend, preventing an epidemic that would have killed about one in 65 of all British women born since 1950. Now up to 80% of these deaths, around 5000 per year, are estimated to be prevented by screening, at a cost per life saved of about £36 000.

There are still many controversies within the programme. There is strong evidence that early screening substantially reduces the death rate throughout life, but recently the age of beginning screening was pushed back from 20 to 25 years.

The UK already has one of the longest screening intervals in the developed world but some say we should go further, arguing that screening 3-yearly is poor value compared to 5-yearly screening.

Cytology remains the gold standard for cervical cancer detection in Europe and the US but relies on subjective interpretation. As many as 300 000 women a year need re-testing due to inadequate smears. Newer methods should make this less of a lottery.

The role of HPV (human papillomavirus) testing is under particularly intensive research. Changes in sexual behaviour mean that up to half of the young women in Britain have been infected with a high-risk strain of HPV by the time they are 30. HPV is present in virtually all cases of cervical cancer and prevalence in high-grade pre-invasive lesions varies from 80 to 95%.

A new vaccine against the dangerous HPV types is a major breakthrough and it is hoped will prevent a great deal of cervical cancer. It appears to be very safe and highly effective in the medium term and widespread programmes for vaccination are being rapidly developed. Some states in the US have even made it mandatory, but critics raise concerns over parental control amid unfounded fears it may encourage adolescent promiscuity.

Taking a broader view, vaccination programmes could be of great value in the developing world where no screening programmes exist, but who will pay for it?

What we know already:

- Fewer than 1000 women die in England each year from cervical cancer, but to prevent one death around 1000 women need to be screened for 35 years, 150 women have an abnormal result, over 80 are referred for investigation, and over 50 have treatment.
- Failure of cervical screening in terms of attendance frequency or inaccurate reporting is the most important single factor that leads to cervical cancer.
- A range of screening strategies are possible. They involve combinations of liquid-based cytology, earlier referral of those with mild dyskaryosis for colposcopy, stratifying referral with HPV testing or screening primarily with HPV testing.

- Information strategies with reassurance are much needed to reduce the unnecessarily high levels of anxiety caused by testing and screening. Women may not understand what 'pre-cancerous' means.
- Reassurance of the prevalence of HPV may help. Around 20% of young women and about 5% of women over 35 are estimated to be infected at any one time.
- HPV vaccination is scheduled to be given to girls in the UK between the ages of 12 and 13 starting from September 2008, with an additional 300 000 girls aged 17 to 18 also receiving it. The current plan is for a 2-year catch-up programme for 15 to 18 year olds from September 2009.

The screening programme

The NHS cancer screening programme currently recommends:
- women will be invited for a first test at the age of 25 years (instead of 20 years)
- cervical screening will be offered every 3 years until the age of 50
- women aged 50–64 years will then be offered screening every 5 years

The new method of liquid-based cytology is currently being introduced to replace conventional Pap smears as systematic literature review suggests it might provide substantial benefits. The technique led to a much quicker reporting time and fewer inadequate tests, i.e. fewer false negatives. In Bristol for example, the rate of inadequate smears fell from around 9% to 1.5%. It is hoped that the new approach will prove cost effective in the longer term reducing inadequate smears and subsequent retesting.

Recent Papers

CERVICAL SCREENING

Cervical screening
Raffle AE
BMJ, 2004; **328**:1272–1273

This editorial challenges the most recent changes in the cervical screening protocol.

The author argues that:
- the difference between 3 yearly and 5 yearly screening is too small to measure, which is why we are having to use estimates
- switching to 3 yearly intervals means nine routine tests by age 50 instead of six
- 3-yearly screening costs 60% to 66% more than 5 yearly, and harm from more over-diagnosis and over-treatment increases
- the estimates from the commissioned studies suggest that in the author's own local programme, 3-yearly screening could at best add one extra woman added to the existing 24 annually in whom death from cervical cancer is prevented. Another 1000 would be added to the list of women with abnormal results

CLINICAL ISSUES

SCREENING

- she agrees that screening under 25s is now unethical regarding the harm to benefit ratio
- stopping screening above 50 years is advocated. She estimates that helping one patient over 50 years due to 5-yearly screening takes 420 000 tests, costing over £8m

With limited resources and other pressing issues, how would you spend the money?

Liquid based cytology in cervical cancer screening
Denton KJ
BMJ, 2007; **335:** 1–2

The success of the cervical screening programme is well established but a change to liquid-based cytology (where cells are washed into a vial of liquid and sampled on to a slide instead of being smeared directly onto a slide) represents the first major change in slide preparation in the last 50 years. The process can be partially automated and the sensitivity to CIN 2 or higher is preserved. It seems to offer an antidote to the variable rates of inadequate conventional smears which have been noted to reach nearly 10% in the UK.

Every country has a slightly different programme in terms of screening intervals, rescreening of negative/inadequate samples, coverage, sensitivity and specificity, and characteristics of the population, all of which influence detection rates. This means the results of even the most rigorous study may not apply directly to other populations.

However, introduction of liquid-based cytology to the UK will be complete during 2008. Its superiority is not based on sensitivity or specificity but reducing poor sampling, increasing capacity, faster reporting, less anxiety and it provides a platform for automation and HPV testing.

Accuracy of liquid based versus conventional cytology: overall results of new technologies for cervical cancer screening: randomised controlled trial
Ronco G, Cuzick J, Pierotti P, *et al.*
BMJ, 2007; **335:** 28

This trial randomised 45 000 women between 25 and 60 years to conventional cytology or liquid-based cytology and found no significant difference in sensitivity for detection of CIN 2 or more. It was more sensitive for CIN 1 but more 'positives' meant it had a lower positive predictive value.

The main advantage seems to be a reduction in the number of unsatisfactory slides and a shorter time to interpretation. The same sample can also be used for HPV testing.

Prevalence of human papillomavirus antibodies in young female subjects in England
Jitl M, Vysel A, Borrow R, *et al.*
Br J Cancer, 2007; **97:** 989–991

Research from the Health Protection Agency tested 1483 women under 29 in England for HPV.
- 10% of girls were infected by age 16.
- 20% tested seropositive for one of the four significant HPV subtypes.
- The rates of infection may be underestimated by up to 50% as not all undergo seroconversion (indicating past or current infection).

The effects of a successful vaccination programme may not be seen for 10–20 years and it may take that length of time to illustrate cost effectiveness. In the meantime it will be crucial to continue cervical screening.

Overview of the European and North American studies on HPV testing in primary cervical cancer screening
Cuzick J, Clavel C, Petry KU *et al.*
Int J Cancer, 2006; **119**: 1095–1101

Meta-analysis of 60 000 women in 11 European and North American studies looked into testing prior to cervical smear for high-risk HPV.
- The HPV test was substantially more sensitive (96% overall and quite consistent) than cytology in screening and detecting CIN 2+ changes and above. This was true for all ages and in every study.
- HPV testing is also easier to perform, highly reproducible, easily monitored and gives an objective rather than subjective result.
- Cytology had a sensitivity of 53% overall which was highly variable in the studies, but better in women older than 50.
- HPV testing was less specific (90.7% versus 96.3%).
- The specificity of both tests increased with the age of women tested, probably because there are more transient HPV infections in younger women, the authors said.
- Overall, HPV testing had a positive predictive value of 15.5% compared to cytology's PPV of 20%.

The authors support the principle of using the most sensitive test first and following up positives with the more specific test. They maintain that HPV should therefore be the sole primary screening test. Despite cytology's higher PPV (20%), its low sensitivity leads to a high proportion of cancers being missed and so they claim it should be reserved for women who test positive for HPV.

This is a distinct possibility in the future, but large projects will be needed to trial this approach and illustrate effects on morbidity and mortality.

SCREENING

Lifetime effects, costs, and cost effectiveness of testing for human papillomavirus to manage low grade cytological abnormalities: results of the NHS pilot studies
Legood R, Gray A, Wolstenholme J *et al.*
BMJ, 2006; **332**: 79–85
and
Effect of testing for human papillomavirus as a triage during screening for cervical cancer: observational before and after study
Moss S, Gray A, Legood R, and the Liquid Based Cytology/Human Papillomavirus Cervical Pilot Studies Group
BMJ, 2006; **332**: 83–85

Three centres participating in an NHS pilot for alternative strategies in cervical screening modelled data on more than 10 000 women aged 25–64 who had borderline and mildly dyskaryotic smears on liquid-based cytology.

- They found that performing HPV testing on this group and referring for immediate colposcopy if positive, and repeating cytology (and HPV testing) after 6 months if negative, was an effective strategy.
- Although more expensive than repeat cytology alone, it saved slightly more lives, due partly to earlier and better targeted colposcopy and reduction in loss to follow up.
- The rate of repeat smears fell by 74%, but referral for colposcopy for low grade abnormalities more than doubled.
- The cost of these colposcopies is the major concern with this as a wider approach – the cost to society is estimated as between £7500 and £30 000 per life year saved.

HPV VACCINATION

Cervical cancer, human papillomavirus, and vaccination
Lowndes CM, Gill ON
BMJ, 2005; **331**: 915

At least 95% of cervical cancer results from infection with 15 or more HPV types. HPV 16 and 18 account for 70% on their own.

Large scale trials on several non-infectious HPV vaccines are now in progress in many sites around the world.

The largest concerns a quadrivalent vaccine (for HPV types 6 and 11 as well as 16 and 18). Over 12 000 women up to the age of 26 years in 90 centres in 13 countries participated in this FUTURE II study. Three doses of vaccine or placebo were given over 6 months.

- Of those free of infection after the full vaccination, 100% were still free of infection at 17 months.
- There were no observed cases of high-grade precancerous change or non-invasive cancer in the vaccinated group.
- There were 21 such cases in the placebo group.
- Of those who did not complete the entire protocol for the trial, e.g. by missing an appointment, and who may therefore have become infected in the first 6 months during the vaccination period, 97% were still uninfected (only one case was infected) at review.

These promising results could save a significant amount in screening costs.

Questions remain of course. How much cancer will be prevented? Should we vaccinate boys? Will boosters be necessary? Will vaccination benefit those already infected?

Mortality benefits could take up to 20 years to show due to the long latent period – the very thing which makes screening possible. Screening should of course continue in the meantime. Hopefully we will be in a position to accelerate the delivery of the vaccine throughout the world.

Analysis of four RCTs by the FUTURE II study group found that protection against CIN 2/3 cytology or carcinoma *in situ* associated with HPV 16/18 continued for at least 3 years. If we look beyond those who are lucky enough to be negative for high-risk HPV at baseline, the overall effectiveness of the vaccine in all women is only 18% (*Evidence-Based Medicine,* 2007; **12**: 168).

Effect of human papillomavirus 16/18 L1 virus-like particle vaccine among young women with preexisting infection: a randomized trial
Hildesheim A, Herrero R, Wacholder S, *et al.*
JAMA, 2007; **298**: 743–753

This study in over 2000 women under 25 in Costa Rica with confirmed HPV in cervical specimens show no improved clearance of HPV 16 or 18 in those receiving three doses of the vaccine. Clearance occurred in about one-third in both groups regardless. The placebo used was a vaccination for hepatitis A.

The results support those of other trials that concluded that HPV vaccines do not slow progression of precancerous change in women who are already infected with HPV.

Challenges of implementing human papillomavirus (HPV) vaccination policy
Raffle AE
BMJ, 2007; **335**: 375–377

The installation of this new approach to preventing cervical cancer will require careful planning and adequate education and meticulous follow up. It will be important to avoid any public confusion or scaremongering for a successful launch.

The UK will begin its programme targeting 12–13 year old girls in 2008.

- The quadrivalent vaccine protects against HPV-16 and HPV-18 which are associated with 70% of cervical cancers as well as HPV-6 and HPV-11 associated with most cases of genital warts. A new bivalent vaccine containing only the first two ingredients is also available.
- More than 80% of borderline and mildly abnormal cytology and low grade histology (CIN grade 1–2) will not be prevented by vaccination.
- Vaccination in the 16–26 year old age group gives only 17% overall protection so the tried and tested cervical screening programme is still more effective in females over 16.
- We still do not know for how long immunity persists. Boosters may be needed in the future. Nor do we know that it prevents the cancers that kill (but this is likely).

CLINICAL ISSUES

SCREENING

- Cost effectiveness will appear if some of the screening frequency can be reduced in the future for successfully vaccinated cohorts.

HPV vaccine and adolescents' sexual activity
Lo B
BMJ, 2006; **332**: 1106–1107

Although HPV vaccination is over 90% effective in preventing new infections and precancerous cervical lesions caused by the HPV types that it covers, some have raised ethical concerns.

With sexual activity starting earlier, the vaccine needs to target those around the age of 11–12 in order to catch adolescents before they acquire infection. In the US where this editorial was written, pro-family lobbies like to seek parental choice in anything that might influence sexual behaviour. Informed consent is usually required from parents and children for minors, and advocates of sexual abstinence claim vaccination will condone or promote sexual activity. However, fear of sexual infection is not thought to be a major reason for abstinence.

Vaccination is no problem if the parents agree. Estimates suggest that about 75% will when properly informed. But if an adolescent prefers vaccination and parents refuse there may be a problem. Additionally, in cases of abuse parents do not act in the child's best interest.

Hopefully as the goal is cancer prevention, some of the legal minefields of contraception (which now has legal precedents in the UK) and abortion will be subverted.

Making vaccination routine, i.e. without extensive discussion, could be short-sighted until any concerns about the vaccine are eliminated.

HPV vaccine is also sorely needed in developing countries where cervical cancer takes many lives. The expense is unaffordable and a series of three injections may not be feasible so a global programme of research and assistance is needed.

CHLAMYDIA

The Challenge

Chlamydia trachomatis infection is the commonest sexually transmitted infection in the UK and indeed the world. It is the most preventable cause of infertility in women but fewer than an estimated 10% of prevalent infections are diagnosed. It has been hoped that screening could reduce pelvic inflammatory disease by up to 50% but there is still a major question mark over the directness of the relationship.

Public awareness of chlamydia and its consequences remains inadequate. The national screening pilot found 14% of under 16 year olds, 10% of 16–19 year olds, and 7% of 20–24 year olds were infected.

In April 2003 the national chlamydia screening programme began throughout England. It is managed nationally by the Health Protection Agency, but the way in which screening is delivered is decided locally and chlamydia screening is not yet part of essential services. The main approach is opportunistic but there is doubt over whether we can be successful with this approach alone. The number of new cases of chlamydia increased by 4% to 113 585 in 2006.

At least amongst GPs, common reasons that hinder the progress of chlamydia screening include a lack of knowledge of the benefits of testing, how to test, lack of resources, and being reticent towards broaching the subject of sexual health in general and testing for chlamydia in particular.

The option is to screen proactively, so in some areas GP registers are being used to send invitations to young adults to be screened. This is the only screening approach that has been shown in randomised trials to reduce the incidence of pelvic inflammatory disease.

What we know already:

- Chlamydia screening programmes have been shown to reduce infection and related morbidity. Treatment with a single 1 g dose of azithromycin is simple and has high compliance.
- At the end of July 2007 – by which time all English trusts were expected to be offering opportunistic chlamydia screening – only 99 of 152 (65%) were doing so.
- Government targets aim to screen 15% of all 15–24 year olds and by September 2007 had only managed 2.5%.
- ClaSS – the chlamydia screening studies project (a multicentre randomised trial based on 27 general practices in the Bristol and Birmingham areas) – found that partner notification by trained practice nurses immediately after the diagnosis was at least as cheap and effective as referral to a specialist centre. This is probably due to the fact that one-third of those referred did not get round to attending the GUM clinic.

Recent Papers

INCIDENCE

Incidence of severe reproductive tract complications associated with diagnosed genital chlamydial infection: the Uppsala Women's Cohort Study
Low N, Egger M, Sterne JAC *et al.*
Sex Transm Infect, 2006; **82**: 212–218

This interesting research suggests that the benefits and cost-effectiveness of chlamydia screening might have been overestimated.

Previous studies of hospital and clinic populations imply that up to 40% of cases of untreated chlamydia progress to PID within a few weeks of infection, and that nearly 25% of women with PID will have an ectopic pregnancy or become infertile. This may be an overestimation according to this research in a cohort of 44 000 Swedish women aged 15–24 in the Uppsala study.

The rate of PID was 5.6% in those who tested positive for chlamydia and was 4% in those who tested negative. Lower figures than expected were also associated with ectopic pregnancy and infertility.

Cumulative incidences of hospital-diagnosed pelvic inflammatory disease, ectopic pregnancy, and infertility by age 35 were 2–4% overall, and 3–7% in those with a positive test for chlamydia. This is reassuring for patients, but if the incidence of complications associated with chlamydia have been overestimated, then current screening programmes may not be as beneficial or as cost-effective as hoped.

Additionally, research is beginning to suggest that infection may resolve itself within a year in asymptomatic patients without doing any damage.

SCREENING

Screening programmes for chlamydial infection: when will we ever learn?
Low N.
BMJ, 2007; **334**: 725–728

This is an excellent paper which barely wastes a sentence as it dismantles the arguments for our current approach to screening in the UK.

The drop in rates of chlamydia that happened in Sweden was a key factor in the growth of screening. But the idea that this was due to the actual screening is a misrepresentation of the facts, Low explains. It led to uncritical acceptance of screening before the benefits and harms were evaluated in RCTs.
- The fall in the rates of chlamydia coincided with the national campaign to prevent HIV which changed sexual behaviour.
- No RCT has evaluated opportunistic chlamydia screening as currently practised.
- Cost effectiveness of screening has been overestimated due to inadequate modelling.
- Even in Sweden, chlamydia has been on the increase since 1995.

Our actual programme does not even follow our own pilot model where GPs were heavily involved in recruitment and screening rates were much higher. So how do we define a screening programme? We have a good definition of 'screening', but what constitutes a 'programme'? Low offers the definition of "a continuing organised service that ensures that screening is delivered at sufficiently regular intervals to a high enough proportion of the target population to achieve defined levels of benefit at the population level while minimising harm".

Chlamydia would seem to be an ideal candidate for screening – it is common, curable, easy to diagnose, often causes no symptoms and it can lead to serious consequences. But if opportunistic programmes are ineffective, why not screen proactively? Even cervical screening only became effective when we gave up on the opportunistic approach.

We are not even that sure about the natural history of the disease. We need to know prevalence and be able to control transmission with partner notification. Perhaps the asymptomatic infections we are detecting do not have the risk of PID that we thought. Studies are indicating that incidences of PID are lower than expected.

Rates of infection are increasing in countries who screen opportunistically implying that the programme is ineffective.

Perhaps we will continue to be unsuccessful without good partner notification or perhaps there is a widespread loss of immunity after treatment. We need to find out if we are doing more good than harm.

Screening for *Chlamydia trachomatis*
Jones R, Boag F
BMJ, 2007; **334:** 703–704

The National Chlamydia Screening Programme in England began in 2001 and uses an opportunistic approach to target sexually active people under 25 years while they are attending a healthcare setting.

There have been many critics of this approach. Pilot studies in general practice were effective in screening 50% of the target group, but in the programme itself more than half the areas achieved a screening rate of less than 5%.

As Low's paper (*above*) establishes, there is a lack of evidence for the whole approach. Studies showing a reduction in PID, in ectopic pregnancy, and in rates of chlamydia, are actually due to an extensive safe sex campaigning going on at the same time as the screening programme was being evaluated.

Chlamydia is the only sexually transmitted infection for which population screening has been implemented. Another approach is proactive screening using a register to identify and summon the target population as is done with cervical screening. It is the alternative model and previously thought to be difficult and unacceptable to some. There are serious question marks over its cost-effectiveness too. But it may be the only way to curb the growth in prevalence.

SCREENING

Cost effectiveness of home based population screening for *Chlamydia trachomatis* in the UK: economic evaluation of chlamydia screening studies (ClaSS) project
Roberts TE, Robinson S, Barton PM, *et al.*
BMJ, 2007; **335**: 291

If opportunistic screening is truly ineffective, what about practice screening using a register as we do in cervical screening?

This part of the ClaSS project was an economic evaluation based on a realistic dynamic model incorporating estimates of partner notification, anticipated uptake levels and a lower incidence of complications from chlamydia than previously believed.

It concluded that proactive population screening for chlamydia was an expensive intervention that probably does not represent good value for money.

Coverage and uptake of systematic postal screening for genital *Chlamydia trachomatis* and prevalence of infection in the United Kingdom general population: cross sectional study
Macleod J, Salisbury C, Low N *et al.*
BMJ, 2005; **330**: 940

Invites went out to 19 773 UK men and women aged 16–39 years to participate in chlamydia screening by posting a urine specimen they collected at home. The authors found that:
- postal screening was feasible but only about 1 in 3 accepted screening
- uptake was lower in the young, in men, in ethnic minorities and in disadvantaged areas
- prevalence of genital *Chlamydia trachomatis* was just below 2.8% for men and almost 3.6% for women
- in those under 25 years, these figures reached around 5% in men and 6% in women
- screening ultimately seems to lead to wider inequalities in sexual health

---

New point of care Chlamydia Rapid Test—bridging the gap between diagnosis and treatment: performance evaluation study
Mahilum-Tapay L, Laitila V, Wawrzyniak JJ, *et al.*
BMJ, 2007; **335**: 1190–1194

A new test – the Chlamydia Rapid Test – could be a valuable tool for the future. It is based on self-collected vaginal swabs and gives a diagnosis within 30 minutes, with a sensitivity of 83.5% and a positive predictive value of 86.7%.

This trial in 1349 mostly asymptomatic women between 15 and 64 years of age validated the test as a practical option for screening. A higher load of chlamydia was obtained than in endocervical swabs or urine sampling, and the rapid results made the test highly acceptable to patients.

It would enable rapid testing, rapid treatment and immediate contact tracing.

SEXUAL HEALTH

The Challenge

In 2005 about 340 million people globally acquired new infections of the four most common curable sexually transmitted infections (gonorrhoea, chlamydia, syphilis, and trichomoniasis) and 4.1 million acquired HIV.

There is a continuing challenge to the nation's sexual health with many sexually transmitted infections (STIs) including chlamydia still on the increase. Attendances at genitourinary medicine (GUM) clinics have doubled in the last 10 years, reaching over a million cases a year. Overall the number of new STIs diagnosed in GUM clinics in the UK rose by 2% from 368 341 in 2005 to 376 508 in 2006. Services are overburdened and failing to deliver high quality open access services. There have been slight falls in diagnoses of syphilis and gonorrhoea recently which at least is an encouraging trend. However, about 30% of people infected with HIV in the UK are diagnosed late (with low CD4 counts) – less than half of those through routine screening. For two decades we have known how to prevent every method of spread of HIV and for two decades we have failed to do it. Educational programmes promoting monogamy, abstinence, delayed sexual intercourse and condoms need to be well resourced.

More people have more sexual partners in their lifetime than ever before. The age of first intercourse gets ever lower and sex education is still patchy and of dubious efficacy. More teenage girls become pregnant in the UK than anywhere else in Europe. Sexually active adolescents seriously underestimate their risks of STI.

Fortunately, deregulation which allowed sales of emergency contraception over the counter has not led to unsafer sex. There has been no increase in use of emergency contraception, no increase in episodes of unprotected sex, but more women now buy it over the counter rather than attending elsewhere.

Partner notification (a.k.a. contact tracing) is hugely important. The stigma attached to STIs makes partner notification difficult. 'Provider-led' strategies where health providers initiate contact, work better than 'patient-led' strategies where the patient sends their partner in for treatment. But there are many problems with delivering this. Lack of specificity of many diagnoses can lead to overdiagnosis, and upsetting the power balance in relationships could incur the risk of domestic violence.

Sexual dysfunction is being increasingly medicalised. The prevalence of 'female sexual dysfunction' disturbingly comes in at 43%, a figure now widely quoted in the media. Figures drop if you do not accept lack/loss of sexual desire as a serious problem. Does female sexual dysfunction actually represent the "corporate sponsored creation of a disease"? This over-medicalisation and over-simplification has caused concern. Changes in sexual desire are the norm – a healthy response to patterns of stress, tiredness and relationship difficulties. According to some, use of the term 'dysfunction' is misleading. Difficulties become dysfunction becomes disease. Doctors treat disease and they like to do it with drugs. It is quicker than paying attention to aspects of causality. Nothing makes the drug companies happier.

Recent Papers

HIV

Reducing the length of time between HIV infection and diagnosis
Dodds C, Weatherburn P
BMJ, 2007; **334:** 1329–1330

This editorial highlights the promotion of the opt-out strategy for HIV testing to speed up early diagnosis and reduce onward transmission. This should expand to primary care settings and other acute settings.

In England and Scotland, prevalence has not reached the Centre for Disease Control's 0.1% threshold for universal testing. Only one-quarter of the undiagnosed HIV is thought to be from non-African-born heterosexuals who do not inject drugs, so widespread testing may not be effective.

Opt-out HIV testing is not even a universal policy in GUM clinics in the UK, and use of point of care testing kits that give appealingly rapid results is uncommon. Intensified targeting should occur before targeting those less likely to have HIV, argue these authors.

Time to move towards opt-out testing for HIV in the UK
Hamill M, Burgoine K, Farrell F, *et al.*
BMJ, 2007; **334:** 1352–1354

It is estimated that one-third of HIV cases in the UK are undiagnosed.

Expanding testing to routine practice unless the patients opt out is one way to improve diagnosis. We are no longer required to do extensive pre-test counselling and more rapid tests can give quicker results. Currently we have no recommendations for this in the UK, although the US has adopted such guidelines. Routine opt-out testing could reduce stigma and increase testing but cost-effectiveness in areas of low prevalence is questionable. Before widespread adoption in facilities who routinely take blood, such as emergency departments and acute admission wards, more data will be needed.

Are condoms the answer to rising rates of non-HIV sexually transmitted infection? No
Genuis SJ
BMJ, 2008; **336:** 185

Levels of education and promotion of condoms have never been higher yet levels of sexually transmitted infection are still increasing. Methods of disease transmission that condoms do nothing to protect against include skin to skin contact and skin to sore contact. In addition, the effectiveness of condoms is continually compromised by compliance issues, incorrect use and mechanical failure.

One of the main problems is that those engaged in particularly risky behaviour rarely use condoms consistently. Even among stable couples where one of the partners is HIV positive, only half use condoms consistently.

What makes people engage in risky sexual behaviours is what really needs to be targeted. The patterns are akin to other self-destructive behaviours such as substance mis-use. Improvements in countries such as Thailand and Cambodia are more likely to be down to changes in behaviour such as fewer partners, safer sex and less use of sex workers following large scale educational campaigns.

Condoms have an important role, but rather than harping on and on about safe sex, a credible public health policy with comprehensive programmes is what is needed.

Are condoms the answer to rising rates of non-HIV sexually transmitted infections? Yes
Steiner MJ, Cates W
BMJ, 2008; **336:** 184

This rebuttal is more condom-centric. They focus on the key role of condoms as our best proven solution for preventing transmission of STIs. Claims of inconsistency can be attributed to limitations in study design. Other critical factors such as actual exposure to infection or incorrect use are under-researched.

However, these arguments are not mutually exclusive as both reviewers basically agree that a wider range of measures than promoting condoms or abstinence is needed.

HERPES

Ethics of screening for asymptomatic herpes virus type 2 infection
Krantz I, Löwhagen G, Ahlberg BM et al.
BMJ, 2004; **329**: 618–621

Universal serological testing for herpes simplex virus type 2 does not seem to be ethical, especially where there is a low prevalence of infection. Sensitivity and specificity of tests are good at 95% and some experts have advocated screening but:

- many of those infected are asymptomatic
- there is no cure and infection is life long and sexually transmissible
- the psychosocial impact on relationships could be catastrophic
- cost-effectiveness of testing is unproven
- positive predictive values in areas of low prevalence will be very low, with false positives reaching 30–40%. In high prevalence groups, around 10% have a false positive
- even antenatal screening is expensive and the benefits for babies unproven

ADOLESCENTS

Sexual health in adolescents
Stammers T
BMJ, 2007; **334**: 103–104

Despite the school sex education programmes, teenage sexual health is getting worse and worse. Looking at soft outcomes such as pupil satisfaction and condom use is all very well but there has been a failure to curb the rise in the 'harder' outcomes of increasing infections and terminations. New research from a teacher-delivered educational programme shows no effect on these outcomes.

A different approach is needed and delaying first intercourse is one of the most important things. 'Saved sex' becomes a more positive and helpful term than abstinence. Teenage sex is more a search for meaning, identity and belonging. Behavioural programmes that promote good decision-making seem to be very helpful whether or not they even mention sex.

Mandatory reporting to the police of all sexually active under-13s
Bastable R, Sheather J
BMJ, 2005; **331**: 918–919

This editorial discusses 2005 government guidance for mandatory reporting of all sexually active young people under 13 to the police and the collection of data in relation to sexually active young people under 16.

These measures have been criticised as insensitive and risk alienating people already in abusive situations by bringing their situation into the realms of criminality. The GMC's guidance is clear: 'confidentiality can be breached without consent only where there is a risk of serious harm to the patient or others'. The legal status of the protocols is unclear but they seem to imply a retreat from the Gillick judgment.

Mandatory reporting may be too blunt an instrument. Young people value the confidentiality. Compromising this could prevent them from asking for help in the first place.

CONTRACEPTION

Cancer risk among users of oral contraceptives: cohort data from the Royal College of General Practitioner's oral contraception study
Hannaford PC, Selvaraj S, Elliott AM, *et al.*
BMJ, 2007; **335:** 651
and
Risk of cancer and the oral contraceptive pill
Meirik O, Farley TMM
BMJ, 2007; **335:** 621–622

Hannaford's paper and accompanying editorial looked at one million women years of data to examine the link between the pill and the risk of cancer.

- Long term follow up of the use of the oral contraceptive in the UK has shown that there is no overall increased risk of cancer in women who have ever used the pill.
- Risk was lower for cancer of the colon, rectum, uterus, and ovaries.
- Risk of breast cancer was similar.
- Some excess risk of cervical cancer persisted 10–15 years after stopping the pill.
- Some risk of brain or pituitary cancer persisted 20 years after stopping but this may be prescription bias as the pill may be used to regulate periods.

It reminds us that the pill is safe with regard to cancer even dating back to when higher dose pills were in common usage. But also that regular cervical cytology is important in women on the pill.

Another meta-analysis of 85% of the known data showed that the risk of cervical cancer actually decays quite quickly and disappears within 10 years. It only occurs in those on the pill for 5 years or more. Worries over cervical cancer are no reason to avoid the pill (*Lancet,* 2007; **370:** 1609–1621).

Emergency contraception
Glasier A
BMJ, 2006; **333:** 560–561

According to the Office for National Statistics, pharmacy sales doubled again in 2004 to reach 50% of total requests by 2005.
Controversies have surrounded the use of emergency contraception.

However, use in most countries is actually pretty low. In the US it is something of an ideological battleground. Supporters claim that 43% of the reported fall in abortion in the US was due to the use of emergency contraception. England and Wales could have expected to prevent 66 500 abortions with the same logic, but in fact the abortion rate has risen. The reduced access to abortion clinics in the US might be a more relevant factor.

In addition, how sure are we that it really works? A high quality trial will always

SEXUAL HEALTH

be unethical. When easily available at home, use more than doubled but three studies failed to show a measurable effect on pregnancy or abortion.

You might as well try it if you do not want a baby, but it is hardly as powerful as those both for or against it seem to claim.

PRESCRIBING RISKS

Documentation of contraception and pregnancy when prescribing potentially teratogenic medications for reproductive-age women
Schwarz EB, Postlethwaite DA, Hung Y-Y, Armstrong MA
Ann Inter Med, 2007; **147:** 370–376

This US study of nearly half a million women in California of childbearing age found that 1 in 6 were prescribed a drug that was potentially teratogenic during 2001. The most commonly prescribed drugs were antibiotics, benzodiazepines, and psychiatric drugs. For almost half of these women there was no mention of any form of contraceptive plan. Some 1% were pregnant within 3 months.

Although use of condoms may not be recorded, it is still very likely that women are inadequately informed of the risks.

CONTACT TRACING

Improved effectiveness of partner notification for patients with sexually transmitted infections
Trelle S, Shang A, Nartey L, *et al.*
BMJ, 2007; **334:** 354

This systematic review of 14 RCTs showed that methods of partner notification were effective in reducing sexually transmitted disease. They looked at techniques used when patients are supplied with drugs to treat their partner or with home testing kits for collecting urine specimens ready for posting. Partner notification decreased persistent or recurrent infections in index cases of chlamydia and gonorrhoea.

A commentary in *Evidence-Based Medicine* (2007; **12:** 147) reminds us that we still do not know how often medications are delivered and taken as prescribed and some healthcare workers may have reservations about prescribing to people that they have not seen.

A *BMJ* editorial notes that strategies such as these are attractive but fail to address the fundamental barriers that patients have in discussing these sensitive matters with their partners, or the potential harms such as violence towards women about which little is known (*BMJ*, 2007; **334:** 323).

ALLERGIES

The Challenge

Approximately 15 million people in England now suffer from allergies, of whom 10 million will experience symptoms in the course of a year. Allergic diseases account for 6% of GP consultations and 10% of primary care prescribing costs. Direct NHS costs for managing allergic problems are estimated at over £1 billion every year.

Conditions include allergic rhinitis, anaphylaxis, asthma, conjunctivitis, eczema/dermatitis, food allergy, urticaria and angioedema. They affect around 30% of the adult population, and 40% of children, making these amongst the commonest diseases in England. The incidence of allergic disease in the UK has trebled in the last 20 years with one-fifth of the population seeking treatment each year. Mixed pictures are commonplace, for example, rhinitis, asthma and eczema can co-exist as 'multi-system allergic disease'. The UK ranks highest in the world for asthma symptoms and near the top for eczema and allergic rhinitis. Only Australia and the US have higher total rates of allergy.

Allergy is increasing in incidence and severity. Until 1990, peanut allergy was rare. By 1996, the prevalence amongst children was one in 200. Now it affects one in 70 children and has trebled in the last 4 years.

What we know already:

- IgE sensitisation and asthma can occur at very low levels of exposure and there is probably an important gene–environment interaction.
- Around one-third of parents of affected children know when and how to use their pre-loaded devices for auto-injecting adrenaline.
- A study of 50 local GPs who had all prescribed auto-injecting devices found only one could work a training device and he suffered from anaphylaxis himself. Just over half did not think that immediately going to hospital is necessary after taking adrenaline for anaphylaxis.

Guidelines

Allergy: the unmet need. *Royal College of Physicians Working Party.* June 2003.
This scathing report on the provision of allergy services is a UK blueprint for better patient care in a burgeoning epidemic.

The report claims there has been a national failure to meet minimum standards of care. There is a major shortage of allergy specialists with only six fully staffed clinics in the UK. This has driven people towards the dubious claims of many complementary therapists and unproven techniques of investigation and treatment.

Allergy is increasing in incidence. Latest projections estimate that approximately one-third of the UK will develop allergy at some point in their lives. It is also increasing in severity. Peanut allergy was rare 10 years ago; now it affects one in 70 children and has trebled in the

ALLERGIES

last 4 years. Further, it is complex. Mixed pictures of, for example, rhinitis, asthma and eczema can co-exist as 'multi-system allergic disease'.

The report makes recommendations for a 'whole system' approach to allergy led by appropriately trained specialists who can lead a nationwide training infrastructure involving regional allergy centres and training in primary care.

Allergy. *The House of Lords Select Committee on Science and Technology.* September 2007 (www.parliament.uk).

This report called for withdrawal of Dept of Health advice from 1998 which advised pregnant women and new parents to avoid peanuts.

In fact this policy is not evidence-based and might be fuelling the rapid increase in peanut allergy by preventing tolerance.

Recent Papers

PREVALENCE

Time trends in allergic disorders in the UK
Gupta R, Sheikh A, Strachan DP *et al*.
Thorax, 2007; **62**: 91–96

This analysis shows that after rising year on year in recent decades, rates of eczema, allergic rhinitis and hay fever seem to have stabilised and may even be falling according to a review of GP data, prescriptions and hospital records. However, admissions to hospital for anaphylaxis have risen by 700%, for food allergy by 500%, and for skin urticaria by 100%. Speculation as to the reasons includes altered sources of allergens as well as changes to medical practice.

Are the dangers of childhood food allergy exaggerated?
Colver A, Hourihane J
BMJ, 2006; **333**: 494–496 and 496–498

This pair of articles debates the question in the title.

Although a growing problem, Colver argues that, spurred on by the media, the dangers of food allergy are overstated and cause unnecessary alarm for families and schools. We are increasingly frightened of our food and yet the prevalence of severe reactions including death may not have increased.

The author estimates that one death per 830 000 children with food allergy occurs per year and that of serious childhood reactions admitted to hospital, only 10% would have benefited from having an adrenaline auto-injector at home.

Asthma is so strongly associated with fatal reactions that absence of asthma should reassure parents and doctors. (All but one of nine children with fatal or near fatal reactions in one study and all but one of 32 adult patients in another had asthma.)

Diagnostic problems do not help. In another study, half the children who tested positive to peanut allergy on skin prick could eat them quite happily. It is also common for parents to blacklist many potential allergens when their child is confirmed allergic to one allergen. In addition, most children outgrow allergy to milk and eggs and periodic retesting with an oral challenge in hospital will help confirm this.

Auto-injectors deliver a heavy weight of responsibility to parents, most of whom lack confidence to use it. Hourihane argues for them to be made available for those that might need to use them. He argues that there is little evidence of the anxiety that it is claimed these devices cause and that a perception of control for the family might be a good thing.

PREVENTION

Environmental and dietary interventions in the first 5 years of life did not reduce risk of asthma and allergic disease. *Evidence-Based Medicine*, 2007; **12**: 19
The following paper is reviewed
Prevention of asthma during the first 5 years of life: a randomized controlled trial
Marks GB, Mihrshahi S, Kemp AS, *et al.*
J Allergy Clin Immunol, 2006; **118**: 53–61

This RCT from Australia looked at controlling allergens in 616 high-risk pregnant women (who had a relative with asthma) with the aim of reducing the risk of developing asthma in their unborn child.

Interventions such as impermeable bed sheets, regular washing of bedding and a diet high in omega-3, as opposed to omega-6, fatty acids were successfully implemented.

At 5 years of age, the children had no reduced risk of asthma or allergic disease.

It is suggested that interventions that target atopy, such as reduction of house dust mite, may require assessment after the age of 5, because later wheezing corresponds to allergic asthma. But this study does not show that primary prevention of allergy is effective with these measures.

Reducing infant exposure to food and dust mite allergens reduced the incidence of asthma and allergy at age 8 years. *Evidence-Based Medicine*, 2007; **12**: 117
The following paper is reviewed
Prevention of allergic disease during childhood by allergen avoidance: the Isle of Wight prevention study
Arshad SH, Bateman B, Sadeghnejad A, *et al.*
J Allergy Clin Immunol, 2007; **119**: 307–313

In this UK RCT, follow up of 120 children over 8 years showed that primary prevention could reduce the development of atopy, allergic asthma, rhinitis and eczema in later childhood. There was no impact on food allergy.

The measures taken were, however, drastic and not to everybody's taste. Lactating mothers and infants in their first year had to strictly eliminate common allergens such as dairy, egg, wheat, nuts, fish and soya. Anti-house dust mite measures were taken too.

ALLERGIES

This is only the second study to show benefit with primary prevention. Both used multiple interventions.

ALLERGY SERVICES

Should UK allergy services focus on primary care?
Levy ML, Sheikh A, Walker S *et al*.
BMJ, 2006; **332**: 1347–1348

The marked increase in prevalence of allergic disease has led to calls for updated allergy services. Now is the time to decide whether it should be primary care that is the key provider of such a service to the UK population.

Multiple allergies affect an estimated 10% of people under 45 years and 5% of older people and are problematic to manage.

These patients could easily end up seeing different specialists rather than one person with expertise in multisystem disease. They might be seeing a gastroenterologist for food allergy and a respiratory physician for asthma and attend ENT clinic for rhinitis.

Diagnosis is made more difficult by the questionable availability and interpretation of the likes of skin prick tests and IgE testing.

There is minimal training in the UK undergraduate and postgraduate programmes. In primary care a local practitioner – a GP with special interest or nurse consultant – could be trained to organise a clinic to serve the whole trust. An overhaul like this will need a major input of resources to make a real difference.

COMPLEMENTARY AND ALTERNATIVE THERAPIES

The Challenge

The public want complementary therapies and the government is committed to patient choice. They are extensively used throughout the world and the British market for complementary and alternative medicine (CAM) is estimated at £1.6 billion a year. One in ten adults in the UK has visited a practitioner of complementary medicine. People clearly have a desire to help themselves and adopt some responsibility for their own care. In many cases they are willing to pay for it. The growth has been possible due to patients contributing to costs – 90% of complementary therapy is privately purchased.

Doctors therefore need a high index of suspicion that their patients may be using alternative medication and make active enquiries to that effect. More research is needed to quantify the risks they are exposing themselves to as neither clinicians nor patients have enough high quality information.

There is a growing lobby for increased integration of complementary and orthodox techniques. Some countries even reimburse the costs of many complementary techniques. Suspicion remains in the medical profession about many of the alternative practitioners and practices but hostility is starting to erode and training has reached the syllabus of many a medical school.

Half of the general practices in England offer some access to complementary or alternative therapy. In one-third of practices, a primary healthcare team member offers the service, usually acupuncture and homeopathy. Each week 10% of GPs either perform acupuncture on someone or refer to someone who will. One randomised trial from primary care using sham acupuncture as a control claimed to reduce GP visits for headache by 25% and reduce sick days and medication use by 15% at a cost of £9000 per QALY. The authors claim that such a good value intervention needs to be widely available for NHS patients. Strangely, however, it is as easy to find studies that claim no such benefit. As ever the personal effect of therapeutic relationships 'cloud' the evidence issues and leaves the door wide open.

Many spurious treatments have now crept in. Often treatments are used for life-threatening or chronic illnesses and lack of regulation has allowed disreputable practitioners to practise quackery and put the public at risk.

Two hundred years ago, Samuel Hahnemann started the homeopathic bandwagon rolling by inventing the concept of treating 'like for like' – a treatment he started on himself. Many mocked but it captured the imagination of royalty who have helped to popularise it in England in particular. There are now as many as half a million UK homeopathy clients and a handful of dedicated hospitals. However, they have not used the time they had to provide high quality evidence of effectiveness, so PCTs are gradually withdrawing NHS funding from homoeopathy. Tunbridge Wells Homeopathic Hospital will close and the Royal London Homeopathic Hospital is in great danger.

There are moves in many countries to properly regulate practices involved in alternative therapies. The Dutch want to make it illegal for anyone other than trained doctors to be allowed to make a medical diagnosis. We may see the takeover of these therapies by registered medical practitioners depending on the legislation adopted. If orthodox medicine controlled access to

COMPLEMENTARY AND ALTERNATIVE THERAPIES

alternative medicine, that is bound to be unpopular with the alternative practitioners. The power struggle may destroy the effect of the interventions in the first place and kill the goose that lays the golden eggs.

What we know already

- A survey from Bath looked at use of complementary medicine by children. Around 18% had tried it in some form and 7% have visited a practitioner – 85% were said to have benefited.
- Parents pursue 'natural treatments' for their children but toxicity of many herbal medicines is unknown. One Birmingham study of 24 creams for atopic eczema found all but 4 adulterated with steroids – mainly the very potent clobetasol, which in the doses recommended risked adrenal suppression.
- In one large Taiwanese study, an estimated 24% of Chinese herbal medicines were shown to be adulterated with conventional pharmacologically active medicines – half of these had two such contaminants.
- Investigations by the Medicines and Healthcare Products Regulatory Agency in the UK, have found that some products being sold as herbal, natural, and safe contain prescription-only drugs, such as sildenafil, tadalafil, finasteride and clotrimazole.
- Saw palmetto is used by 2 million men in the US to treat benign prostatic hyperplasia. A high quality double-blind randomised trial in 225 men over 1 year convincingly refuted previous suggestions of a benefit on prostatic size, urinary flow rate and quality of life.
- Herbal products suspected of interacting with warfarin include garlic, ginseng, ginkgo biloba, feverfew, ginger and St John's Wort.
- St John's Wort is recognised as a treatment for depression, but users suffer possible decreases in the bioavailability of conventional drugs – there are insufficient data to either quantify the interaction for this or any other herbalist medication.
- The principal finding of a systematic review of 22 trials on the pharmacokinetics related to use of St John's Wort, was that the studies were small and the methodology of poor quality; much better research is needed.
- A UK postal survey found 19% of warfarin patients reported taking one or more complementary medicines. Only 5% definitely felt that the herbal medicine could interfere with other prescribed drugs. Only 4% had discussed use of these products with their GP.
- Very few patients using herbal medications receive warnings of the possible adverse effects.

New regulations

Regulation of herbal medicine and acupuncture: proposals for statutory regulation. *Dept of Health*, March 2004.

The House of Commons Select Committee on Science and Technology recommended statutory regulation for acupuncturists and herbalists in the UK in November 2000.

Proposals for this were issued in March 2004 by the Department of Health with recommendations for a council that sets standards and investigates practitioners.

An estimated 4000 practitioners are not regulated by other bodies. The idea is that they would need to undergo professional development and be up to date with developments in medicine. Voluntary regulation is thought to be sufficient for the likes of aromatherapy and reflexology. Homeopaths may opt for statutory regulation.

The Medicines and Healthcare products Regulatory Agency (MHRA) has published a consultation document on the regulation of unlicensed herbal remedies.

Statutory regulation of herbal medicine and acupuncture: Report on the consultation. *Dept of Health*, February 2005.
This report analysed responses from the debate on the regulation of alternative therapies.

Trust, assurance and safety – the regulation of health professionals in the 21st century. *Dept of Health*. 2007.
This is the first report to expand on the calls for regulation since 2000 (www.official-documents.gov.uk/document/cm70/7013/7013.pdf).

Recent Papers

REGULATION

Should NICE evaluate complementary and alternative medicine?
Franck L, Chantler C, Dixon M
BMJ, 2007; **334**: 506

This half of a *BMJ* 'Head to Head' debate argues that NICE should indeed evaluate CAM.

The authors credit these interventions as treatment for mind, body and spirit whose outcomes are often framed as 'feeling better' rather than cure. They tell us that most people see complementary therapies as an adjunct rather than a substitute for conventional medicine. They note that NICE has incorporated some of these therapies into their own guidance, while admitting that these recommendations have not been subject to the same rigorous evaluation.

They go on to explain why a NICE investigation has not taken place – inadequate methods of evaluation, dependency on the individual therapist and impossibility of blinding. Or maybe they are just displaying attitudinal bias, or perhaps it is just a lack of resources. Whatever the reason they claim the result is unequal access to complementary therapies which, better employed, might be a window to drug savings.

They find it "surprising" that NICE has not been asked to bestow its wisdom. Quite how anyone should decide a spirit is feeling better, they leave up to NICE.

With an argument this vapid, they leave their competitor little to do for victory.....

COMPLEMENTARY AND ALTERNATIVE THERAPIES

Should NICE evaluate complementary and alternative medicines?
Colquhoun D
BMJ, 2007; **334:** 507

This is a well-presented thesis explaining that resources are not infinite and that NICE has enough on its plate. If NICE were to apply its normal criteria, almost all complementary and alternative medicine would be removed from the NHS with immediate effect. That may be no bad thing, but even NICE has incorporated some aspects into their own guidelines and has better things to do with its 240 employees and limited resources that wallow in these mud pits.

Homeopathy has had 200 years to produce some evidence. Acupuncture and traditional Chinese medicine has had thousands of years. There is still little convincing evidence. A billion dollars spent on the National Center of Complementary and Alternative Medicine in the US has failed to prove the effectiveness of any alternative method. Many of the more sensible practitioners of the arts even admit this.

We can still sympathetically offer some of these pleasing feelgood interventions in support and palliative care, without the need to subscribe to "early 19th century hocus pocus".

Mapping the alternative route
Day M
BMJ, 2007; **334:** 929–931

For a long time complementary therapy was seen as a gentle alternative to conventional medicine but high profile health complications have occurred, notably with toxic herbs.

The lack of regulation remains a worry. Anyone can set themselves up as a counsellor or therapist and regulation is always on the agenda. Any therapist of any kind must be expected to know their limits of competence.

Plans for regulation which were announced by the government in 2000 have been very quiet until 2007 when the Department of Health finally released a White Paper to regulate acupuncture and Chinese and herbal medicines.

The job will probably fall to the Health Professions Council, but they have the statutory regulation of counsellors, psychologists and similar therapists on their 'to do' list first.

How will they assess competency where efficacy is not established? The main job is to protect the public so safety will come first. Practitioners will need to understand the potential harms they might do.

One critic – Professor Ernst – is against regulation claiming that it endorses these valid approaches. Regulating placebo therapies seems ridiculous.

Individualised herbal recipes takes us into even trickier waters. No therapeutic benefit but a huge opportunity for interaction and toxicity. However, by 2011, changes to the Medicines Act mean that herbal medicine practitioners having one-to one consultations with patients must be part of a statutory register.

ACUPUNCTURE

Characteristic and incidental (placebo) effects in complex interventions such as acupuncture
Paterson C, Dieppe P
BMJ, 2005; **330**: 1202–1205

This excellent overview discusses how it may not be meaningful to split complex interventions into characteristic and incidental elements in order to analyse them with a biomedical model and ideally, a randomised controlled trial.

The authors explain that this will lead to what they describe as false negative results. Complementary treatments contain a spectrum of treatment factors which add 'incidental effects' (placebo effects or contextual factors such as the credibility of the intervention or consultation style of the practitioner) to any 'characteristic effects' of the intervention (specific effects of the actual process).

Unlike the Western biomedical model whereby the diagnosis precedes treatment, Chinese diagnosis is a rolling process buttressed at each of the many patient–practitioner meetings with measures such as pulse and tongue diagnoses and feedback on the effects of needling. This process is likely to elicit a direct effect in terms of a 'meaning response'. It continually reinforces itself and accommodates new concerns whether physical, emotional or social – a trouble shared is a trouble halved. The spell is weaved while self-confidence and self-awareness increases. The difference is not so much a function of the practitioner as a function of the different theoretical models.

A sham control procedure should include all the peripheral effects except for classical needling.

Complex interventions such as physiotherapy lie in a middle ground. The physiotherapist's assessment rather than a biomedical diagnosis starts the ball rolling. This may be explained to the patient in terms of a weakness of a particular muscle or ligament and the care package prescribed around that.

Acupuncture in patients with tension-type headache: randomised controlled trial
Melchart D, Streng A, Hoppe A *et al.*
BMJ, 2005; **331**: 376–382

This large study of 270 patients described the 'sham' intervention of superficial needling of non-acupuncture points as 'minimal acupuncture'.

The credibility of the real and 'sham' acupuncture were both rated very similarly by patients and both these interventions were equally and significantly effective in reducing the number of days with tension headache compared to a further control of no acupuncture of any kind for 12 weeks.

The point locations for traditional Chinese acupuncture did not appear relevant. The possibility for potent placebo effects is heightened where there is an exotic conceptual framework with frequent practitioner contact which includes a repeated ritual and high expectations.

The same team produced similar results for migraine (*JAMA,* 2005; **293**: 2118–2125).

COMPLEMENTARY AND ALTERNATIVE THERAPIES

Acupuncture and knee osteoarthritis: a three-armed randomized trial
Scharf H, Mansmann U, Streitberger K *et al*.
Ann Intern Med, 2006; **145**: 12–20

This study showed a symptomatic benefit of acupuncture in osteoarthritis of the knee in 53%. With over 1000 participants, the study was large and well-designed. All received six sessions of physiotherapy and anti-inflammatory drugs. They also had either 10 consultations with a doctor, 10 sessions of real acupuncture, or 10 sessions of sham acupuncture.

Sham and real acupuncture worked equally well. Each was effective in more than half the patients compared to standard treatment which only helped 29%.

As ever it is not entirely clear whether the needling or the provider contact are the real cause of the benefit.

Acupuncture as an adjunct to exercise based physiotherapy for osteoarthritis of the knee: randomised controlled trial
Foster NE, Thomas E, Barlas P
BMJ, 2007; **335**: 436

Some recent trials have concluded that acupuncture for osteoarthritis of the knee is more effective than placebo, but no trial has investigated the additive benefit of acupuncture in combination with a recognised treatment such as exercise-based physiotherapy.

This study in 37 UK physiotherapy centres randomised 352 adults over 50 with knee osteoarthritis, to exercises plus adjunctive treatment with true acupuncture or non-penetrating acupuncture (a credible control). Using a no-treatment control group was not considered given the known benefit of advice and exercise. Patients were told they were receiving "one of two methods of acupuncture" in up to 6 sessions over 3 weeks.

Follow up was made on several occasions during the 12 months and acupuncture failed to show any improvements in pain scores. If anything the non-penetrating side showed some improvement in pain and unpleasantness.

So according to this large high quality trial, it is safe but not of benefit.

A randomized clinical trial of acupuncture compared with sham acupuncture in fibromyalgia
Assefi NP, Sherman KJ, Jacobsen C *et al*.
Ann Intern Med, 2005; **143**: 10–19

This study of 100 patients with fibromyalgia compared twice-weekly acupuncture for 12 weeks with 1 of 3 sham treatments – acupuncture for the wrong diagnosis (irregular periods), needling at non-acupuncture points, or faking it with toothpicks. The three sham techniques were pooled and blinding was adequate.

Real acupuncture fared no better than sham.

HERBALISM

Regulating herbal medicines in the UK
Ferner RE, Beard K
BMJ, 2005; **331**: 62–63

This editorial points to three important clinical criteria for licensing herbal medicines – efficacy, safety and quality of manufacture. Evidence is hard to come by and we still have treatments from the 16th century whose claims are not proven one way or the other. The European Union takes the view of registering drugs that have a 'long history' of use. In this context, this means 30 years, half of which should have been in the EU. They argue that longstanding use and experience is a plausible surrogate for efficacy and only safety needs to be considered. The US considers these medicines dietary supplements and outlaws unproven claims of therapeutic effect.

The UK seems likely to go down the route of using the Herbal Medicines Advisory Committee to advise government.

Herbal medicine: buy one, get two free
Ernst E
Postgrad Med J, 2007; **83:** 615–616

This paper draws our attention to three distinct types of herbal therapy.

Phytotherapy is a single extract with a number of pharmacological ingredients, e.g. St John's Wort (*Hypericum perforatum*). It is tested as a single entity and examined with the principles of evidence-based pharmacotherapy.

Secondly, the over-the-counter herbals industry peddles dietary supplements unsupported by evidence or clinician contact.

Thirdly, traditional herbalism is practised by herbalists who have received a boost from the evidence for phytotherapy, but have outdated disease models such as 'damp' and 'cold' which requires a treatment to be 'dry' or 'hot'. Only two RCTs have ever been published, and both failed to show superiority over placebo.

Ernst reminds us of our duty to speak out and not to be scared of the politically correct lobbyers. We have to warn our patients of potential harm.

A systematic review of randomised clinical trials of individualised herbal medicine in any indication
Guo R, Canter PH, Ernst E
Postgrad Med J, 2007; **83:** 633–637

The non-standard nature of tailor-made herbal recipes, used in Chinese, Ayurvedic and European herbal medicine, means that they need a high standard of proof (given the potential for harm) before such practices can be endorsed.

A review of all the evidence from RCTs found only 3 out of 1300 studies from which it was possible to draw any meaningful conclusions about these individualised treatments, dished out for any intended benefit or outcome.

COMPLEMENTARY AND ALTERNATIVE THERAPIES

- Only one of the three studies found results better than placebo, but crucially the individualised treatment was inferior to standardised treatment for IBS, indicating that claims by herbalists for the superiority of this approach are disingenuous.
- No evidence of benefit for osteoarthritis of the knee or prevention of chemotherapy-induced vomiting was found.

The authors conclude that individualised herbal medicines cannot be recommended for any indication. They comment that researchers should take care in blinding and the optimism of their interpretation when it comes to claiming results.

At least these trials demonstrate that rigorous RCTs are feasible. Regulation now needs to be brought to bear on practitioners to ensure that they identify red flag symptoms for referral.

Herbal supplements did not relieve vasomotor symptoms of menopause in women.
Evidence-Based Medicine, 2007; **12:** 78
The following paper is presented
Treatment of vasomotor symptoms of menopause with black cohosh, multibotanicals, soy, hormone therapy, or placebo: a randomized trial
Newton KM, Reed SD, LaCroix AZ, *et al.*
Ann Intern Med, 2006; **145:** 869–879

The Herbal Alternatives for Menopause Trial – HALT – found that herbals supplements, such as black cohosh, multibotanicals, and dietary soy, have no effect on vasomotor symptoms. Conventional hormone therapy on the other hand reduced symptoms.

The study was well-designed, blinded, randomised and controlled and had several treatment groups.

HYPNOTHERAPY

Gut-directed hypnotherapy for irritable bowel syndrome: piloting a primary care-based randomised controlled trial
Roberts L, Wilson S, Singh S *et al.*
Br J Gen Pract, 2006; **56:** 115–121

The alleviation of symptoms with gut-directed hypnotherapy in IBS has been found in the past to be useful in centres of secondary care. This primary care study looked into 101 patients, aged 18–65 years, with a diagnosis of IBS resistant to conventional management for greater than 6 weeks. The intervention was five sessions of hypnotherapy in addition to usual care.

Compared to usual management alone there were significant improvements in pain, diarrhoea and quality of life in the hypnotherapy group at 3 months, but no sustained effect was shown. The authors tell us that the lack of long-term benefit will preclude introduction of this intervention in a more widespread way.

HOMEOPATHY

Are the clinical effects of homoeopathy placebo effects? Comparative study of placebo-controlled trials of homoeopathy and allopathy
Shang A, Huwiler-Muntener K, Nartey L *et al.*
Lancet, 2005; **366**: 726–732

> This review looked into the implausibilities of homeopathy and matched 110 double-blind trials of homeopathy against 110 for conventional medicine for the same condition. Small study sizes and less rigorous methods inflated apparent effectiveness and the authors found evidence of publication bias for both methods.
>
> Unlike conventional medical trials, however, the authors found weak evidence for a specific effect of homeopathy which was consistent with the idea that it functions as a placebo.

MAGNETS

Magnet therapy
Finegold L, Flamm BL
BMJ, 2006; 332: 4

> Selling medical magnets is a billion dollar global business. They are advertised to cure everything from pain to cancer. The studies which claim therapeutic effects fall prey to both familiar and unique biases. Specifically, experiments are difficult to blind. Real magnets might stick to keys in your pocket giving the game away or bracelets might feel a tiny drag subconsciously picked up when near ferromagnetic surfaces.
>
> The harm, however, is very real. The neglect of illness which 'proper' medical science has something to offer is serious and financial harm is profound.
>
> The massive magnetic fields of MRI scanners show neither ill nor harmful effects.
>
> Patients should be advised that magnet therapy has no proven benefits.

COMPLEMENTARY AND ALTERNATIVE THERAPIES

DYSPEPSIA AND *HELICOBACTER PYLORI*

The Challenge

Dyspepsia is a chronic condition endemic in the UK, affecting 40% of people annually and costing the NHS around £1 billion per year. The term covers a number of indigestion symptoms such as epigastric pain, heartburn and acid reflux, sometimes with feelings of bloating and nausea. The vast majority of cases are self-managed and do not present to the GP.

Gastro-oesophageal reflux disease – GORD – is now looked upon as a chronic condition necessitating long-term therapy in most patients, focussing attention on symptoms rather than injury to oesophageal mucosa.

Drugs for these conditions account for the largest prescribing costs in the NHS.

Helicobacter pylori infection causes most duodenal ulcers (95%) and gastric ulcers (70%). It is also likely to cause around 9% of dyspepsia cases where no ulcers are detected. For dyspepsia without alarm symptoms, to 'test and treat' for *Helicobacter pylori*, or to give a proton pump inhibitor empirically, is more economical than referral for endoscopy.

Proton pump inhibitors are perceived as very safe and have become one of the most frequently prescribed classes of drug in the world in a very short time. In 2006 expenditure was £425 million in England alone. Although they are overprescribed, they are also available over the counter in the UK.

What we know already:

- Testing for *H. pylori* in primary care reduces demand for open access endoscopy but by nowhere near as much as the 70% hoped for. A study in randomised patients aged under 55 years from 47 practices using serology testing found only 19% fewer referrals in the intervention group.
- The urea breath test is the most accurate way to detect *H. pylori*, with a sensitivity of 95% and a specificity of 95%. But the stool antigen test is almost as good. Serology is much less specific.
- Treating patients for *H. pylori* infection is more likely to benefit those whose main symptom is gastritis than those with acid reflux as their most prominent symptom.
- Eradication treatment fails in 10–20% of cases and failure is more likely in smokers, according to a meta-analysis of 13 trials.
- There is an association between acid suppression therapy, particularly with PPIs, and *Clostridium difficile* infection. Less than 1 case per 100 000 in 1994 has become 22 per 100 000 in 2004.
- One week of treatment with omeprazole, clarithromycin and amoxicillin is as effective as 2 weeks in eradication of *H. pylori* in patients with duodenal ulcer.
- Smoking and high dietary salt worsens reflux but tea and coffee do not according to a large study of Norwegians quizzed about their lifestyle habits.
- Mortality from gastric cancer in Europe has fallen by around 50% between 1980 and 1999.

Guidelines

A NICE guideline, *Dyspepsia – management of dyspepsia in adults in primary care*, was issued in August 2004, revised July 2005.

Key recommendations include:

- review medication for possible causes of dyspepsia, such as NSAIDs or nitrates
- urgent referral for endoscopy regardless of age when symptoms are accompanied by 'alarm symptoms' of chronic gastrointestinal bleeding, progressive unintentional weight loss, difficulty swallowing, persistent vomiting, iron deficiency anaemia, or epigastric mass
- for patients without any alarm features, routine endoscopic investigation is not necessary but in those over 55 years, endoscopy is useful if symptoms persist for 4–6 weeks despite initial interventions especially if there has been a previous gastric ulcer, or increased concern about the risk of gastric cancer
- initial therapeutic strategies for dyspepsia are empirical treatment with a proton pump inhibitor (PPI) or 'test and treat' – testing for and treating *Helicobacter pylori*
- NICE recommends *H. pylori* eradication in *H. pylori*-positive patients who have peptic ulcer disease and endoscopically determined non-ulcer dyspepsia
- patients who have GORD should be offered a full-dose PPI for 1 or 2 months. Recurrence of symptoms should be managed by the lowest 'on demand' dose of PPI that is effective

Recent Papers

ERADICATING *HELICOBACTER PYLORI*

Who benefits from *Helicobacter pylori* eradication?
Delaney BC
BMJ, 2006; **332**: 187–188

Definitions of dyspepsia and GORD vary and have led to the terms having poor predictive value for pathology. NICE therefore recommends a common pathway for heartburn and epigastric pain.

- We know now that eradication of *H. pylori* is highly effective in reducing recurrence of proven duodenal ulcer with an NNT of 2.
- Testing for *H. pylori* and treating if found is cost-effective for those with dyspepsia.
- According to the CADET–Hp study, test and treat is more effective than just suppressing acid with a PPI. The MRC–CUBE trial reported in 2006 that this strategy is similar in cost-effectiveness to just using a PPI, having equal QALYs and costs, but resulted in a small but significant improvement in dyspepsia symptoms at 1 year.
- Even when there is no obvious cause to the dyspeptic symptoms and endoscopy is negative for ulcer and oesphagitis, eradication therapy is still pretty effective. The NNT increases to around 15 but no treatment is any better. With the burden of these chronic relapsing conditions, these smaller benefits may be cost-effective and good evidence has at least convincingly refuted early suspicions that eradication might make GORD worse.

What about going one stage further and screening asymptomatic people for *H. pylori* in order to seek and destroy? The study by Lane *et al.* (below) showed benefit with an NNT of 30 to prevent one consultation. Where prevalence is low – only 15% screened positive – accurate tests such as the urea breath test should be used as half of all serology results would be false positives. The cost–benefit is not clear but NICE currently leaves space for eradication as a treatment option in uninvestigated dyspepsia.

Impact of *Helicobacter pylori* eradication on dyspepsia, health resource use, and quality of life in the Bristol helicobacter project: randomised controlled trial
Lane JA, Murray LJ, Noble S *et al.*
BMJ, 2006; **332**: 199–202

This community study looked at the value of *H. pylori* screening in over 10 000 unselected people between 20 and 59 years old.

Positives were given eradication treatment and had 35% fewer consultations for dyspepsia over the next 2 years. They also had 30% fewer regular symptoms. This study showed the effectiveness and feasibility of screening but the increased cost of the medication seemed to make the 'test and treat' approach currently more economically appealing.

OVER-PRESCRIPTION

Overprescribing proton pump inhibitors
Forgacs I, Loganayagam A
BMJ, 2008; **336**: 2–3

Between 25% and 70% of prescriptions for PPIs have dubious indications and it is estimated that £100 million could be saved from the NHS budget each year. They account for 90% of the drug budget for dyspepsia despite the availability of cheaper drugs.

There is plenty of evidence that primary care is not entirely to blame. Hospital prescribing in several countries is not guideline-orientated either. Decision making and treatment plans for the medication they prescribe are communicated inadequately to GPs.

Studies have shown that up to 1 in 4 long term users may be able to stop the drug with no consequences. The authors point to clear overuse. The superior efficacy and high safety of such drugs is not an excuse, however. They are associated with an increase in prevalence of pneumonia and *Campylobacter* enteritis as well as doubling the risk of infection with *Clostridium difficile* amongst other rarer side effects.

Inappropriate prescribing of proton pump inhibitors in primary care
Batuwitage BT, Kingham JGC, Morgan NE, Bartlett RL
Postgrad Med J, 2007; **83**: 66–68

This attempt to make primary care doctors prescribe PPIs less inappropriately did not amount to much. They used a gentle intervention – a letter circulated to local GPs giving the findings of their audit of medical admissions to hospital and offering advice regarding prescribing PPIs.

It had no influence on prescribing habits when they repeated the process 6 months later. Not even a trend. Roughly half the PPIs were deemed inappropriate on each occasion. Some were prescribed with aspirin or NSAIDs 'just in case', some for non-specific abdominal symptoms such as vomiting for uncertain cause, but most for a problem that had long since resolved.

Perhaps they learned something about how GPs think, so maybe it was not a total waste of time. They suggest that maybe guidelines (which they were reading) might be too restrictive. Or maybe GPs are too lazy to take a full history? Maybe next time they will wait until they are asked.

They do note that financial rather than educational incentives can be effective, however. The bottom line is that too often, too many GPs perceive them as a harmless remedy for any digestive problem and we need to tighten evidence-based practice to avoid needless waste.

On-demand maintenance therapy with proton pump inhibitors is as effective as continuous therapy for non-erosive GORD. *Evidence-Based Medicine*, 2007; **12:** 177
The following review is presented
Systematic review: maintenance treatment of gastro-oesophageal reflux disease with proton pump inhibitors taken 'on-demand'
Pace F, Tonini M, Pallotta S, *et al*.
Aliment Pharmacol Ther, 2007; **26:** 195–204

How can we reduce our prescribing? This review gives one option, noting that 16 studies including 14 RCTs found that taking PPIs on-demand was as effective as taking them continuously in patients with non-erosive GORD. Those with more severe disease benefited from daily maintenance.

If the condition is erosive but only mildly so, the review suggests daily maintenance at half the initial treatment dosage.

DYSPEPSIA AND *HELICOBACTER PYLORI*

UROLOGY

The Challenge

Recognition and treatment of childhood UTI in general practice is variable and especially difficult in those under 1 year. Lack of specific urinary symptoms, difficulty in urine collection, and contamination of samples cause problems which lead to failure to make a bacteriological diagnosis, missed diagnosis or treatment delays. Fortunately, most children have a single episode and recover promptly.

Easily treatable infections are thought to cause renal scars in young children that can lead to hypertension, renal failure and some renal transplants in adulthood. Scars can be detected immediately on scanning with dimercaptosuccinic acid (DMSA) and lead to prophylactic treatment. There is little or no risk of new renal scars developing in children aged 4 and older.

Current imaging, prophylaxis, and prolonged follow-up strategies place a heavy burden on patients, families, and NHS resources and carry risks without evidence of benefit. Therefore such scanning has recently been de-emphasised by the 2007 NICE guidelines after variability in implementation. This updates the 1991 Guideline from the Royal College of Physicians (1991) on treatment of childhood UTI.

Dipsticks positive for leucocyte esterase and nitrite are useful indicators of infection but more work is needed to help us interpret their predictive power and stratify it by age and method of collection.

Dealing with a urinalysis dipstick which is positive for blood alone also presents a dilemma for doctors. This seems like it might this be a good screening test for bladder cancer, but reports to date have recommended abandoning testing for microhaematuria.

Estimated GFR has now crept into primary care consciousness. It has become the standard method used to identify and monitor patients with reduced renal function in the UK and other countries. It is hoped that recognition of low levels and appropriate management of patients with chronic kidney disease will reduce cardiovascular events and slow further deterioration in renal function in these patients.

Overactive bladder seems to be undertreated in the UK. One-sixth of adults over 18 report symptoms of overactive bladder and the effects on quality of life can be profound. Many do not seek help.

What we know already:

- UTI affects at least 3.6% of boys and 11% of girls.
- Studies imply that GPs have been missing three-quarters of UTIs in infants and half in children overall.
- The extent to which GPs think it acceptable to use antibiotics 'blindly' on children without confirming UTI is unknown.
- Phase-contrast microscopy is simple and improves diagnosis of bacteriological UTI.
- Estimated GFR, calculated using the '4-v MDRD' based prediction formula, is now routinely reported by biochemistry laboratories alongside serum creatinine results (except in non-validated patient groups).

- Systematic review finds that pelvic floor muscle training, comprehensively taught, increases cure in stress, urge and mixed incontinence. Combining this with bladder training is better than pelvic floor training alone.
- Anticholinergic drugs are often prescribed first line in primary care to reduce detrusor muscle contraction. Systematic review does show them to be effective in overactive bladder but not very.
- Electrical stimulation for urge incontinence and some surgical options have also been shown to be effective.

Recent Papers

UTI IN CHILDREN

Urinary tract infection in primary care
Mangin D, Toop L
BMJ, 2007; **334:** 597–598

Increasing evidence of resistance to trimethoprim may influence prescribers to change their first line antibiotic, but such microbiologically determined resistance rates do not equate directly to treatment failure. This editorial recommends that clinical assessment of failure to get better, after say 4 days of treatment, is a much more important guide to treatment. Similarly urine dipsticks do not reliably predict the response to antibiotic treatment.

Diagnosis and management of urinary tract infection in children: summary of NICE guidance
Mori R, Lakhanpaul M, Verrier-Jones K
BMJ, 2007; **335:** 395–397

New guidance from NICE updates the 1991 guidelines.

This summary outlines the assessment and treatment of UTI in children. Key aspects of treatment include:
- specific guidance is given based on positivity of leucocyte esterase and nitrite downplaying use of antibiotics if nitrite is negative
- dipstick urine testing is to be used first line for children over 3 years
- urine microscopy and culture is preferable for children under 3 years
- immediate referral to secondary care of children under 3 months with UTI
- treatment of simple lower UTI in children over 3 months with 3 days of antibiotics
- no routine prescribing of antibiotic prophylaxis
- no routine imaging to detect vesico-ureteric reflux
- only send for ultrasound if UTI is atypical or younger than 6 months
- DMSA scan is considered only in children under 3 and only in recurrent or complicated infection

The authors note strongly held views by some clinicians regarding imaging strategies, but claim that current evidence shows no such benefit. The most useful intervention is prompt diagnosis and treatment and the guidelines emphasise this less invasive approach.

A letter by Coulthard gives a different side to the story and claims the NICE guidelines may not represent a consensus. He refers to "highly restrictive secrecy agreements" during the consultation process that has led to what he sees as errors in the guidelines – a result of "inadequate" review of the literature. He accuses the authors of misusing statistics and using flawed logic to represent selective opinions. He clearly values DMSA screening and prophylactic antibiotics and does not welcome the consensus view they claim to represent. It is a strong letter which may be a testament to NICE getting any new guidelines out at all (*BMJ*, 2007; **335:** 463).

Management of urinary tract infection in children
Watson AR
BMJ, 2007; **335:** 356–357

The 1991 UK guidelines emphasised that UTI and vesico-ureteric reflux can cause scarring of the kidneys leading to hypertension and chronic renal failure. Enthusiasm for extensive investigation has waned after DMSA scans found parenchymal defects that do not develop into scarring and many scars are present without reflux. Most children only have one infection and have a normal urinary tract.

Our daily work needs to concentrate on considering the diagnosis in the first place, taking a good history including a family history (as vesico-ureteric reflux can have a 30% familial incidence) and persevering with trying to get good urine samples for dipstick and if necessary culture. Microscopy for white cells and bacteria gives a strong indication of UTI but expertise has greatly diminished in this area.

The author of the editorial notes that the relegation of imaging strategies will be controversial but the new focus on simpler methods may improve detection.

UTI IN ADULTS

Developing clinical rules to predict urinary tract infection in primary care settings: sensitivity and specificity of near patient tests (dipsticks) and clinical scores
Little P, Turner S, Rumsby K *et al.*
Br J Gen Pract, 2006; **56:** 606–612

Despite the frequency of this diagnosis, independent predictors of UTI are still poorly validated in primary care.

This study of over 400 women with suspected UTI found that only nitrite, leucocyte esterase and blood independently predicted infection. A dipstick decision rule using these three variables was moderately sensitive (77%) and specific (70%) and PPV was 81%. If all three tests were negative, the NPV was 65%.

Response to antibiotics of women with symptoms of urinary tract infection but negative dipstick urine test results: double blind randomised controlled trial
Richards D, Toop L, Chambers S
BMJ, 2005; **331**: 143

A small study in New Zealand randomised 59 women with symptoms of UTI but a negative dipstick to either 3 days of trimethoprim or placebo.

- Trimethoprim shortens dysuria in women with symptoms of uncomplicated UTI and negative dipstick result by a median time of 2 days. The NNT is 4.
- A negative dipstick test for leucocytes and nitrites did not predict response to antibiotic treatment.
- These results support the practice of empirical antibiotic use guided by symptoms, meaning that the minimisation of antibiotic use remains a dilemma.
- An infectious cause for the symptoms is likely in these circumstances, which is not being diagnosed with our usual methods.

CHRONIC KIDNEY DISEASE

Formula estimation of glomerular filtration rate: have we gone wrong?
Giles PD, Fitzmaurice DA
BMJ, 2007; **334**: 1198–1200

Chronic kidney disease sufferers have increased risk of cardiovascular disease. A test that reliably detects early kidney disease may provide a point of intervention for cardiovascular and kidney disease. That test is eGFR (estimated glomerular filtration rate). Since 2005 in the UK, the National Service Framework for renal services has required labs to routinely report eGFR as part of their biochemistry findings. Laboratories produce formula-based estimates and primary care has been asked to establish registers of those with eGFR worse than 60 l/min/1.73m².

This article challenges the formula used. They admit that the formula is accurate enough to stage patients with known kidney disease and a low GFR. However, the creation of registers has allowed a new screening test to slip in by the back door. This has occurred without reference to the usual strict criteria for appraising such things. Without evaluating the balance of harm to benefit for individuals tested. And without knowing the sensitivity and specificity of the test or the positive and negative predictive values.

Estimated GFR has enormous variation between individuals and underestimates renal function in people without kidney disease. This risk of false positives is high, which would be all very well if the next test up was a simple one. But the next 'test' is referral to a renal clinic and free entry on to a register that might influence your chance of getting life insurance in the future. Routine measurement lacks a good scientific basis, will pressurise specialist services and create unnecessary anxiety.

The authors conclude that using eGFR to screen for chronic kidney disease in primary care deserved much more careful evaluation than it got.

A response tells us that the intention was not to be a screening programme as much as testing those at risk, including patients with diabetes and hypertension.

UROLOGY

This would then achieve one of the aims of the guidelines – reducing late referral of people who are heading for dialysis (*BMJ*, 2007; **334:** 1287). What that is if it's not screening beats me!

PROSTATIC SYMPTOMS

Lower urinary tract symptoms in men
Chapple CR, Patel AK
BMJ, 2007; **334**: 2
and
Self management for men with lower urinary tract symptoms: randomised controlled trial
Brown CT, Yap T, Cromwell DA *et al.*
BMJ, 2007; **334**: 25

Watchful waiting has long been established as a safe alternative to resection of the prostate in lower urinary tract symptoms of voiding, storage and post-voiding, such as occur in benign prostatic hypertrophy. Just advising on lifestyle modification, however, is unlikely to do much to improve symptoms.

Self-management has many more components and this study in secondary care showed it to be significantly more beneficial than usual care. It included education about the causes and natural course of lower urinary tract symptoms and also reassurance about prostate cancer, advice on fluid management, toileting and bladder retraining. Crucially, there was a cognitive ingredient to promote behavioural change by teaching problem solving and goal setting in three small group sessions.

Some 140 men, mean age 63 years were randomised.

- At 3 months, treatment failure occurred in 10% of the self-management group and 42% of the standard care group.
- Symptomatic improvements were sustained up to 1 year.
- The effect was twice that of pharmacotherapy compared with placebo in randomised trials.

Possible biases included:

- selection bias – only those with the time and motivation may attend such a trial
- lack of objective assessment of flow rate (as outcome was by symptom score)
- a higher proportion of the self-management group had a university education (45% vs. 24%)

The authors suggest a large multicentre trial to confirm these apparently large benefits.

HAEMATURIA

Long-term outcome of hematuria home screening for bladder cancer in men
Messing EM, Madeb R, Young T et al.
Cancer, 2006; **107**: 2173–2179

Of 3500 men over 50 who tested their urine repeatedly for haemoglobin over a 19 year period, 16% were investigated for haematuria and 8% of those were diagnosed with bladder cancer.

Relatively, the numbers of high and low grade cancers found were similar, but for the high grade tumours only 15% of the patients found by screening had muscle invasion compared to 60% of the unscreened group. After 14 years, 20% of these unscreened patients were dead but none of those detected by screening had died. The authors note that testing for haematuria could be a sensitive method for detecting bladder cancers and seems to improve survival.

The diagnostic value of macroscopic haematuria for the diagnosis of urological cancer in general practice
Bruyninckx R, Buntinx F, Aertgeerts B et al.
Br J Gen Pract, 2003; **53**: 31–35

How strong a predictor of serious illness is haematuria? Cases of haematuria presenting to general practice were assessed for incidence of urological cancers in this study taking in around 1% of the entire Belgian population.

- The positive predictive value of haematuria for these cancers in patients over 60 years was 22% for men and 8% for women.
- In the under 60s, predictive values were in single figures.
- No urological cancer was found in the age group under 40 years.

The authors conclude that thorough investigation for urological cancer is indicated in men older than 60 years with macroscopic haematuria.

In patients of either sex under 60 years of age, watchful waiting can be justified.

Time to abandon testing for microscopic haematuria in adults?
Malmström P
BMJ, 2003; **326**: 813–815

The paper reviews the controversial significance of microhaematuria by assessing current evidence in this poorly researched area where little consensus exists.

- In several studies, cancers were detected no more often than in controls.
- Microhaematuria is rare in renal cancer making renal biopsy difficult to justify.
- In men with prostatic symptoms due to BPH, one-third tested positive for microhaematuria but this did not correlate with any feature of the condition so was not helpful in assessment.
- The only disease for which microhaematuria might be considered an early stage is bladder cancer.
- Although new bladder cancer often presents with painless macroscopic haematuria, we do not know the time interval whereby we might pick it up at a microscopic stage.

- Cancers referred at the microscopic stage are around 5% of referrals, but there is no evidence that cancers are less advanced when picked up at this stage.
- The preclinical stage may be too brief, leaving primary screening for microhaematuria with too low a sensitivity.

INCONTINENCE

Epidemiology, prescribing patterns and resource use associated with overactive bladder in UK primary care
Odeyemi I, Dakin H, O'Donnell R
Int J Clin Pract, 2006; **60**: 949–958

This study aimed to clarify incidence and prevalence of overactive bladder by analysing cases of 69 000 symptomatic patients in UK general practice.
- Prevalence was 4 per 1000 people.
- 28% were prescribed anticholinergics of which one-fifth tried more than one medication.
- 59% were referred to secondary services.
- 2.8% underwent urinary tests/investigations.
- 0.2% were seen by a continence nurse.

This study indicated that overactive bladder may be underdiagnosed, under-referred and undertreated in the UK.

The sensitivity and specificity of a simple test to distinguish between urge and stress urinary incontinence
Brown JS, Bradley CS, Subak LL *et al.*
Ann Intern Med, 2006; **144**: 715–723

A simple questionnaire called the 3IQ asks two incontinence questions to distinguish between stress and urge incontinence, which is important for deciding whether to recommend pelvic floor exercises or urge suppression exercises.

The first question asks if urine has leaked in the last 3 months (even a small amount). Those answering positively are asked if the leakage occurs when there was physical activity or a sense of urgency or both. The third asks about the circumstances when it occurs most often to get an idea of whether this is stress, urge or missed incontinence.

The tests were fairly accurate in predicting urge incontinence (sensitivity 0.75, specificity 0.77) and stress incontinence (sensitivity 0.86, specificity 0.60) and, although not perfect, could be a useful tool in primary care settings.

Clinical and cost-effectiveness of a new nurse-led continence service: a randomised controlled trial
Williams KS, Assassa RP, Cooper NJ *et al.*
Br J Gen Pract, 2005; **55**: 696–703

This UK trial randomised nearly 4000 women and men to input from a continence nurse practitioner or usual care. The 8 week intervention included advice on diet and fluids, bladder training, pelvic floor awareness and lifestyle advice. It showed significant improvement in symptoms of incontinence, frequency, urgency, and nocturia, which were sustained at 6 months. Satisfaction was high and the service is likely to be a cost-effective model in this under-reported condition.

IMMUNISATION

The Challenge

Delays in primary immunisation compromise child health.

Most people wrongly believe that doctors and scientists are equally divided over the safety of MMR – an impression thought to be created by the media. The original study from Wakefield *et al.* in 1998 had poor methodological quality and there has been a dearth of evidence to support it. A Cochrane review in 2005 also agreed there was no credible evidence to connect MMR with autism or, for that matter, Crohn's or any other serious disease. Despite this, parental confidence in vaccination has been rocked. There is uncertainty over whether to trust the media or the medical profession and they worry about any adverse consequences of their decision. Tragic consequences became inevitable and measles, mumps, rubella have all had recent resurgences.

So has *Haemophilus influenzae* type B. The impact of vaccination campaigns is not always predictable. The Hib infection rates in the UK fell dramatically after the introduction of childhood immunisation in 1992. However, since 1998 there was a marked resurgence of cases in children, most of whom were fully vaccinated, doubling every year. Adult Hib antibody levels had dropped and so did population 'herd' immunity. There were fewer chances to become naturally immune. Parents and grandparents, an older unimmunised group who mix with kids, became vulnerable. This led to introduction of a booster after the first birthday which should in time permit herd immunity and prevent further increases in infections. It shows how important high quality surveillance is.

Although infections with hepatitis B are asymptomatic in 70%, carrier status is high and the complications of the disease are difficult to treat. They are, however, easy to prevent with a highly effective vaccine. So with 260 million people chronically infected globally, is it finally time to introduce universal immunisation against hepatitis B in the UK?

With global migration, the case is getting stronger all the time and already over 150 countries have instituted a universal neonatal hepatitis B programme. At least 55% of the world's children now receive the three doses of the hepatitis B vaccine. The UK is one of the few developed countries to have chosen a selective approach for high risk cases, but changes in populations need fluid strategies. Full economic evaluations need to be made and continually revisited to compare vaccination costs of a universal programme with the burden of the chronic disease.

Rotavirus causes one-third of all hospital admissions for diarrhoea and leads to about 600 000 deaths per year – 6% of deaths in the under fives. In the UK, 1 in 40 children are admitted to hospital for rotavirus infection in their first 5 years. Vaccines new to the market can be very effective in preventing rotavirus diarrhoea.

What we know already:

- Childhood schedules have recently been updated to reflect current requirements: a pentavalent vaccine – DTaP/Hib/IPV – is given in infancy at 2, 3 and 4 months at the same time (but a different site) as the meningococcal C vaccine
- Inactivated polio vaccine replaces the old sugar cube, possible due to the near elimination of polio worldwide, and the pertussis ingredient has changed from a whole cell vaccine to

---

an acellular vaccine with up to five components (and yet a much lower antigenic load) which causes fewer adverse reactions
- Uptake of MMR is around 88% but drops by the second dose to 74%; after a single dose, 5–10% of children are not fully protected against measles
- Extended vaccination policies such as varicella zoster, rotavirus, hepatitis B and meningitis B could be future possibilities
- Concerns about mercury-containing thiomersal, previously used as a preservative in vaccines caused a lot of panic; best evidence in 1000 children found no consistent evidence of an adverse effect on their brains up to the age of 10 years

Recent Papers

MMR

Effects of a web based decision aid on parental attitudes to MMR vaccination: a before and after study
Wallace C, Leask J, Trevena LJ
BMJ, 2006; **332**: 146–149

We now know that the alleged association with autism is totally without evidence to support it. Yet the harm is done.

Accessing a website with a series of questions designed to inform parents about the pros and cons of MMR has been shown capable of improving parental attitude to the vaccine.

Although it encouraged significantly more to be 'pro-vaccination', to a lesser extent it fed the negative attitudes of those who already were against the vaccine. They continued to dwell on outdated concerns and so avoided any risk of guilt in the event of any adverse outcome.

Concerted efforts to broach concerns have led to an apparent contradiction. Despite an information explosion, parents still choose to believe they have inadequate or biased information. This must come down to a mistrust of doctors and/or politicians and the media. We need to look seriously at our communication strategies regarding decisional conflicts such as this. Tools like the one in this study may be part of the solution for a minority to whom it appeals.

Think mumps
Godlee F
BMJ, 2005; **330**: 1132–1135

This editorial reminds us of the many vaccine scares over the years and the devastating impact of antivaccine activism.

With the mumps outbreak continuing in 2005 as it did in 2004, the author notes that the epidemic is ironically indicative of the success of UK vaccination policy. Cases are mainly in 19–23 year olds who were not exposed to mumps as children due to the success of MMR introduction in 1988, and who missed out on the second dose for various reasons (the second dose was introduced in 1996).

IMMUNISATION

Mumps must now be part of the differential diagnosis for a generation of doctors who have never seen a case. There is no treatment, however, beyond isolating the infected and vaccinating the susceptible.

TUBERCULOSIS

Stopping routine vaccination for tuberculosis in schools
Fine P
BMJ, 2005; **331**: 647–648

From autumn 2005 the routine BCG vaccination of schoolchildren against tuberculosis stopped. This change comes as notifications of tuberculosis in England and Wales are at their highest level since 1983.

There are good reasons. Changes in epidemiology, unsubstantiated fears of co-infection with HIV and localisation of TB in immigrant communities mean the time is right to come into line with vaccination policy in many other countries. Imported disease declines with time and has not led to increases in the risk for the indigenous population. BCG vaccination will now be offered to infants in communities with an average incidence of tuberculosis of at least 40 per 100 000 and to unvaccinated families from countries of similar incidence.

Most people born in the UK now will not receive BCG. As most will not be exposed to mycobacteria, tuberculin testing will become more efficient in detecting infection.

HEPATITIS B

Hepatitis B vaccination
Pollard AJ
BMJ, 2007; **335**: 950

The UK has no such universal immunisation programme for hepatitis B, but now the BMA had added its voice to lobby the Department of Health to look at this again.

The low incidence of the disease we have enjoyed in the UK could be coming to an end thanks to travel and immigration. The vast majority of cases come from abroad. Already 180 000 people in the UK are chronically infected with hepatitis B and 3.3% of legal migrants are thought to be chronically infected.

Our current policy of targeting high risk groups such as drug users and also the perinatal period in babies born to hepatitis B-positive mothers is effective. An extension of this strategy to families with at least one parent from an endemic country could be difficult to meet politically, although is done in the Netherlands.

The easiest way to protect everyone is the method used widely in Europe – adding hepatitis B immunisations to the current UK schedule and making the pentavalent vaccine a hexavalent one.

An alternative is to add it to the new HPV vaccine to rapidly create a cohort of immune individuals, in this case girls.

ROTAVIRUS

Efficacy of human rotavirus vaccine against rotavirus gastroenteritis during the first 2 years of life in European infants: randomised, double-blind controlled study
Vesikari TM, Karvonen A, Prymula R, *et al.*
Lancet, 2007; **370**: 1757–1763

> This study tested a new live attenuated oral vaccine – Rotarix – which is active against one strain of rotavirus and found that:
> - the two doses of the vaccine were given on average at 11 weeks and at 20 weeks
> - rotavirus gastroenteritis reduced by 87% over one season, falling a little further over two seasons to 79%
> - it prevented 92–100% of hospital admissions for rotavirus and was particularly effective against severe infection
> - protection was offered against other strains and there was a 72% reduction in hospital admissions for gastroenteritis of any cause
> - intussusception had led to the withdrawal of the first rotavirus vaccine but no increased risk was noted here
>
> It shows potential for reducing the burden of gastroenteritis in children and could be added to routine immunisation schedules. Testing is now needed in developing countries where other obstacles may exist such as malnutrition and potential for breaks in the cold chain.

VARICELLA

A varicella-zoster virus vaccine reduced the burden of illness of herpes zoster in older adults. *Evidence-Based Medicine*, 2005; **10**: 177
The following paper is reviewed
A vaccine to prevent herpes zoster and postherpetic neuralgia in older adults
Oxman MN, Levin MJ, Johnson GR *et al.*
N Engl J Med, 2005; **352**: 2271–2284

> This double-blind study was the first study to look at a vaccine that avoids re-expression of a latent virus. It found that a single dose of herpes zoster virus in those over 60 years with a history of varicella, reduced the risk of zoster by 51% and of post-herpetic neuralgia by 67% over 5.5 years.
>
> It was very safe and the commentary argues for a universal immunisation programme as the morbidity saved, particularly in those over 60 years, is considerable. The NNT of 59 looks unappealing but it is explained that even if it was 100% effective the NNT would still be 30.

Loss of vaccine-induced immunity to varicella over time
Chaves SS, Gargiullo P, Zhang JX, *et al.*
N Engl J Med, 2007; **356**: 1121–1129

> The US has vaccinated children against chickenpox since 1995, but their recommendations have recently added a booster dose after discovering that immunity wanes after a single dose of live attenuated vaccine.

IMMUNISATION

Some 10% of children had "breakthrough chickenpox" and this was more likely if they were between 8 and 12 years old and more than 5 years from their vaccination. Disease was more severe the further from the vaccination they were.

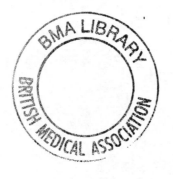